Mental Health Case Studies in Paramedic Practice

Mental Health Case Studies in Paramedic Practice

Edited by

Joanne Augustus, Yuet Wah Patrick, Paula Gardner, and Paul K. Miller

Open University Press

Open University Press
McGraw Hill
Unit 4
Foundation Park
Roxborough Way
Maidenhead
SL6 3UD

email: emea_uk_ireland@mheducation.com
world wide web: www.mheducation.co.uk

Executive Editor: Hannah Church
Editorial Assistant: Molly Overend
Content Product Manager: Graham Jones

A catalogue record of this book is available from the British Library

ISBN-13: 9780335253326
ISBN-10: 0335253326
eISBN-13: 9780335253333

Typeset by Transforma Pvt. Ltd., Chennai, India

O10273 ACL 2026

Praise page

"The joy of this book is that it brings together evidence, real life examples, practice underpinned by pedagogical knowledge to help practitioners better understand mental health and equip them for real life practice. Providing compassionate evidence based care for individuals in relation to mental health is not an option its an essential skills required by paramedics as well as all health practitioners. This book provides a framework to help you on that journey to refine your interactions, understanding and compassion for individuals."

Professor Brian Webster-Henderson OBE,
Deputy Vice Chancellor, University of Cumbria, UK.

"This book presents an important and novel perspective on a key area for the health and care system, emergency responding in a context of mental health challenges across the population. Paramedics work in an arena of high complexity, supporting people at their most vulnerable, with immediate physical and psychological needs. This collection of case studies reminds us that compassionate, trauma-informed care requires focus on the mind, and its body ... holistic care, is much more than corporeal repair."

Professor Eileen F. S. Kaner, Professor of Public Health &
Primary Care Research, Population Health Sciences Institute,
University of Newcastle upon Tyne, UK.

"This book offers valuable insight into mental health care, supported by a series of well-constructed and engaging case studies. The inclusion of reflective elements and end-of-chapter questions is particularly effective in reinforcing learning and enabling readers to critically consider how the content applies to professional practice. Each chapter is thoughtfully developed and intellectually stimulating, and the comprehensive reference lists provide clear opportunities for further exploration and deeper engagement with the subject matter."

Samantha McCabe-Hogan, Course Lead for PG Enhanced Level Practice,
School of Health and Social Care, Sheffield Hallam University, UK.

"This is a really relevant and up-to-date text that reflects modern paramedic practice and the mental health needs of people we care for today. The case studies are well set in context, making them easy to relate to and useful for those working in emergency and urgent care

settings. It helps build understanding of often complex situations and offers practical insight for clinicians. A valuable and much-needed contribution to the field."

Daniel Finnerty, Principal Lecturer in Allied Health,
Wrexham University, UK.

"An excellent resource for all those involved in prehospital care and paramedicine. A well-structured book with pertinent vignettes providing examples of mental health case studies and how best to deal professionally with what can be complex situations at times. This is the book that paramedics have been waiting for and should be the go to resource when dealing with mental health calls."

Meirion Williams, Senior Lecturer in Advanced Clinical Practice,
University of South Wales, UK.

"I am delighted to recommend this unique and informative text, **Mental Health Case Studies in Paramedic Practice.** ***This is the one of the first of its kind to advance knowledge underpinned by applied clinical reasoning to address mental health presentations in pre-hospital care. Its strength lies in its sensitive and in-depth case study approach embracing a breadth of populations which is suitable for all those invested in paramedic education and practice. The purpose of the text is to highlight the importance of thoughtful, and evidence based person-centred professional judgement. I am grateful to Jo Augustus and her co-authors for bringing this much needed work to support those who care for people on their prehospital journey when at their most vulnerable and in need of thoughtful and considered practice."***

Professor Joy Duxbury OBE, Professor of Mental Health Nursing,
Director of Research Institute of Health, University of Cumbria, UK.

What is lost does not leave us.
It settles into how we listen,
how we wait,
how we learn to hear again.

– Jo Augustus

For Brian and Jackie Augustus, always present, in memory, in influence, and in love.

– Jo Augustus

For Pamela Miller, whose patience and dedication continue to astonish me every single day. But particularly her patience.

– Paul K. Miller

For Jacob, Cameron, Joseph, and Ella and to the belief that mental health deserves care, compassion, and conversation.

– Paula Gardner

Contents

About the editors x

How to use this book xi

List of abbreviations xii

Glossary of key terms xiv

1 INTRODUCTION: FOUNDATIONS OF MENTAL HEALTH IN PARAMEDIC PRACTICE 1
Jo Augustus

2 NEURODEVELOPMENTAL DISORDERS, NEURODIVERSITY, AND EARLY CRISIS CARE 17
Jo Augustus and Paul K. Miller

3 NEUROCOGNITIVE DISORDERS, CONSENT, AND CRITICAL INTERVENTION 53
Emma Brookes and Paul K. Miller

4 MENTAL HEALTH AND LONG-TERM CONDITIONS: CHRONIC ILLNESS, COMPLEXITY, AND SOCIAL ISOLATION 85
Emily Holland, Gemma Goadsby, Yuet Wah Patrick, and Jo Augustus

5 WOMEN'S MENTAL HEALTH: MATERNITY 113
Susan Rhind, Sarah Hilton, Yuet Wah Patrick, and Jo Augustus

6 WOMEN'S HEALTH AND WELLBEING: GENDERED CARE NEEDS 135
Jane-Louise Reid and Yuet Wah Patrick

7 SEVERE AND ENDURING MENTAL ILLNESS: PSYCHOSIS, SCHIZOPHRENIA, AND EATING DISORDERS 157
Jo Augustus and Kaitee Robinson

8 SELF-HARM AND SUICIDALITY: PARAMEDIC RESPONSES TO RISK AND DISTRESS 180
Seb Brown, Corina Downing, Paula Gardner, and Jo Augustus

9 ACUTE BEHAVIOURAL DISTURBANCE AND SUBSTANCE-RELATED PRESENTATIONS: ASSESSMENT, SAFETY, AND INTERVENTION 212
Ashley Stewart, Paula Gardner, and Jo Augustus

10 CONCLUSION: INTEGRATING EVIDENCE, COMPASSION, AND POLICY INTO PARAMEDIC MENTAL HEALTH PRACTICE 239
Jo Augustus

Index 243

About the editors

Jo Augustus is a Senior Lecturer specialising in mental health, urgent and emergency care, and paramedic education apprenticeships at the University of Cumbria. Her work bridges clinical practice, research, and teaching, with a strong focus on compassion, equity, and reflective practice. She writes to support clinicians navigating complexity at the front line.

Paula Gardner is Principal Lecturer in paramedic apprenticeships at the University of Cumbria and an experienced registered paramedic. A recognised leader in paramedic education, she brings extensive expertise in workforce development, mentorship, and programme leadership. Her work champions compassionate, evidence-informed practice, with particular interests in mental health, human factors, and suicide prevention.

Yuet Wah Patrick is Senior Lecturer in paramedic science at the University of Gloucestershire and an experienced registered paramedic. She has worked clinically and in education, mentoring students and championing inclusivity. Her interests include legal/ethical practice, social inequalities, and enhancing paramedic education via research and practice.

Paul K. Miller is an Associate Professor in social psychology at the University of Cumbria and has, to date, published on a wide range of topics, largely in allied health, psychotherapy, and clinical medicine. These have recently included interpersonal communication, decision-making, stigma and stigmatised identities, workplace cultures, neurodiversity, and dementia.

How to use this book

Mental Health Case Studies in Paramedic Practice is designed to advance applied knowledge, clinical reasoning, and ethical competence in the management of mental health presentations within pre-hospital care. It is suitable for undergraduate and postgraduate paramedic education, as well as continuing professional development.

The text adopts a case-based pedagogical model. Each chapter integrates a clinically grounded narrative with relevant pathophysiology, legal and ethical analysis, and evidence-informed management guidance. Learning is reinforced through multiple-choice questions, structured clinical reasoning prompts, and reflective exercises aligned with Health and Care Professions Council Standards of Proficiency.

The multiple-choice questions assess higher-order application of knowledge. Guided reasoning questions are intended to scaffold structured, defensible decision-making in time-critical and ethically complex contexts. Reflective components support professional accountability and portfolio development.

This is a multi-authored volume. Although the chapters adhere to a broadly consistent structural framework, each reflects the disciplinary expertise and interpretive lens of its contributors. Variations in emphasis are deliberate and reflect the multifaceted nature of contemporary paramedic practice.

The cases presented intentionally incorporate clinical uncertainty, incomplete information, and competing ethical considerations. This reflects the operational realities of pre-hospital care. The purpose of the text is not prescriptive algorithmic instruction, but the cultivation of proportionate, lawful, and person-centred professional judgement.

List of abbreviations

ABCDE	Airway, Breathing, Circulation, Disability, Exposure
ABD	acute behavioural disturbance
ACS	acute coronary syndromes
ADHD	attention-deficit/hyperactivity disorder
AMHP	approved mental health professional
AMTS	Abbreviated Mental Test Score
APH	antepartum haemorrhage
ATMIST	Age, Time, Mechanism, Injuries, Signs, Treatment
BPSD	behavioural and psychological symptoms of dementia
CAMHS	Child and Adolescent Mental Health Services
COPD	chronic obstructive pulmonary disease
C-SSRS	Columbia-Suicide Severity Rating Scale
CVD	cardiovascular disease
CYP	children and young people
ECA	emergency care assistant
ECG	electrocardiogram
ECHR	European Convention on Human Rights
ED	emergency department
EDI	equality, diversity, and inclusion
GABA	γ-aminobutyric acid
GP	general practitioner
HCPC	Health and Care Professions Council
HEMS	Helicopter Emergency Medical Service
HPA	hypothalamic-pituitary-adrenal axis
IPPA	Identify, Plan, Protect, Act (risk framework)
IVF	in vitro fertilisation
JRCALC	Joint Royal Colleges Ambulance Liaison Committee
LBD	Lewy body dementia
MAPPA	Multi-Agency Public Protection Arrangements
MARAC	Multi-Agency Risk Assessment Conferences
MCA	Mental Capacity Act 2005
MDT	multidisciplinary team
MEED	Medical Emergencies in Eating Disorders guidance
MEWS	Maternity Early Warning Scores
MHA	Mental Health Act 1983 (as amended 2007)
MSE	mental state examination
NCD	neurocognitive disorder
NEWS2	National Early Warning Score 2
NHS	National Health Service
NICE	National Institute for Health and Care Excellence

PHQ-9	Patient Health Questionnaire-9
PMDT	Prehospital Maternity Decision Tool
PPH	postpartum haemorrhage
PreRT	pre-rapid tranquilisation
PTSD	post-traumatic stress disorder
SBAR	Situation, Background, Assessment, Recommendation
SLE	systemic lupus erythematosus
SMI	severe and enduring mental illness
UTI	urinary tract infection
VTE	venous thromboembolism

Glossary of key terms

Acute behavioural disturbance (ABD): A rapid-onset state characterised by extreme agitation, aggression, confusion, and physiological instability. Often associated with substances, mental illness, or medical causes. Considered a medical emergency requiring careful risk assessment, de-escalation, and close monitoring.

Approved mental health professional (AMHP): A specially trained professional (often a social worker, nurse, psychologist, or occupational therapist) authorised under the Mental Health Act 1983 to make decisions regarding detention for assessment or treatment.

Assessment of capacity: A structured evaluation under the Mental Capacity Act 2005 to determine whether a person can understand, retain, weigh, and communicate information related to a specific decision at a specific time.

Behavioural and psychological symptoms of dementia (BPSD): A term used to describe non-cognitive symptoms associated with dementia, including agitation, aggression, anxiety, depression, hallucinations, wandering, and sleep disturbance. These symptoms often reflect unmet needs, distress, pain, or environmental factors rather than deliberate behaviour and are common triggers for emergency service involvement.

Bio-psycho-social model: A holistic framework that understands mental health through the interaction of biological, psychological, and social factors. Central to contemporary paramedic assessment.

Capacity and consent: *Capacity* refers to a person's ability to make a specific decision at a specific time, based on their ability to understand, retain, weigh relevant information, and communicate a decision. *Consent* is the voluntary agreement to assessment or treatment given by a person with capacity. In the UK, capacity and consent are governed by the Mental Capacity Act 2005, which supports least-restrictive, person-centred care.

Cognitive assessment: A structured process used to evaluate a person's cognitive functioning, including orientation, attention, memory, language, and executive skills. In pre-hospital care, cognitive assessment is used to identify acute confusion, delirium or cognitive impairment, inform capacity assessments, and guide clinical decision-making rather than to establish a formal diagnosis.

Crisis Resolution and Home Treatment Team (CRHTT): A specialist mental health service providing urgent assessment and intensive home-based support as an alternative to hospital admission.

Cultural safety: An approach recognising the impact of culture, power, inequality, and discrimination on healthcare experiences. Requires reflective practice, anti-racism, and avoidance of stereotyping.

De-escalation: A set of communication and environmental strategies used to reduce agitation, promote calm, and prevent escalation during mental health crises.

Delirium: An acute and fluctuating change in consciousness, attention, and cognition, often due to an underlying medical condition. It is important for paramedics to distinguish delirium from psychiatric symptoms.

Dementia: An umbrella term describing a group of progressive conditions characterised by a decline in cognitive function that is sufficient to interfere with daily activities. Dementia commonly affects memory, attention, language, reasoning, and behaviour, and is caused by neurodegenerative, vascular, or other neurological processes. It is not a normal part of ageing.

Detention: Under the Mental Health Act 1983, a legal process allowing a person to be held in hospital for assessment or treatment when they pose a risk to themselves or others due to a mental disorder. Paramedics often encounter Section 135 or 136 situations involving police.

Ecological systems theory: Bronfenbrenner's model describes how individuals are influenced by interconnected systems (micro-, meso-, exo-, macro-, and chronosystems). Helps paramedics understand the contextual influences behind crisis presentations.

Equality, diversity, and inclusion (EDI): A commitment to delivering fair, non-discriminatory, and culturally safe care. In mental health, this includes recognising how racism, poverty, sexism, disability, and LGBTQ+ identities shape experiences of distress.

Holistic assessment: An approach that considers the whole person – including physical, mental, emotional, social, and environmental factors – when planning care.

Liaison psychiatry/mental health liaison team: A service based in emergency departments providing rapid assessment, risk formulation, and treatment planning for patients presenting with mental health needs.

Mental Capacity Act (MCA) 2005: Legislation guiding decision-making for individuals who may lack capacity. Includes the presumption of capacity, support to make decisions, best-interest decisions, and the least restrictive option.

Mental Health Act (MHA) 1983 (amended 2007): The primary legislation governing the assessment, treatment, and safeguarding of individuals with mental disorder who require compulsory care.

Neurocognitive disorders: A clinical classification used to describe conditions in which there is acquired impairment of one or more cognitive domains, such as memory, executive function, attention, or language. Neurocognitive disorders include delirium, mild neurocognitive disorder, and major neurocognitive disorder (dementia), and may arise from neurodegenerative disease, vascular pathology, infection, trauma, or metabolic causes.

NICE guidelines: Evidence-based recommendations from the National Institute for Health and Care Excellence that shape clinical practice, including mental health conditions, self-harm, dementia, and behaviour that challenges.

Non-conveyance decision: A clinical decision not to transport a patient to hospital following assessment. In mental health contexts, this requires robust risk formulation, safety planning, and multidisciplinary coordination.

Paramedic wellbeing: A professional responsibility (HCPC Standards of Proficiency) requiring practitioners to maintain their own psychological and physical health. Includes awareness of burnout, PTSD, compassion fatigue, and vicarious trauma.

Person-centred care: A therapeutic approach focusing on the person's values, lived experience, preferences, and strengths, rather than solely on symptoms or diagnosis.

Pre-hospital care: The assessment, treatment, and management of patients in the period before arrival at definitive care, typically delivered by ambulance clinicians in a community, domestic, public, or custody setting. Pre-hospital care emphasises early recognition of risk, stabilisation, safeguarding, and appropriate referral or conveyance decisions.

Psychosis: A condition involving hallucinations, delusions, disorganised thinking, or loss of reality testing. Can arise from mental illness, substance use, or organic causes.

Right Care, Right Person (RCRP): A national agreement ensuring that mental health-related calls receive healthcare-led responses instead of default police attendance. Places greater emphasis on paramedic mental health capabilities.

Risk assessment: Structured evaluation of risks such as suicide, self-harm, harm to others, exploitation, neglect, or vulnerability. Central to paramedic mental health practice.

Safeguarding: Processes to protect children and adults at risk of abuse, neglect, or exploitation. Mental health crises may indicate underlying safeguarding concerns.

Self-harm: Intentional injury to oneself, with or without suicidal intent. NICE describes it as a marker of emotional distress requiring compassionate, non-judgemental assessment.

Suicidal ideation: Thoughts of ending one's life, ranging from passive death wishes to active plans. Requires sensitive exploration and immediate safety planning.

Trauma-informed practice: An approach acknowledging the prevalence of trauma and avoiding re-traumatisation. Focuses on safety, choice, empowerment, trust, and collaboration.

Triage: The process of prioritising patient care based on clinical urgency. In mental health, this includes identifying risk, agitation level, behavioural disturbance, and need for specialist involvement.

Vulnerable adult: An adult who, due to illness, disability, mental health needs, or social circumstance, may be unable to protect themselves from harm. Paramedics frequently encounter vulnerability during crisis presentations.

1 Introduction: Foundations of mental health in paramedic practice

Jo Augustus

Paramedic practice has undergone substantial transformation over the last three decades, shifting from an emergency-transport profession to a clinically autonomous, decision-making role integral to urgent and emergency care. Mental health presentations now form a significant proportion of the ambulance workload, with paramedics frequently assessing risk, supporting people in acute psychological distress, and navigating increasingly complex multi-agency pathways. As UK health systems evolve and the legal, policy, and societal landscape changes, there has never been a more critical time for paramedics to develop specialist competencies in mental health assessment, communication, and person-centred care.

The authors situate mental health as a core component of contemporary paramedic practice. It integrates theoretical frameworks, evidence-based approaches, legislative considerations, and authentic case studies designed to promote professional judgement, reflective capacity, and confidence. The book adopts a life-course perspective, recognising that mental health needs do not arise in isolation but unfold across developmental stages, social contexts, and personal histories. By examining children, adolescents, adults, older adults, and people with severe and enduring mental health conditions, the chapters highlight the diversity of presentations encountered by paramedics and the importance of tailoring care to the individual. This book is a multi-authored volume, with each chapter written by clinicians and academics working across different areas of paramedic and mental health practice. While the chapters follow a broadly consistent structure, each has been written in the author's own voice and reflects their clinical perspective and pedagogical approach. This includes variation in case discussions, reflective elements, and Further Learning materials. The aim is not to present a uniform textbook formula, but to reflect the diversity and complexity of contemporary paramedic practice.

This introductory chapter sets the conceptual foundations for the book, beginning with the evolution of paramedic practice and the contemporary definition of mental health. It then explores the theoretical principles underpinning the person-centred, bio-psycho-social, and ecological approaches to assessment. Key policy developments, including Right Care, Right Person (RCRP), are examined to highlight the shifting responsibilities and expectations placed upon ambulance services. The chapter also addresses the centrality of equality, diversity, and inclusion (EDI), reflecting social movements such as Black Lives Matter and the increasing recognition of structural inequity within mental health systems. Finally, the chapter introduces the book's pedagogical approach, emphasising the value of case-based learning, reflective practice, and practitioner wellbeing.

The evolution of paramedic practice

The paramedic profession has transitioned from a narrow focus on emergency transport to a broad, multifaceted role that integrates assessment, clinical reasoning, health promotion, mental health care, and multi-agency collaboration. Early models of paramedic practice were derived from military trauma systems, with an emphasis on rapid extrication and conveyance. However, as patient needs changed and public expectations grew, health policy, regulation, and education began to reshape the profession. Several factors underpin this evolution:

1. *Expansion of clinical autonomy and education*. The development of degree-level qualifications, postgraduate routes, specialist roles, and advanced practice has created a more analytically capable and clinically confident workforce. Paramedics are now expected to:
   - deliver autonomous assessment and management
   - undertake complex decision-making
   - apply evidence-based practice
   - work across organisational boundaries
   - provide psychosocial support during mental health crises

   This aligns with the HCPC Standards of Proficiency (2023), which emphasise critical thinking, risk management, safeguarding, communication, and personal wellbeing.

2. *Increasing mental health demand*. International and UK research shows mental health presentations constitute a growing proportion of ambulance callouts. A scoping review by Emond, O'Meara, and Bish highlighted that mental health-related presentations are now an increasingly significant part of pre-hospital workload, yet paramedics often feel underprepared (Emond et al., 2019). Similarly, Abbaspour et al. (2020) found a high incidence of post-traumatic stress disorder (PTSD) and psychological distress among pre-hospital emergency medical service workers exposed to traumatic events and mental health crises. These psychological impacts influence clinical performance, staff retention, and quality of care.

3. *Role expansion through policy*. New models of care such as crisis response cars, mental health joint response units, and urgent community teams position paramedics as critical partners in mental health crisis pathways. NHS England's Right Care, Right Person (2023) formally shifts responsibility for mental health crises away from policing and towards health-led responses. This further embeds paramedics within mental health assessment networks.

In summary, paramedic practice now requires a deep understanding of mental health, trauma, inequality, and human experience well beyond the confines of biomedical emergency response.

Defining mental health: A contemporary perspective

Mental health is more than the absence of illness. It encompasses emotional regulation, resilience, social connectedness, and the ability to navigate daily life. The World Health Organization describes mental health as foundational to well-being, agency, and participation (WHO, 2022). Mental ill-health (e.g. depression, psychosis, anxiety, eating disorders, substance-related crises) reflects a disturbance in cognition, behaviour, or emotional regulation (APA, 2022).

Mental health presentations are deeply individual. Symptoms may be shaped by:

- biological vulnerabilities
- trauma and life experiences
- social disadvantage or discrimination
- physiological changes across the life span
- environmental stressors
- cultural identity and belonging

For paramedics, mental health assessment therefore demands not only clinical knowledge but also empathy, curiosity, cultural humility, and an awareness of structural factors influencing crisis (Augustus et al., 2022).

Person-centred care

Person-centred care is foundational to all paramedic practice. It emphasises seeing the patient as a person with preferences, values, relationships, and a unique narrative. It contrasts with traditional, diagnosis-driven models that focus solely on risk or symptoms. Person-centred approaches involve:

- building trust
- listening actively
- validating emotional experience

- supporting autonomy and choice
- collaborating on decisions
- avoiding judgement or coercion where possible

Scott (2023) highlights that emergency staff must reject stigmatising (i.e. difficult, disruptive) language and instead adopt compassionate, humanising approaches to mental health crises.

The bio-psycho-social model

Developed by Engel, the bio-psycho-social model recognises that mental health arises from dynamic interactions between:

- *Biological factors*: genetics, neurochemistry, physical illness.
- *Psychological factors*: thoughts, trauma, coping, emotion regulation.
- *Social factors*: housing, relationships, discrimination, poverty.

This framework (Engel, 1977) helps paramedics interpret complex presentations holistically. For example:

- A patient with chronic obstructive pulmonary disease (COPD) experiencing panic attacks may be responding to breathlessness, medical uncertainty, and social isolation.
- An adolescent self-harming may be coping with trauma, bullying, neurodiversity, or identity-related stress.
- A person with schizophrenia experiencing relapse may have been affected by medication non-adherence, drug use, social deprivation, or loss of support networks.

Ecological systems theory

Bronfenbrenner's ecological model expands the bio-psycho-social framework to consider multiple interconnected systems (Table 1.1). This model is valuable for paramedic assessment, as mental health crises rarely result from single factors. It encourages practitioners to piece together the broader story influencing distress (Augustus et al., 2022).

Bronfenbrenner's ecological systems theory illustrates how an individual's mental health is shaped by multiple interacting environments, from immediate relationships to wider societal systems. For paramedics, this model is particularly valuable because it helps make sense of complex crises in which clinical symptoms may be deeply linked to social disadvantage, discrimination, trauma, family conflict, or gaps in service provision. For example, a young person self-harming may be influenced not only by personal distress but also by school pressures (mesosystem), family instability (microsystem), or wider societal stigma (macrosystem). By using this model, paramedics can broaden their assessment beyond the presenting problem, strengthening

Table 1.1: Ecological systems theory

Layer	Description	Paramedic relevance
A. Microsystem	Immediate relationships (family, peers)	Collateral histories, safeguarding
B. Mesosystem	Links between microsystems	Tensions between school and family, carer strain
C. Exosystem	Wider systems (services, workplaces)	Breakdowns in community support, social care gaps
D. Macrosystem	Societal values, culture, inequality	Racism, stigma, austerity, sexism
E. Chronosystem	Life transitions over time	Bereavement, ageing, illness, trauma

person-centred practice and enabling more meaningful referrals and safety planning (Bronfenbrenner, 2009).

Adapting Bronfenbrenner's ecological systems model for paramedic practice

At the centre is the person (patient, family member, or paramedic), surrounded by interacting layers of influence.

- Person/Individual
- Who? The patient (and sometimes the paramedic)
- What to consider?
  - Physical health (e.g. pregnancy, COPD, diabetes)
  - Mental health (e.g. psychosis, anxiety, eating disorder)
  - Neurodiversity, communication style, language, coping strategies
  - Beliefs about illness, help-seeking, and services

Reflective Question: 'What do I know about this person's mental and physical health, strengths and vulnerabilities – not just their "presenting complaint"?'

A. *Microsystem*: Immediate relationships and encounters

- Family, partner, children, friends, carers.
- Interactions with paramedics, call handlers, police, midwives, ED staff.
- School, college, workplace on that day.

Examples:

- A young woman in labour whose partner is panicking – a paramedic's calm communication can stabilise the whole microsystem.
- A teenager in crisis where parents minimise symptoms or are themselves distressed.

B. *Mesosystem*: Connections between services

- Links between home, GP, community mental health team, maternity services, social care, school, and ambulance service.
- Quality of communication and handover between services.

Examples:

- Poor liaison between community perinatal team and maternity triage → woman repeatedly rings 999.
- Good GP and perinatal mental health follow-up → paramedic can safely use alternative pathways.

***Reflective Question*:** 'Which other services are involved or should be? How well are they joined up?'

C. *Exosystem*: Wider health and social system

- Local availability of services: crisis teams, perinatal mental health teams, refuges, drug and alcohol services.
- Ambulance service policies, response targets, referral pathways.
- Housing, benefits, asylum processes, school exclusion policies.

Examples:

- A woman in temporary accommodation who repeatedly calls 999 because she cannot access routine midwifery care.
- A person in psychosis who waits 12+ hours in the corridor of the emergency department (ED) because of bed shortages.

D. *Macrosystem*: Culture, law, and social norms

- Stigma surrounding mental illness, self-harm, psychosis, neurodiversity.
- Racism, sexism, ableism; cultural expectations of motherhood, masculinity, 'strength'.
- National policy: Mental Health Act, Equality Act, NICE guidance, NHS priorities.

Examples:

- Black women more likely to experience coercive responses and poorer maternity outcomes.
- Cultural beliefs about shame and honour influencing disclosure of domestic abuse or suicidal thoughts.

***Reflective Question*:** 'How might culture, stigma, or discrimination be shaping what I'm seeing – and how I respond?'

E. *Chronosystem* (the element of time and its influence on a person's development): Time, life events and service change

- *Life course*: childhood adversity, previous birth trauma, migration, bereavement.

- *Onset and course of illness*: first episode of psychosis vs. long-term severe mental illness (SMI).
- Major events: COVID-19, cost-of-living crisis, service reorganisations.

Examples:
- A woman with previous traumatic blood blister-like aneurysm now in labour again, highly anxious when paramedics arrive.
- Paramedic burnout after repeated exposure to perinatal loss.

Equality, diversity, and inclusion

Mental health cannot be separated from broader questions of equality, diversity and inclusion (EDI). Evidence consistently shows that structural inequalities such as racism, sexism, ableism, homophobia, transphobia, class-based discrimination, and the cumulative effects of poverty significantly shape mental health outcomes, access to care, trust in services, and overall wellbeing. Social movements such as Black Lives Matter have accelerated public understanding of systemic racism and highlighted longstanding disparities in detention rates, crisis pathways, and clinical outcomes for people from racialised communities. For paramedics, these issues are not abstract; they influence everyday interactions, levels of distress, histories of trauma, and the degree of trust patients may place in emergency responders. Recognising inequality is therefore not an add-on, but a fundamental part of safe, person-centred paramedic practice.

Paramedics frequently encounter individuals whose distress is exacerbated by social marginalisation, from neurodivergent children who have experienced exclusion from education to older adults facing loneliness, to LGBTQ+ individuals living with minority stress, to women presenting with undiagnosed perinatal mental health needs. Understanding how discrimination and disadvantage accumulate over the life course helps paramedics interpret behaviour more compassionately and create more meaningful therapeutic alliances. The principles of EDI also protect practitioners from unintentionally replicating harm, ensuring that care remains culturally safe, trauma-informed, and humanising.

Key EDI considerations for paramedics include:

- Awareness of structural racism and its impact on crisis pathways, coercive practices, and mistrust of services.
- Understanding intersectionality, recognising that individuals may experience multiple layers of discrimination simultaneously.
- Using culturally safe communication, avoiding assumptions, and adapting language where appropriate.
- Recognising minority stress, particularly for LGBTQ+ individuals, neurodivergent people, and those living with disabilities.
- Working sensitively with interpreters, carers, and cultural advocates to enhance understanding and rapport.

- Identifying the social determinants of poverty, housing instability, and unemployment that may be driving distress.
- Reflecting on personal bias, implicit attitudes, and professional power dynamics that affect decision-making.

Policy context: Right Care, Right Person

The introduction of the National Partnership Agreement: Right Care, Right Person (RCRP) represents a major shift in how mental health crises are managed across England (NHS England, 2023). Historically, police services have responded to a wide range of mental health-related incidents, often due to gaps in health and social care provision. However, this has led to inappropriate criminalisation, inconsistent decision-making, and situations where individuals in psychological crisis receive inadequate or non-clinical responses. Right Care, Right Person aims to ensure that individuals experiencing mental ill-health are met by the service best equipped to meet their needs, typically healthcare professionals. For paramedics, this means being increasingly central to mental health crisis responses and ensuring decisions are clinically informed, compassionate, and lawful.

Right Care, Right Person has significant implications for ambulance services (Table 1.2). Paramedics must be confident in mental health assessment, capacity evaluation, risk formulation, and referral pathways, as the absence of police attendance removes a historical safety net. At the same time, the policy aligns with paramedic expertise: paramedics are skilled communicators, used to working in unpredictable environments, and trained in de-escalation and safeguarding. The policy also encourages stronger boundaries between health and policing roles, reinforcing the responsibility of the healthcare system to provide safe, effective, and rights-based crisis care (NHS England, 2023).

Table 1.2: Implications of RCRP for paramedics

Area	Impact
Workforce demand	Increased volume of mental health-related ambulance callouts
Decision-making	Greater reliance on paramedic clinical judgement regarding risk and conveyance
Collaboration	Closer links with crisis teams, liaison psychiatry, and approved mental health professional (AMHP) services
Safeguarding	Expanded responsibilities for vulnerability assessment, capacity evaluation, and safety planning
Documentation	More detailed recording of risk, rationale, consent, and multidisciplinary liaison

Note: This book's case studies are explicitly aligned with RCRP principles.

Key implications of RCRP for paramedic practice include:

- Increased mental health-related demand, with paramedics attending a greater volume of crises previously handled by police.
- Enhanced clinical decision-making responsibilities, particularly around risk assessment, capacity, consent, and conveyance.
- A need for robust multidisciplinary collaboration, including timely liaison with crisis teams, AMHPs, social care, and liaison psychiatry.
- Greater emphasis on de-escalation skills, therapeutic communication, and trauma-informed practice.
- Clear documentation requirements, ensuring legal, ethical, and professional reasoning is transparent.
- Understanding thresholds for police involvement, especially where there is imminent harm, crime, or weapon risk.
- Increased accountability, as the default police response is removed, highlighting the importance of paramedic training and confidence.

Paramedic wellbeing: A professional priority

Paramedic wellbeing is a crucial component of safe and sustainable mental health practice. Mental health crises are often emotionally intense, unpredictable, and traumatic, not only for the person experiencing the crisis but also for the clinician providing care. Research demonstrates that paramedics face disproportionately high levels of workplace stress, burnout, exposure to violence, compassion fatigue, and symptoms of PTSD. International studies (e.g. Abbaspour et al., 2020; Alghamdi et al., 2023) indicate that up to half of prehospital clinicians may be experiencing moderate to severe psychological distress at any given time. These pressures influence clinical judgement, communication, team dynamics, and the likelihood of errors, making wellbeing a patient-safety issue as well as a personal one.

The HCPC Standards of Proficiency (2023) emphasise the responsibility of practitioners to maintain their own physical and emotional health, seek supervision, recognise personal limits, and manage the psychological demands of the role. In mental health contexts, emotional resilience is especially important. Paramedics must process intense interpersonal encounters, navigate ethical dilemmas, and manage the weight of risk often without closure or follow-up. Without support, these pressures can accumulate, contributing to burnout or withdrawal from the profession. A wellbeing-centred culture is therefore essential, where staff are empowered to access reflective practice, debrief sessions, mentorship, training, and organisational support.

Key wellbeing considerations for paramedics working in mental health include:

- Regular reflective practice, allowing clinicians to process emotionally demanding cases.
- Access to structured debriefing, particularly after complex or high-risk incidents.

- Recognising early signs of burnout, compassion fatigue, dissociation, and emotional exhaustion.
- Seeking supervision or mentorship, aligned with HCPC expectations for professional support.
- Maintaining boundaries, ensuring that empathy does not give rise to emotional over-identification.
- Prioritising physical health, sleep, and recovery, especially during periods of high workload.
- Organisational cultures that value psychological safety, encouraging transparency, peer support, and help-seeking.

Each chapter of the book includes reflective prompts and wellbeing considerations in order to promote safe practice.

The case study as a learning tool

Case-based learning is an essential pedagogical approach within paramedic education, enabling learners to connect theoretical knowledge to the realities of frontline mental health care. Unlike abstract descriptions of symptoms or protocols, case studies offer authentic, context-rich scenarios that mirror the complexity, uncertainty, and emotional intensity of real-world practice. They encourage students to step into the practitioner role, examining not only what decisions are made, but why they are made, how those decisions are justified, and what ethical, cultural, or interpersonal factors must be considered. Case studies also create space for emotion, reflection, and critical thinking skills that are central to effective, person-centred paramedic practice. Throughout this book, cases are designed to reflect diverse populations, varied clinical presentations, and the multi-agency nature of mental health crisis work. They provide a safe and supported environment for learners to analyse, question, and rehearse decision-making, ultimately promoting confidence, competence, and professional identity formation.

Case-based learning helps paramedic students to:

- Apply theory to practice, making connections between mental health concepts, legislation, and real-world presentations.
- Appreciate the complexity of crisis situations, including overlapping physical, psychological, and social factors.
- Explore communication strategies, practising de-escalation, active listening, empathy, and rapport-building.
- Engage with ethical and legal decision-making, including capacity, consent, risk, safeguarding, and duty of care.
- Critically analyse clinical judgement, developing reasoning skills around conveyance, referral, non-conveyance, and safety planning.
- Reflect on emotions, bias, and professional behaviour, supporting self-awareness, cultural humility, and trauma-informed practice.

- Understand the role of multidisciplinary collaboration, including liaison psychiatry, AMHPs, crisis teams, and police under RCRP principles.
- Recognise the pressures, ambiguities, and time-critical nature of paramedic practice, helping students prepare for real-world uncertainty.

Mental health models in paramedic practice

Table 1.3 outlines four key conceptual models – biomedical, bio-psycho-social, ecological systems, and person-centred care – that underpin contemporary paramedic approaches to mental health. For paramedics, these models provide different lenses for interpreting complex presentations, such as acute psychosis, anxiety, self-harm, and behavioural disturbance. Understanding the strengths and limitations of each enables practitioners to adapt their assessment and decision-making according to the individual and the situation. For example, although the biomedical model offers clarity around diagnosis and pharmacology, it may overlook trauma or structural inequality; conversely, the ecological model or the bio-psycho-social model supports holistic reasoning but requires greater time and cognitive effort. By comparing models side-by-side, paramedics can better appreciate how theory informs practice and why a flexible, person-centred approach is essential in mental health care.

Skills required for mental health crisis assessment aligned to HCPC Standards

Table 1.4 highlights the core competencies expected of paramedics when managing mental health crises, mapped explicitly to the HCPC Standards of Proficiency (2023). These skills extend far beyond clinical assessment and include therapeutic communication, culturally safe practice, reflective self-awareness, and legal literacy relating to the Mental Health Act 1983 (MHA), Mental Capacity Act 2005 (MCA), and safeguarding. For paramedics, this table

Table 1.3: Comparison of mental health models in paramedic practice

Model	Strengths	Limitations
Biomedical	Clear diagnostic criteria; links to medication	Can overlook trauma, context, inequality
Bio-psycho-social	Holistic; integrates psychological and social factors	Requires more time and training
Ecological systems (Bronfenbrenner)	Recognises structural and societal influences	Complexity can challenge rapid assessment
Person-centred	Builds trust; improves outcomes	Requires emotional labour from clinician

Table 1.4: Skills required for mental health crisis assessment (aligned to HCPC, 2023)

Competency area	Expected paramedic capabilities
Communication	Active listening, validation, rapport-building
Risk assessment	Suicide/self-harm, harm to others, vulnerability, safeguarding
Legal literacy	MHA, MCA, safeguarding duties, RCRP
Cultural safety	Anti-racist, inclusive, trauma-informed approaches
Clinical decision-making	Conveyance vs. non-conveyance, referral pathways
Wellbeing awareness	Recognising emotional strain, seeking supervision

reinforces that mental health care is an integral part of their professional scope, not an optional extension. It also emphasises the emotional labour involved in crisis work and the importance of practitioner wellbeing, supervision, and resilience. By reviewing these competencies, paramedics can identify their own strengths and development needs, supporting safe, compassionate practice across diverse and unpredictable mental health scenarios (HCPC, 2023).

The bio-psycho-social model

The bio-psycho-social model emphasises that mental health presentations arise from interconnected biological, psychological, and social influences. For paramedics, this visual reinforces the importance of holistic assessment, recognising, for example, how medication side effects (biological), trauma histories (psychological), or homelessness (social) can directly shape a person's behaviour and risk (Engel, 1977). In fast-paced, high-pressure environments, paramedics may feel compelled to focus on immediate symptoms; however, this model encourages deeper enquiry and curiosity, helping practitioners to avoid assumptions or pathologising behaviour that may be rooted in unmet needs. The bio-psycho-social approach aligns with NICE guidance, HCPC standards, and trauma-informed practice, supporting more accurate judgement, more compassionate care, and more effective multi-agency collaboration.

Adapting the bio-psycho-social model for paramedic practice

The bio-psycho-social (BPS) model provides a holistic framework that helps paramedics understand not just *what* is happening to a patient, but *why* it is happening and *what factors* may influence their presentation, safety, and recovery. Originally developed by Engel (1977), the model emphasises that health is shaped by biological, psychological, and social influences that interact dynamically. In paramedic practice where clinicians often meet people at moments of acute crisis, using the BPS model enriches assessment, supports person-centred care, and improves clinical judgement.

A. *Biological factors: What is happening in the body?* Paramedics routinely assess biological contributors, but the BPS model encourages going beyond symptoms to understand underlying mechanisms.

Key considerations:

- Current physical condition, e.g. pregnancy, infection, dehydration, diabetes.
- Injury, pain, fatigue, medication adherence, side effects, intoxication or withdrawal.
- Co-morbidities that may mask or mimic mental health symptoms, e.g. hypoglycaemia, hypoxia, sepsis, thyroid disorders.
- Neurodevelopmental or neurocognitive differences influencing responses.

Paramedic examples:

- Breathlessness could be panic, but could also be a pulmonary embolism, asthma, anaemia, or sepsis.
- Confusion may indicate delirium, hypoxia, trauma, medication effect, or psychosis.
- Pain in labour or miscarriage interacts with emotional response and cultural meaning.

***Reflective Question*:** 'What biological changes or risks might explain or interact with the patient's presentation?'

B. *Psychological factors: What is happening in the mind?* Psychological influences often shape how symptoms are interpreted, described, and coped with. For paramedics, recognising these factors is crucial for safe decision-making.

Key considerations:

- Mood, anxiety, trauma history, distress, coping strategies.
- Fear, pain, shame, guilt, stigma influencing help-seeking.
- Cognitive state – alertness, orientation, insight, hallucinations, intrusive thoughts.
- Birth trauma, perinatal mental health concerns, grief reactions.
- Neurodiversity, e.g. sensory overload, communication preferences.

Paramedic examples:

- A distressed patient after pregnancy loss may appear calm or withdrawn, e.g. shock, dissociation.
- A person in psychosis may refuse care not due to hostility, but through fear or perceptual disturbance.
- Pain and fear in labour – altered breathing, panic, miscommunication.

***Reflective Question*:** 'How is the patient feeling emotionally, and how might this affect their communication or decisions?'

C. *Social factors: What is happening around this person?* Social determinants are especially important in paramedic work, where crises often arise from inequalities, unsafe environments, and unmet needs.

Key considerations:
- Housing, poverty, digital exclusion, transport, language barriers.
- Family dynamics, caregiving responsibilities, domestic abuse.
- Cultural beliefs around illness, birth, mental health, or death.
- Migrant status, NHS charging concerns, health literacy.
- Breakdown of community or maternity services; lack of continuity of care.
- Access to GP, mental health teams, perinatal services.

Paramedic examples:
- A woman who cannot access antenatal care due to language/digital barriers is more likely to call 999.
- A young person in crisis after family conflict.
- A patient refusing conveyance due to childcare responsibilities or insecure immigration status.

Reflective Question: 'What social or cultural factors are shaping risk, access, communication, or expectations today?'

Putting the three domains together: Why it matters for paramedics

In the pre-hospital setting, biological, psychological, and social factors interact rapidly. Understanding these interactions helps paramedics:

- Distinguish physical emergencies from psychological distress and recognise when both are present.
- Perform safer risk assessments, including suicide, safeguarding, and capacity.
- Take a trauma-informed approach, reducing fear and improving communication.
- Recognise inequalities that influence antenatal care, mental health crises, or repeat 999 calls.
- Plan appropriate referral pathways, including urgent care, perinatal mental health teams, crisis services, social care, or safeguarding.

Example: A woman experiencing preterm labour

- *Biological*: pain, bleeding, contractions, risk of postpartum haemorrhage (PPH).
- *Psychological*: fear, grief, shock, dissociation.
- *Social*: limited English, no antenatal care, digital exclusion, immigration concerns.

A holistic understanding improves interpretation, communication, and safety.

A paramedic-friendly BPS reflection tool

Quick BPS check: Five questions

1 *Biological:* What physical conditions or risks may be driving the presentation?
2 *Psychological:* What emotions, thoughts, or trauma responses are influencing communication or decisions?
3 *Social:* What environmental or cultural factors could be shaping risk or help-seeking?
4 *Interaction:* How are these domains influencing each other?
5 *Action:* What pathways, safety measures, or follow-up does this combination require?

Conclusion

The themes explored throughout this introductory chapter highlight the profound transformation of contemporary paramedic practice and the centrality of mental health within that evolution. Paramedics are no longer confined to the traditional remit of emergency transport; instead, they operate as autonomous clinicians navigating complex, emotionally charged, and socially layered presentations. Mental health is now recognised as a routine component of urgent and emergency care, shaped by biological, psychological, social, and structural influences that require sensitive, holistic assessment. The interplay between the bio-psycho-social model, Bronfenbrenner's ecological systems theory, and person-centred care underscores the importance of understanding individuals within the overall context of their lives, rather than through diagnostic labels alone. This introduction also highlights the growing emphasis on trauma-informed approaches, cultural humility, and anti-discriminatory practice, reflecting developments such as Black Lives Matter and the recognition of enduring inequalities within mental health systems. Together, these frameworks encourage paramedics to adopt a reflective, curious, and compassionate stance, acknowledging the humanity of every patient encountered.

At the same time, national policy shifts – most notably Right Care, Right Person – reinforce the expanding responsibilities placed upon ambulance services as health-led responders to mental health crises. This requires enhanced legal literacy, collaborative working across multidisciplinary teams, and greater confidence in risk assessment, capacity evaluation, and nuanced decision-making. This introduction also foregrounds the emotional labour inherent in mental health care, drawing on evidence that paramedics experience significant psychological strain, burnout, and exposure to trauma. Consequently, practitioner wellbeing emerges as an essential professional competency, integral to safe and sustainable practice. Case-based learning is positioned as a valuable pedagogical tool throughout this book, enabling students to apply theory to realistic, complex scenarios; to engage critically with the ethical, interpersonal, and organisational dimensions of practice; and to develop clinical reasoning grounded in empathy, evidence, and reflective judgement. Collectively, these themes set the foundation for a text that aims not only to build knowledge, but to support the development of thoughtful, resilient, and person-centred practitioners equipped to respond to the full spectrum of mental health needs encountered in pre-hospital care.

References

Abbaspour, S., Tajik, R., Atif, K., Eshghi, H., Teimori, G., Ghodrati-Torbati, A., et al. (2020). Prevalence and correlates of mental health status among pre-hospital healthcare staff. *Clinical Practice and Epidemiology in Mental Health, 16*, 17–23.

Alghamdi, A., Alharbi, M., Alshibani, A., Allohidan, F., Alabdali, A., and Aljerian, N. (2023). Evaluation of the psychological distress and mental well-being of pre-hospital care providers in Saudi Arabia during COVID-19. *British Paramedic Journal, 8*(1), 1–8.

American Psychiatric Association (APA) (2022). *Diagnostic and Statistical Manual of Mental Disorders* (DSM-5-TR). Washington, DC: APA Publishing.

Augustus, J., Patrick, Y.W., and Gardner, P. (2022). *An Introduction to Mental Health in Paramedic Science.* London: Open University Press.

Bronfenbrenner, U. (2009). *The Ecology of Human Development: Experiments by nature and design.* Cambridge, MA: Harvard University Press.

Emond, K., O'Meara, P., and Bish, M. (2019). Paramedic management of mental health related presentations: A scoping review. *Journal of Mental Health, 28*(1), 89–96.

Engel, G.L. (1977). The need for a new medical model: A challenge for biomedicine. *Science, 196*(4286), 129–136.

Health and Care Professions Council (HCPC) (2023). *Standards of Proficiency: Paramedics.* London: HCPC. https://www.hcpc-uk.org/standards/standards-of-proficiency/paramedics/ (accessed 25 November 2025).

NHS England (2023). *National Partnership Agreement: Right Care, Right Person.* https://www.gov.uk/government/publications/national-partnership-agreement-right-care-right-person (accessed 25 November 2025).

Scott, T. (2023). *Mental Health: Intervention skills for the emergency services.* Cham: Springer.

World Health Organization (WHO) (2022). *Mental health.* https://www.who.int/news-room/fact-sheets/detail/mental-health-strengthening-our-response (accessed 25 November 2025).

2 Neurodevelopmental disorders, neurodiversity, and early crisis care

Jo Augustus and Paul K. Miller

Introduction

Children and young people (CYP) with mental health needs and neurodevelopmental conditions form an increasingly routine part of contemporary paramedic practice. Neurodivergence including autism, attention-deficit/hyperactivity disorder (ADHD), intellectual disability, developmental language disorders, and specific learning differences is estimated to affect approximately 15–20% of the population (Singer, 2019; Baron-Cohen, 2019). Prevalence data for childhood ADHD range globally from 5% to 7%, with many young people continuing to experience impairments well into adolescence and adulthood (Thomas et al., 2015; Salari et al., 2023). At the same time, demand for assessment and treatment has intensified, with children across the UK frequently experiencing long waits for Child and Adolescent Mental Health Services (CAMHS) appointments, neurodevelopmental assessments, and specialist community support (NHS Digital, 2023; Children's Commissioner, 2023). In this context, paramedics are often the first healthcare professionals to respond when a neurodivergent child reaches crisis.

Throughout this chapter, the authors use the term 'neurodevelopmental conditions' to describe a range of clinically recognised presentations, while also drawing on the concept of *neurodiversity*, which frames neurological differences as valid forms of human variation rather than deficits (Kapp et al., 2013; Chapman, 2019). This dual perspective is important. Many CYP and their families experience distress, risk, or impairment that requires meaningful intervention; however, these challenges are often shaped or intensified by environmental demands, sensory overload, unmet support needs, and systemic inequities rather than by the child's neurology alone (Crane et al., 2019). For paramedics, working with neurodivergent CYP therefore requires moving beyond purely symptom-focused approaches to consider how context, communication, sensory environments, and lived experience shape a young person's presentation.

The pre-hospital environment and neurodivergent CYP

The pre-hospital environment can be uniquely complex for neurodivergent CYP. Ambulances, crowds, bright lights, sudden noise, and rapid questioning can lead to sensory overload, shutdown, or behaviour that challenges (Alisic et al., 2017; Nicolaidis et al., 2015). Research highlights that behaviours often interpreted as aggression or refusal may instead be expressions of anxiety, pain, trauma, or difficulty processing information under stress (Rodríguez-Armendariz et al., 2024). Simple adjustments such as reducing sensory load, slowing communication, offering predictability, and allowing processing time have been shown to improve engagement and safety during emergency encounters (Lombardi et al., 2024). These adaptations require clinicians to adopt a flexible, trauma-informed approach, balancing clinical urgency with attunement to the child's sensory, emotional, and communicative needs.

Children and young people rarely present in isolation – they exist within families, peer groups, schools, and communities that profoundly influence wellbeing and help-seeking. Many families navigating neurodevelopmental pathways experience fragmented support, school exclusions, or long waits for assessment and intervention (Children's Commissioner, 2023; YoungMinds, 2023). When a young person's needs escalate and no timely alternatives exist, families may turn to emergency services not because of acute medical risk but because all other avenues have been exhausted. Paramedics therefore operate not only as clinicians but as mediators within systems that often feel overwhelming, under-resourced, or impenetrable.

NICE guidelines relevant to autism (NICE, 2021a), ADHD (NICE, 2018), self-harm (NICE, 2022), and crisis care for CYP set out evidence-based recommendations for assessment, de-escalation, and referral. Yet guidelines cannot fully account for the realities of pre-hospital encounters: the distressed 13-year-old in a supermarket car park, the adolescent who communicates more effectively through text or gesture, or the young person whose distress is rooted in trauma or sensory overload. This chapter therefore encourages readers to critically examine how decision-making whether to convey, how to communicate, how to assess risk, or when to involve other agencies can either uphold or drift away from a person-centred ethos.

This chapter aims to support paramedic students and practising clinicians to deepen their understanding of how neurodevelopmental differences influence assessment, communication, distress, and safety in the pre-hospital setting. Through theory, lived-experience perspectives, and detailed case studies, we will explore how neurodiversity intersects with mental health, trauma, and social inequality. Importantly, the chapter also recognises the emotional labour inherent in responding to CYP in crisis. Sustaining compassionate, person-centred practice requires attention to paramedic wellbeing, reflective practice, and supervision essentials rather than optional extras in this challenging area of care.

What is trauma-informed practice?

Trauma-informed practice for paramedics involves recognising that many patients have past or ongoing experiences of trauma that can shape how they respond during emergencies. It requires approaching every interaction with an emphasis on safety, choice, collaboration, trust, and empowerment, avoiding actions that could inadvertently re-trigger distress. For paramedics, this means using calm communication, reducing sensory and environmental stressors, explaining procedures before doing them, and prioritising dignity during assessment and intervention. By understanding how trauma affects behaviour, cognition, and physiological responses, paramedics are better able to deliver compassionate, person-centred care particularly in mental health and neurodivergent presentations.

Understanding neurodevelopment and neurodiversity

Neurodevelopmental disorders: Overview

The term 'neurodevelopmental disorders' describes a variety of conditions that arise during the developmental period and affect personal, social, intellectual, and/or occupational functioning (Morris-Rosendahl and Crocq, 2020; Tal-Saban et al., 2025). Dominant contemporary classification systems, the latest revisions of the *Diagnostic and Statistical Manual of Mental Disorders* (DSM-5-TR) and the *International Classification of Diseases* (ICD-11), provide descriptive frameworks for understanding how these disorders manifest (rather than categorical diagnoses thereof), inherently recognising that neurological development fluctuates considerably between individuals, and produces distinct variations in how individuals process information, communicate with others, and engage with their environments (APA, 2022; WHO, 2022). The most common of these disorders are described below.

Autism spectrum condition (ASC) is, at its core, characterised by atypical methods of addressing social communication and interaction, alongside restricted and/or repetitive patterns in behaviour, interests, or activities (Miller et al., 2025a; Nicolaidis et al., 2015). These features present across a broad spectrum, with considerable variation between autistic individuals. Sensory processing differences are common, involving heightened or diminished sensitivity to many environmental stimuli including light, sound, touch, taste, and smell (Bowden and Miller, 2025). Many autistic people also experience difficulties conceptualising and communicating emotions, with alexithymia (an alienation from one's own feelings) considerably more common than among the general population (Kinnaird et al., 2019; Miller et al., 2025b).

The core difficulties that autistic people experience with simply 'being in the world', and isolation from it, are core factors in why their rates of diagnosed depression and anxiety disorders are significantly above general population norms (Moore et al., 2022; O'Nions et al., 2024).

Attention-deficit/hyperactivity disorder (ADHD) involves persistent patterns of inattention, hyperactivity, and impulsivity affecting functioning across a variety of contexts (Popit et al., 2024). Individuals may present with predominantly inattentive features, predominantly hyperactive-impulsive features, or a more balanced combination of both (Cortese et al., 2025; Salari et al., 2023). It is a defining clinical characteristic of ADHD that these difficulties in sustaining focus, organising tasks, and regulating behaviour are the result of neurological differences in executive function and self-regulation rather being indicative of volitional conduct (APA, 2022; WHO, 2022), although this does not always afford affected individuals exception from social judgement to the contrary (Kalokyri, 2025). More recent research has also increasingly identified a relationship between ADHD and pain sensitivity, particularly indicating a potential vulnerability to chronic pain that can be mistaken for 'catastrophising' (Brown et al., 2025).

Intellectual disability is characterised by the DSM-5-TR and the ICD-11 in terms of significant limitations evident in general intellectual functioning and adaptive behaviour (APA, 2022; WHO, 2022). Originating (by definition) during the developmental period, these limitations affect the conceptual, social, and practical skills of the individual. Considerable variations in presentation, however, mandate careful attention to provision of corollary social, occupational, and emotional support (Dagnan et al., 2023; Mahoney et al., 2021; Pallisera et al., 2021).Communication and developmental language disorders, meanwhile, specifically affect an individual's understanding and/or use of symbolic interaction systems, predominantly spoken and/or written language, facial expressions, and gestures (APA, 2022; WHO, 2022). Ranging from fluency disorders such as stuttering to more totalising difficulties with social interaction, these can create barriers to socialisation and general quality of life that may prove highly distressing for the affected individual and often require carefully tailored communication therapies (Duinmeijer et al., 2025; Ekström et al., 2023).

Specific learning disabilities (SLDs) address differences in acquiring and using core skills in one or more of reading, writing, and mathematics. Dyslexia, probably the most well-known of these, affects reading and written language processing. This variously involves difficulties with accurate and fluent word recognition and sentence-level decoding that typically derive from phonological processing challenges (Catts et al., 2024). Dysgraphia impacts upon writing, including fine motor control, letter formation, spelling, and grammar (Chung et al., 2020). Dyscalculia involves persistent problems with comprehending and acquiring numerical concepts, 'number facts', and mathematical procedures (Ergan, 2025). It should be noted that SLDs are not typically indicative of general intellectual capacity; indeed, they are in part defined by their discordance with an affected individual's broader cognitive level (Chung et al., 2020).

However, individuals with SLDs routinely encounter stigma that extrapolates their specific disability to a more general sense of 'incapacity', with potentially serious consequences for their self-esteem and mental health (Ergan, 2025; Haft et al., 2022).

Dyspraxia, or developmental coordination disorder (DCD), affects an individual's motor coordination and planning, with impacts upon fine and gross motor skills and their organisation of movement sequences (APA, 2022; WHO, 2022). Common interpretations of their conditions as simple clumsiness, slowness, and inaccuracy often lead affected individuals to have a diminished self-concept and significant anxiety in social situations (Elsherif, 2025). Relatedly, Tourette's syndrome and related tic disorders are characterised by sudden, rapid, recurrent motor movements or vocalisations that are experienced as involuntary (Johnson et al., 2023). The severity and frequency of tics typically fluctuate over time and commonly intensify during periods of stress, fatigue, or heightened emotion. While individuals may sometimes be able to suppress tics temporarily, typically to the ends of avoiding social stigma, this requires considerable effort and often results in subsequent increases in tic expression (Gill and Kompoliti, 2020; Pring et al., 2025).

Co-occurrence and intersection

A critical consideration for this chapter is that neurodevelopmental conditions seldom present in isolation. The boundaries between different conditions are often indistinct, with considerable overlap and high rates of co-occurrence. An individual may be both autistic and have ADHD (Hatch et al., 2023), ADHD routinely co-presents with a SLD (Faedda et al., 2019), and dyspraxia is disproportionately common in individuals with autism (Massoni, 2025). Moreover, Tourette's syndrome co-occurs with both ADHD and autism (Carias and Wevrick, 2019; Gill and Kompoliti, 2020). This intersection reflects the complex nature of neurological development. It also underscores the extraordinary difficulties that individuals with neurodevelopmental conditions can experience in everyday life.

A small number of such issues around independence, social stigma, self-worth, and mental health are documented above with respect to each of the named conditions. Where the conditions 'stack', the attendant social and psychological problems typically multiply. Trauma histories are disproportionately represented among these populations, often relating to experiences of bullying, social exclusion, or repeated encounters with environments not designed to accommodate difference (Accardo et al., 2025; Bitsika et al., 2022a, 2022b; Vargas-Salas et al., 2025). Sleep difficulties similarly affect many individuals, particularly CYP, and can compound other challenges (Kirkpatrick et al., 2019; Paggetti et al., 2025; Uygur, 2025). Depression, anxiety, and suicide rates are all elevated, again particularly in CYP (Accardo et al., 2025; Kazda et al., 2022; O'Nions et al., 2024; Wilson and Gullon-Scott, 2024). These are key matters of awareness for any frontline healthcare practitioner.

The neurodiversity paradigm

The neurodiversity paradigm largely frames neurological differences, and particularly autism and ADHD, as natural human variation rather than deficits requiring correction (Botha et al., 2022; Kapp et al., 2013; Nordby et al., 2023). This perspective shifts emphasis from medical pathology to that upon the environments, systems, and societal expectations that create barriers or facilitate inclusion for people who experience the world in different ways (Black et al., 2024).

This tension between medical and social models in paramedicine reflects broader debates within disability studies and has substantive implications for healthcare practice (Rahman et al., 2024). Medical models in this domain risk reducing complex, contextually embedded experiences to symptom checklists, potentially overlooking how systemic factors including inaccessible environments, inflexible institutional practices, and societal stigma contribute to distress (Crane et al., 2019). Conversely, strengths-based approaches risk minimising genuine suffering or dismissing legitimate needs for clinical intervention and support (Chapman, 2019). A balanced understanding for paramedics needs to recognise that while neurological diversity merits respect and accommodation, some individuals do experience their conditions in ways that are profoundly disenabling and require meaningful emergency healthcare responses (Lombardi et al., 2024).

In this respect, lived-experience voices increasingly inform service design and delivery through co-production and patient and public involvement and engagement (PPIE) frameworks (Miller et al., 2025b). Contemporary research indicates that receiving an autism diagnosis can fundamentally reshape how individuals contextualise life experiences, legitimise needs for accommodations, reduce anxieties about self-presentation, and facilitate access to formal and informal support networks through shared identity (Botha et al., 2022; Dagnan et al., 2023; Miller et al., 2025a, 2025b). These insights underscore the importance of attending to how neurodivergent individuals understand and articulate their own experiences rather than imposing predetermined clinical interpretations.

For pre-hospital care, the neurodiversity paradigm has direct practical implications. Communication approaches must accommodate diverse processing styles and preferences, recognising that some individuals might communicate more effectively through text, gesture, or alternative modalities than through rapid verbal exchange (Nordby et al., 2023; Rahman et al., 2024). Sensory environments matter profoundly in this respect; bright lights, sirens, crowded spaces, and sudden movements can trigger overwhelming sensory experiences (Crane et al., 2019; Miller et al., 2025b). This can indicate an order of distress that could be read as catastrophising, where this might not inherently be the case (Nicolaidis et al., 2015). Offering choice and control wherever clinically feasible respects autonomy and reduces experiences of powerlessness that may echo previous trauma (Black et al., 2024). Trauma-informed practice becomes essential, recognising that many neurodivergent individuals carry histories of invalidation, coercion, or harm within healthcare and other institutional settings (Alisic et al., 2017; Crane et al., 2019; Garratt, 2023). Adapting practice to accommodate neurodivergent needs is not an optional extra but a fundamental requirement of person-centred, equitable care.

Child and adolescent developmental considerations

Typically, emotional regulation develops progressively through childhood and adolescence, moving from reliance on external co-regulation, where caregivers provide comfort, validation, and emotional scaffolding, towards increasingly autonomous self-regulation strategies (Silvers, 2022). For neurodivergent CYP, this developmental process may follow different timelines or require sustained co-regulation support beyond typical age expectations (Betts and Patrick, 2006; Duinmeijer et al., 2025; Tal-Saban et al., 2025). Standard developmental challenges around planning, impulse control, risk assessment, and emotional regulation may, moreover, be amplified, creating particular vulnerabilities during a crisis (Betts and Patrick, 2006; Black et al., 2024; Kalisch et al., 2024). In such situations, recognising current regulatory capacity and adapting communication accordingly become critical; expecting self-regulation from a distressed CYP who requires co-regulation, for example, will likely exacerbate the situation rather than ameliorate it (Kalisch et al., 2024; Silvers, 2022).

Family and carer contexts profoundly shape how neurodivergent CYP experience and navigate crises (Bitsika et al., 2022a, 2022b; Black et al., 2024). Families may have extensive expertise about their child's communication needs, sensory sensitivities, effective de-escalation strategies, and trauma history. However, families themselves may be exhausted, traumatised, or experiencing breakdown of usual coping mechanisms by the time any external help is called (Kalisch et al., 2024; Schneider et al., 2019). Attending to family dynamics without making assumptions about competence, functioning, or intent requires any healthcare practitioner to simultaneously appreciate that families are typically the experts on their children, and that family stress or dysfunction may itself contribute to the presenting crisis. Creating space for family voices while maintaining focus on the young person's immediate safety and wellbeing can help navigate this inherent tension.

Clinical presentations in pre-hospital settings

Mental health presentations common in neurodivergent CYP

Anxiety represents one of the most prevalent mental health presentations among neurodivergent CYP, for whom rates of diagnosed anxiety disorders are considerably above population norms (Accardo et al., 2025; Miller et al., 2025a; O'Nions et al., 2024). Panic presentations among neurodivergent CYP may also arise variously from sensory overload, social demands exceeding available processing capacity, and/or disruptions to routine and predictability (Fielding et al., 2025; Kalisch et al., 2024). For autistic individuals, difficulties processing ambiguous social information and intolerance of uncertainty can also contribute substantially to anxiety (Moore et al., 2022). Shutdowns occur when sensory or emotional demands overwhelm regulatory capacity, resulting in withdrawal, reduced responsiveness, and apparent disconnection. Whereas meltdowns involve observable distress and agitation, shutdowns represent a retroflexed collapse of regulatory functioning (Phung et al., 2021). Much like impulse control issues in ADHD (Cortese et al., 2025), both require recognition as neurological responses to overwhelming circumstances, rather than volitional behaviour.

What may thus appear as challenging behaviour in neurodiverse CYP frequently represents (mutually) misunderstood communication. Presentations that a paramedic may interpret as aggression, knockback, or non-compliance often communicate unmet needs, pain, fear, or sensory distress in atypical ways (Rodríguez-Armendariz et al., 2024). A young person who pushes away assessment equipment may be experiencing tactile hypersensitivity; physical resistance may signal trauma responses or comprehension difficulties (Bowden and Miller, 2025; Kalisch et al., 2024). As previously noted, bullying victimisation is disproportionately experienced by neurodivergent CYP (Accardo et al., 2025), potentially amplifying distress during pre-hospital encounters where any sense of pressurised 'interrogation' is experienced.

Suicidal ideation and self-harm occur at markedly elevated rates among neurodivergent adolescents (Crane et al., 2019). Self-harm may, however, serve multiple atypical functions within this group, including emotional regulation and/or response to overwhelming sensory experiences. For some neurodivergent young people with difficulties articulating internal states, self-harm becomes a key means of expressing psychological pain (Kinnaird et al., 2019; Miller et al., 2025a). Any assessment must, therefore, attend to both immediate risk and underlying contributors, not least social isolation and systemic barriers to appropriate support (NICE, 2022).

Somatisation issues such as abdominal pain, headaches, and sleep disturbances frequently accompany anxiety, sensory overload, and emotional dysregulation (Kirkpatrick et al., 2019; Uygur, 2025). These presentations may complicate triage decision-making, particularly when young people struggle to articulate relationships between physical symptoms and psychological states. The relative prevalence of alexithymia among neurodiverse – and particularly autistic – youth can somewhat inevitably compound this diagnostic challenge (Bloch et al., 2021; Kinnaird et al., 2019). Similarly, the prospective relationship between ADHD and pain sensitivity merits particular attention, with evidence indicating a potential vulnerability to chronic pain disproportionate to conventional stressors (Brown et al., 2025).

Sensory and environmental factors

The pre-hospital environment presents multiple sensory challenges that can trigger or escalate distress in neurodivergent CYP. Ambulance sirens, flashing and/or bright lights, equipment alarms, radio communications, and crowded scenes create intense auditory and visual stimulation (Bond et al., 2025; Lombardi et al., 2024; Miller et al., 2025b), while unexpected touch, textures of equipment, and smells of medical supplies may provoke hypersensitive responses (Isaacs et al., 2020). These sensory factors can directly impact triage, communication, and cooperation capacity. A young neurodiverse person experiencing corollary sensory overload may be unable to respond to questions, follow instructions, or tolerate examination (Passarello et al., 2022). What may appear as lack of cooperation may reflect a genuine inability to process multiple simultaneous demands, particularly given that sensory processing differences demonstrate clear relationships with anxiety in autistic individuals (Miller et al., 2025a; Moore et al., 2022). Sensory distress can also escalate rapidly; a child who initially appears calm may reach a 'tipping' point as cumulative sensory input exceeds processing capacity (Fielding et al., 2025; Kinnaird et al., 2019).

Contemporary evidence-based approaches to clinical work involve environmental modification wherever possible. Reducing unnecessary noise by lowering radio volumes, minimising unrelated conversations, and avoiding sirens unless operationally essential decreases auditory load (Bond et al., 2025; Lombardi et al., 2024). Dimming lights, avoiding shining torches at faces, and positioning away from flashing emergency lights manage visual sensitivity (Bond et al., 2025). Warning before touching, explaining what touch will involve, and offering choices about who provides care respects bodily autonomy. Providing time and space, allowing the young person to remain in familiar surroundings until movement becomes clinically necessary, and minimising personnel present all reduce overwhelming stimulation (Lombardi et al., 2024). These adaptations require little specialist equipment, only clinical awareness and procedural flexibility.

Communication differences

Neurodivergent CYP often process language literally and/or struggle with figurative speech, implied meanings, and ambiguous instructions (Duinmeijer et al., 2025; Ekström et al., 2023). Idiomatic expressions such as 'we'll take a quick look' or 'just relax' can create confusion when interpreted at face value. Delayed processing means responses may not be immediate; silence may reflect time required to process information rather than lack of attention. It is well noted in broader sociolinguistics that a socially normative discomfort with silence can induce many to 'interject' after a fairly short period of non-talk (Miller, 2013). This action, typically based on the assumption of mishearing or misunderstanding, however well-intentioned, often has the latent function of disrupting and resetting the cognitive processes of a speaker who was not yet ready to speak (Grimwood and Miller, 2014). The upshot thereof is sustained misunderstanding, with yet further stress caused to the neurodiverse individual. Echolalia (the often-rhythmic repeating of words or phrases of another person), although found awkward in conventional conversation by most, can serve multiple functions for a neurodiverse child, including processing time, expressing agreement, or managing anxiety (Cohn and Harrison, 2025;

Cohn et al., 2024). Selective mutism, meanwhile, occurs when anxiety or sensory overload renders speech impossible despite intact language capacity (Duinmeijer et al., 2025). Both are easily read *in situ* as being 'difficult' at best.

In the broader sense of communication, more in line with Erving Goffman's sense of 'presentation of self' (Goffman, 1959), it is imperative to address the issue of 'masking' among neurodivergent youth. This involves a battery of techniques used to suppress natural communication patterns in order to present as 'more neurotypical', which in turn requires substantial effort that steadily depletes cognitive resources for engaging with any form of social engagement (Bowden and Miller, 2025; Miller et al., 2025b). Effective maskers, typically of the later-diagnosed order, can sustain that mask under considerable stress. When the masking fails, however, sudden changes in self-presentation may be mistaken for psychological deterioration rather than recognised as exhaustion of regulatory capacity (Quigley and Gallagher, 2025).

In terms of assisting neurodivergent youth, practical strategies for a paramedic can include using simple, concrete language without idioms or ambiguity (Powell and Bradley, 2025); providing one instruction at a time, allowing processing time, and checking understanding by asking the young person to demonstrate what has been requested improves clarity. Visual aids including written instructions, pictures, and gestures supplement verbal communication. Slowing pace, reducing non-essential talking, and minimising questions to those immediately necessary reduces cognitive load (Kalisch et al., 2024). Offering reassurance through predictability, explaining what will happen next, maintaining consistency between what is said and done, and honouring choices wherever possible, build trust (Cortese et al., 2025; Doherty et al., 2023). Where verbal communication is limited, attending to non-verbal cues, offering alternative methods including text or pointing, and accepting that silence may represent the only available response respect diverse communication needs (Duinmeijer et al., 2025).

Safeguarding and risk assessment

Safeguarding and risk assessment constitute essential components of person-centred care when supporting individuals with neurodevelopmental conditions across the life course. Paramedics must assess decision-making capacity in accordance with the Mental Capacity Act 2005, while for CYP, *Gillick competence* provides guidance regarding the extent to which a child can provide informed consent based upon maturity and understanding (Department of Health and Social Care, 2009). A biopsychosocial perspective proves particularly valuable, recognising how cognitive presentations, emotional distress, and social vulnerability interact to shape risk profiles (Rahman et al., 2024). Family dynamics, an existing Education, Health, and Care Plan (EHCP), previous diagnoses, and the possibility of undiagnosed neurodevelopmental needs all provide crucial contextual information (NICE, 2021a, 2021b).

Considering differential diagnoses remains equally important. Behaviours such as selective mutism, shutdowns, and repetitive movements may reflect autistic distress rather than behavioural refusal (NICE, 2021a), while catatonia may be mistaken for anxiety or withdrawal (NICE, 2013). Similarly, ADHD-related impulsivity can heighten short-term risk-taking or emotional dysregulation and may be misinterpreted as acute behavioural disturbance (NICE, 2018). Evidence-based practice therefore requires gathering collateral information, applying structured assessment tools where available, and recognising when acute deterioration may indicate an underlying medical cause. Paramedics are frequently the first to attend an incident and may be the first to recognise concerns about a child's welfare. In line with locally agreed procedures, they can raise these concerns with social care, the police, a GP, or another appropriate health professional (JRCALC, 2025). Effective safeguarding is strengthened through timely multidisciplinary team involvement ensuring coordinated interventions that prioritise safety, dignity, and wellbeing (NICE, 2021b; HCPC, 2023).

NICE guidelines relevant to CYP neurodevelopmental conditions

NICE provides robust, evidence-based guidance relevant to neurodevelopmental and mental health presentations in CYP. For autism, NICE guidance emphasises early recognition, adjustments for communication differences, and coordinated multidisciplinary team (MDT) working (NICE, 2021a). For ADHD, NICE outlines the need for structured assessment, behavioural support, and awareness of impulsivity and emotional regulation difficulties (NICE, 2018). These guidelines highlight that behaviours often interpreted as defiance or emotional volatility may instead represent cognitive overload, sensory overwhelm, or distress, requiring sensitive adaptation in pre-hospital assessment.

Other relevant guidelines include self-harm (NICE, 2022), depression in CYP (NICE, 2019), anxiety disorders (NICE, 2005, 2018), and challenging behaviour linked to learning disability or autism (NICE, 2021b). For urgent presentations, NICE guidelines NG10 (2015) and NG53 (2016) emphasise least-restrictive care, de-escalation, and recognition of neurodevelopmental needs when responding to distress or aggression. These documents collectively promote integrated care involving CAMHS, paediatricians, schools, early help teams, and social care, an essential consideration for paramedics navigating complex family, developmental, and safeguarding needs.

Decision-making in pre-hospital care

Decision-making in pre-hospital care requires balancing risk, proportionality, and respect for the child's autonomy. Conveyance to hospital is appropriate when there is immediate risk to life, medical instability, significant self-harm, safeguarding concerns, or uncertainty regarding the safety of the home environment. NICE self-harm guidance emphasises that CYP presenting after self-injury or suicidal ideation require thorough psychosocial assessment and not solely physical monitoring (NICE, 2022).

Community alternatives may be more appropriate when the crisis results from neurodevelopmental distress that can be resolved through environmental adjustments, sensory regulation, or family-led support. Many regions operate CAMHS crisis services or paediatric liaison teams that can provide same-day review. NICE stresses that children and young people should be supported in the least restrictive environment, with care close to home wherever safely possible (NICE, 2016, 2021a).

Risk stratification tools, for example within CYP self-harm pathways, should support rather than replace clinical judgement. The HCPC Standards of Proficiency (2023) state that paramedics must use evidence-based frameworks while maintaining person-centred reasoning. Understanding neurocognitive influences helps prevent misinterpretation, for example, recognising an autistic shutdown rather than assuming refusal to engage, or distinguishing ADHD impulsivity from suicidal intent.

Working with parents, guardians, schools, and social care

Collaborative working is essential in the care of CYP with neurodevelopmental conditions. NICE emphasises shared decision-making as a core principle across guidelines for ADHD, depression, autism, and self-harm (NICE, 2018, 2019, 2021a, 2022). Parents and guardians provide invaluable insights into their child's sensory profile, communication style, and triggers for distress, enabling paramedics to develop a more accurate and person-centred interpretation of behaviour.

Non-judgemental, empathetic communication supports families during crisis situations, reduces escalation, and fosters trust. Schools contribute critical contextual information, particularly when an EHCP is in place. Safeguarding responsibilities must be balanced with confidentiality; the Children Act 2004 requires agencies to share information where there is risk of harm, and NICE (2015) reinforces this principle in its safeguarding-related recommendations.

Collaborating effectively with schools, social care, and mental health professionals ensures continuity of care and avoids fragmented responses, particularly important for neurodivergent CYP who may be sensitive to disruption, uncertainty, or unfamiliar environments.

Person-centred approaches

Person-centred care is essential when supporting CYP with neurocognitive conditions. NICE autism and learning disability guidelines emphasise adapting communication, reducing sensory overload, offering choices, and creating predictable, supportive environments (NICE, 2015, 2021a, 2021b). These approaches align with trauma-informed principles, recognising that many CYP have experienced exclusion, misunderstanding, or distress within healthcare or education settings.

Paramedics can support safety and engagement by respecting communication preferences, offering visual aids, slowing the pace of interaction, and making predictable, step-by-step explanations. Collaborative safety planning guided by the young person's own coping strategies and preferences helps preserve autonomy and psychological safety. The HCPC (2023) requires paramedics to practise in a way that respects diversity, upholds dignity, and avoids discriminatory assumptions, all of which are crucial when supporting neurodivergent CYP.

Trauma-informed and neuroaffirming care reduces escalation, prevents re-traumatisation, and ensures that interventions remain compassionate, proportionate, and grounded in evidence-based understanding of neurocognitive needs.

Case study 1: Autism, anxiety, and meltdown

Case study 1: Narrative

It is a Saturday afternoon in early spring when a paramedic crew is dispatched to a 'child behaving erratically' at a large indoor shopping centre. On arrival, they find a 13-year-old girl, Mia, seated on the floor near the entrance to a bright, noisy food court. She is rocking back and forth, hands pressed tightly over her ears, tears streaming down her face. Her mother is crouched beside her, visibly distressed and attempting to comfort her. Several bystanders are gathered, some whispering, others filming on their phones. One mall security guard appears frustrated, repeating, 'You need to calm down or you'll have to leave'.

Mia has a known diagnosis of autism spectrum disorder, sensory hypersensitivity, and co-occurring generalised anxiety. Her mother explains that they had visited one shop after another to buy school shoes, and although Mia seemed fine initially, the combination of bright lighting, crowds, loud music, and constant movement gradually overwhelmed her. When a coffee machine suddenly hissed behind her, she dropped to the floor, began crying, and appeared unable to process what was being said to her. Her mother reports that this is a 'meltdown', not a panic attack, and that Mia often loses the ability to speak in these moments.

The paramedic crew immediately recognises the complexity of the scene: competing demands from the bystanders, a distressed parent, an autistic young person in shutdown, and a chaotic environment that is perpetuating her distress. They reposition themselves to block the view of onlookers, ask security to create space, and lower their voices. One paramedic kneels nearby – not too close – offering slow, minimal speech: 'Mia, it's okay. We're going to make things quieter'. The other dims the lights, asks for the overhead music to be temporarily reduced, and encourages her mother to stay within Mia's line of sight. Gradually, with reduced sensory load, Mia's breathing begins to slow.

Assessment and clinical reasoning

The paramedics begin a quiet, paced assessment. A key clinical question is whether this is:

- an autistic sensory meltdown,
- a panic attack,
- an episode of behavioural distress, or
- a response to a medical cause such as hypoglycaemia, infection, or pain.

The crew note the precipitating sensory triggers, Mia's covering of her ears, her loss of verbal communication, and rocking movements are consistent with an autistic meltdown rather than a panic attack, where hyperventilation, fear of collapse, and catastrophic thinking may predominate (NICE, 2013). The crew also check her capillary glucose, temperature, and heart rate to exclude medical contributors. Her mother confirms Mia has eaten, slept well, and has no recent illness.

Risk assessment is approached sensitively. Although Mia is not engaging verbally, the paramedics do not interpret this as refusal but as communication overload, consistent with NICE autism guidance that highlights the need for adaptation and patience (NICE, 2021a). They assess for self-injury risk, noting she is not harming herself or attempting to flee. Her mother reports no recent concerns about suicidality or self-harm. The crew takes time to observe her body language: fists unclenching, breathing slowing, posture softening.

Communication strategies shift to visual and environmental supports: offering a card that says 'Do you want to move somewhere quieter?, and providing two clear choices – stay seated or walk with mum. Mia nods towards walking with her mother. They move to a quieter corridor, dimmer and less crowded, which reduces her anxiety further.

Application of NICE guidelines

NICE guideline NG170 (autism in under 19s) highlights the need for predictable communication, sensory adjustments, and avoiding unnecessary medical interventions unless clinically indicated (NICE, 2021a). The paramedic crew's approach aligns closely with these principles: reducing sensory input, lowering verbal demand, and offering structured choices.

The situation also intersects with NICE guideline NG225 on self-harm, which emphasises developmentally appropriate assessment, compassion, and shared decision-making (NICE, 2022). Although Mia is not self-harming, the guidance's emphasis on non-judgemental communication and emotional validation is directly applicable.

Additionally, elements of NICE guideline NG10 (violence and aggression) apply, particularly around the importance of de-escalation, avoiding physical restraint, and recognising sensory overload as a trigger for distress (NICE, 2015). The crew's avoidance of coercive measures aligns with least-restrictive principles.

Finally, NICE urgent and emergency care guidance underscores the importance of keeping CYP in familiar environments wherever possible, using family expertise to guide care, and considering alternatives to hospital if safe and appropriate (NICE, 2016).

Neuroaffirming approaches in paramedic practice

Neuroaffirming approaches recognise neurodiversity as a natural and valuable form of human variation rather than a deficit or disorder, emphasising dignity, autonomy, and respect for the individual's sensory, communication, and cognitive style. In pre-hospital care, this means shifting from a 'fixing' mindset to one that supports the person's needs in ways that reduce distress and enhance safety. For paramedics, neuroaffirming practice may include offering clear, direct communication without metaphors; allowing extra time for processing and responses; minimising sensory overload by dimming lights, reducing noise, and avoiding unnecessary touch; and providing choices that support autonomy, such as asking permission before examinations or explaining each step before it happens. Neuroaffirming approaches also involve recognising masking and camouflaging behaviours, validating the person's communication style (whether verbal, written, or non-verbal), and avoiding pathologising language. In crisis situations, paramedics can apply neuroaffirming principles by using predictable routines, grounding techniques, and visual prompts, all of which help reduce anxiety and promote a sense of control. By embedding these approaches into everyday practice, paramedics contribute to more inclusive, equitable, and person-centred care for autistic and otherwise neurodivergent individuals across the life span.

Key neuroaffirming strategies for paramedics

Neuroaffirming approaches: Key principles

Neuroaffirming practice recognises neurodivergence, which includes autism, ADHD, dyslexia, dyspraxia, and other cognitive differences, as natural human variation rather than pathology. It focuses on supporting the person's communication, sensory, cognitive, and emotional needs in ways that uphold dignity, autonomy, and safety.

Practical strategies for paramedics:

- Use clear, concrete language and avoid metaphors, sarcasm, or ambiguous phrasing.

- Allow more processing time and avoid pressuring the patient to respond quickly.
- Reduce sensory overload by lowering lights, reducing sirens when safe, limiting physical touch, and avoiding crowded spaces.
- Offer predictability by explaining each step before you do it, using calm, structured communication.
- Provide choices (e.g. 'Would you prefer to step into the ambulance or sit here while we talk?').
- Validate communication preferences, whether verbal, written, typed, or gestural.
- Recognise signs of masking, and do not interpret monotone voice, avoidance of eye contact, or flat affect as non-cooperation.
- Be aware of sensory aids (noise-cancelling headphones, weighted items, fidget tools) and avoid removing them unless absolutely clinically necessary.
- Acceptance of differences, understanding variations in individual challenges and strengths.

These strategies promote safer, empathetic, and more inclusive care and help reduce escalation during mental health or acute distress presentations.

Decision-making and MDT pathway

The decision now centres on conveyance versus community-based support. Mia's presentation has stabilised, her vital signs are normal, and there is no evidence of medical deterioration. Her mother feels confident she can manage once Mia is out of the shopping centre. The paramedics explore available support pathways:

- Contacting the local CAMHS crisis line for same-day advice.
- Liaising with the school SEND team regarding sensory adjustments for the following Monday.
- Providing written psychoeducation for managing meltdowns in public environments.
- Signposting to local autism support organisations.

A key consideration is that the emergency department (ED) can be overwhelming and traumatising for autistic CYP (NICE, 2021a). Without medical need or acute mental health risk, conveyance may escalate rather than resolve distress.

Through collaborative discussion and ensuring Mia is offered the opportunity to assent via nods, the crew agree on a non-conveyance plan. They offer a GP referral, provide safety advice, outline signs that would warrant re-contacting services, and encourage follow-up with CAMHS if meltdowns are increasing or associated with self-injury or anxiety attacks.

Case study 1: Lessons

This case highlights several learning points about person-centred care in neurodiversity-informed paramedic practice. The decisions that supported Mia's wellbeing included reducing sensory overload, using minimal verbal communication, involving her mother as an expert partner, and prioritising psychological safety. These align with the bio-psycho-social and neuroaffirming approaches encouraged throughout this book.

Potential deviations from person-centred care might include assuming Mia was 'refusing' to cooperate, misinterpreting her behaviour as deliberate, or prioritising crowd expectations over her sensory and emotional needs. A pathologising or behaviourist framing could easily have escalated the scene.

The neurodiversity paradigm emphasises that autistic distress is not a sign of disorder but a response to an environment that overwhelms sensory, cognitive, and emotional capacities. In practice, this means paramedics must look beyond outward behaviour to understand the internal experience and modify the environment accordingly. Applying this lens enabled the paramedics to support Mia safely, compassionately, and in a way that preserved her dignity.

Supporting autistic adults in paramedic care

Autistic adults may experience crisis triggers such as sensory overload, changes in routine, communication mismatch, pain misinterpretation, or difficulties expressing internal states (alexithymia). Paramedics can support autistic adults by reducing environmental stimuli (noise, bright lights, multiple voices), allowing extra processing time, and using clear, literal language free of idioms or ambiguity. NICE autism guidance (2021a) recommends adapting assessment to the person's sensory and communication profile, avoiding forced eye contact, and asking whether the individual has their own coping strategies, such as stimming, weighted items, or specific phrases that aid regulation. During distress, behaviours such as shutdown, pacing, echolalia, or heightened agitation may be misinterpreted as non-compliance. A person-centred and trauma-informed approach therefore requires contextualising behaviours within the individual's neurocognitive profile and avoiding escalation. Paramedics should consider co-occurring conditions including anxiety, depression, ADHD, chronic pain, and gastrointestinal issues which are common in autistic adults. MDT involvement (e.g. crisis services, autism liaison teams, or social care) and collaborative safety planning are crucial, particularly when communication barriers or social isolation are present.

Case study 2: ADHD, impulsivity, and risk

Case study 2: Narrative

At 9:10pm on a Friday evening, a paramedic crew is dispatched to a residential area following a police request for medical support. Officers have detained a 16-year-old boy, Jay, under Section 136 of the Mental Health Act following reports of dangerous behaviour. Witnesses stated that Jay climbed onto the roof of a local youth centre after an argument with peers and was seen consuming an unknown quantity of over-the-counter medication. Police intervened when he began shouting, throwing objects into the street, and threatening to 'end it all'. When the crew arrives, Jay is sitting on the pavement beside a police car, his hands shaking, eyes wide, speech rapid, and mood swinging between anger, fear, and tearfulness.

Jay has a diagnosis of ADHD combined presentation, with a history of impulsivity, difficulties regulating emotions, and previous involvement with youth offending services. His mother, who arrives shortly after, explains that earlier in the day he was suspended from school following a confrontation with a teacher. She reports escalating conflict with peers, recent withdrawal from his football club, and suspected experimentation with cannabis and energy drinks. She also shares concerns about online bullying and that Jay has been refusing his ADHD medication for several weeks.

The police describe the scene: Jay was extremely reactive, ran into the road twice, shouted that his life was 'pointless', and then impulsively took tablets 'without thinking'. They report that he complied only after prolonged negotiation and that they deliberately avoided restraint to prevent escalation. Jay is now calmer, but his thoughts remain disorganised, and he expresses ambivalence about living, saying: 'I don't know what I'm doing half the time'.

The paramedics recognise the complexity of his neurodevelopmental, psychosocial, and emotional needs, as well as the intensity of the crisis. The ongoing police presence, mother's heightened anxiety, and neighbourhood onlookers all create a charged environment requiring sensitive, skilled intervention.

Assessment and clinical reasoning

ADHD in adolescence is associated with impulsivity, emotional dysregulation, and executive-functioning difficulties, all of which can exacerbate risk-taking behaviours (NICE, 2018). The paramedics therefore interpret Jay's actions within this developmental and neurocognitive context, resisting the temptation to frame his behaviour as deliberate or manipulative. Instead, they consider:

- Impulsivity contributing to sudden ingestion of medication without suicidal planning.
- Hyperarousal from conflict escalating into unsafe behaviours.
- Executive dysfunction reducing his ability to weigh consequences or regulate emotions.

- Peer conflict and bullying intensifying feelings of shame and threat.
- Possible substance misuse lowering inhibition thresholds.
- School exclusion elevating vulnerability and stress.
- Safeguarding concerns, including possible exploitation or coercion by peers.

They conduct a full set of physiological observations, assess for overdose symptoms (tachycardia, agitation, nausea, altered consciousness), and review the medication packets retrieved by police. Jay denies wanting to die but states, "I just wanted everything to stop'. This distinction between impulsive acts and sustained suicidal intent is crucial and is highlighted in NICE guidance for self-harm and ADHD management (NICE, 2018, 2022).

The crew modulates their communication: short, concrete sentences, reduced verbal load, avoiding confrontational questioning, and allowing pauses for processing. They validate Jay's distress while maintaining structure: 'We're going to check your body is safe, and then we'll work out the next step together'.

The police officers step back at the crew's request, reducing social pressure and helping Jay settle. This collaborative approach reflects best practice in crisis negotiation with neurodivergent young people.

Evidence-based management

NICE guidance NG87 (ADHD) emphasises that impulsivity and emotional dysregulation increase the likelihood of risky behaviours, substance misuse, and self-harm, and recommends multi-agency support, early crisis planning, and consistent routines (NICE, 2018). The paramedics apply these principles by addressing both the immediate medical risk and the underlying neurocognitive drivers.

For the potential overdose, both NICE (2022) and the Joint Royal Colleges Ambulance Liaison Committee (2025) state that a CYP who has ingested substances, including impulsive or unclear intent, requires psychosocial assessment and often acute medical review. Jay's inconsistent account and ongoing agitation indicate a need for hospital conveyance for blood tests, observation, and mental health evaluation.

The crew also uses collaborative safety planning, explaining clearly:

- why hospital is recommended,
- what will happen in the ED,
- that his mother can accompany him,
- that restraint will not be used unless his safety requires it, and
- that this is not a punishment but a way to ensure he is medically safe.

This aligns with trauma-informed principles and NICE guidance emphasising compassionate, non-judgemental responses to distress (NICE, 2021a, 2022).

MDT involvement

Jay's ongoing care needs extend beyond the acute event. Effective management requires coordinated MDT involvement, including:

- CAMHS crisis team for urgent mental health review, risk assessment, and safety planning.
- School safeguarding lead to address peer conflict, bullying, and educational placement following suspension.
- Social care if there are concerns about neglect, exploitation, or the home environment's ability to keep Jay safe.
- Youth offending services or youth workers if his risk-taking escalates or links to peer group coercion.
- GP and ADHD specialist services to review medication adherence, optimisation, and side-effect concerns.
- Voluntary sector services (e.g. youth mentors, neurodiversity organisations) to support emotional regulation and positive identity development.

The crew documents the interaction thoroughly, ensuring accurate handover to ED staff. They also encourage the police to share their body-worn footage event summary, which can be invaluable for CAMHS assessments.

Case study 2: Lessons

This case highlights multiple challenges and opportunities when providing person-centred care for neurodivergent adolescents. Supporting factors included adapting communication for executive-functioning differences, recognising impulsivity as a neurodevelopmental feature rather than intentional defiance, and reducing environmental pressure by asking police to step back. These practices align with the neurodiversity paradigm, which frames ADHD as a difference rather than a deficit, and emphasises the need for environments and services to adapt to neurocognitive profiles.

Areas of potential difficulty include the risk of stigma, such as misinterpreting risk-taking as attention-seeking or criminality. Equally, assumptions about substance misuse or behavioural difficulty can overshadow emotional pain or trauma exposure, an example of diagnostic overshadowing noted across CYP mental health literature (NICE, 2018, 2022). Equity issues also arise: neurodivergent adolescents are disproportionately excluded from school, overrepresented in youth justice pathways, and at heightened risk of coercive interventions, particularly when police are involved. These systemic factors must be acknowledged in reflective practice.

Overall, the case underscores the importance of integrating evidence-based guidance with compassionate, neuroaffirming practice. Paramedics and police, working collaboratively, can prevent escalation, reduce harm and provide young people like Jay with safe, dignified, and developmentally informed care.

Supporting adults with ADHD in paramedic care

Adults with ADHD may present with impulsivity, emotional dysregulation, heightened stress responses, and executive functioning difficulties that influence how they navigate a crisis. Paramedics can support these individuals by adopting a calm, structured communication approach giving information in short, sequential steps and avoiding overwhelming verbal input or rapid decision demands (JRCALC, 2025). Hyperarousal may be mistaken for aggression or intoxication, so grounding techniques and reassurance can help regulate distress. NICE guidance emphasises the importance of recognising ADHD-related risk behaviours, including impulsive self-harm, substance use, and difficulties with planning or evaluating consequences (NICE, 2018). A bio-psycho-social approach requires paramedics to consider contributing factors such as trauma history, unmet sensory needs, medication adherence, and social stressors, while MDT options, including crisis teams, GP follow-up, or community mental health support, should be explored collaboratively. Maintaining a non-judgemental stance is essential, as stigma often leads adults with ADHD to feel blamed for behaviours that reflect neurocognitive processing differences.

Professional considerations for paramedics

Self-care and emotional labour

Paramedic work with children and young people experiencing neurocognitive crises requires sustained emotional labour. Scenes involving sensory overload, distressed families, police presence, or behavioural escalation can evoke anxiety, frustration, sadness, or uncertainty for clinicians. Responding to meltdowns, impulsivity, shutdowns, suicidality, or parental distress places significant emotional and cognitive demands on practitioners. These experiences accumulate over time and can contribute to compassion fatigue, burnout, or feelings of diminished professional efficacy if not addressed proactively (HCPC, 2023).

Self-care must therefore be integrated into everyday practice rather than treated as an optional add-on. Evidence-based strategies include micro-breaks between high-intensity calls, controlled breathing or grounding exercises during difficult scenes, and peer support immediately after challenging interactions. Trauma-informed principles apply not only to patients but also to practitioners; acknowledging emotional reactions without self-judgement allows paramedics to regulate their own responses, enhancing clinical clarity and preserving compassion.

Structured debriefing is essential. Informal 'hot debriefs' on scene help crews process immediate reactions, while formal reflective practice sessions enable deeper exploration of ethical tensions, communication challenges, and emotional impact. Supervision – whether clinical, pastoral, or peer-led – provides a safe space to examine unconscious biases, refine neuroaffirming approaches, and consider the broader systemic pressures shaping decision-making. These practices align closely with the HCPC Standards of Proficiency (2023), which emphasise reflective capability, emotional resilience, and the importance of maintaining wellbeing to ensure safe and effective care. Building personal routines of rest, boundaries, support-seeking, and professional development helps paramedics sustain their capacity to respond with empathy and professionalism.

Legal, ethical, and professional issues

Responding to neurocognitive crises in CYP requires careful navigation of consent, capacity, safeguarding, and shared decision-making. Paramedics must determine whether a young person can provide informed consent or assent, drawing on concepts such as *Gillick competence*, which recognises that a child under 16 may have sufficient understanding to make certain decisions independently (Department of Health and Social Care, 2009). For older adolescents, the Mental Capacity Act 2005 guides assessments of decision-specific capacity, emphasising a presumption of capacity unless proven otherwise. Neurodevelopmental conditions alone do *not* diminish capacity; instead, communication adjustments, sensory regulation, and additional processing time may be required to enable meaningful participation.

Ethical decision-making must balance autonomy with safeguarding duties under the Children Act 2004. Paramedics are legally required to share relevant information when there is risk of harm or neglect, even when a young person requests confidentiality. Clear explanation of these limits builds trust and reduces fear that disclosure will automatically lead to punitive action. Ethical care also demands respect for diversity, avoidance of stigma, and a commitment to neuroaffirming language that validates rather than pathologises behaviour (HCPC, 2023).

Record-keeping is another core professional responsibility. Documentation should detail communication adaptations used, explanations given to CYP and families, risk assessments, and the rationale for decisions, including conveyance or non-conveyance. Records must reflect not only clinical findings but also the young person's preferences and sensory needs, and the parent or guardian's perspective. Such transparency supports continuity of care across the MDT – particularly CAMHS, paediatric services, and social care – ensuring that future practitioners understand the context of the crisis and the decisions that were made.

Shared decision-making is fundamental. Even during crisis, CYP should be offered choices wherever safely possible, such as preferred communication formats, who should accompany them, or whether they need quieter spaces. The HCPC (2023) emphasises the duty to involve service users in decisions affecting their care, and this remains true even when distress limits verbal communication. Person-centred practice requires patience, flexibility, and an understanding that behavioural expressions are often communication of unmet needs.

Working within systems pressures

Paramedics increasingly operate within systems characterised by limited CAMHS capacity, fluctuating thresholds for referral, and variable local provision for crisis support. These pressures influence clinical decisions and can leave families feeling unsupported or 'passed between services'. Understanding these constraints is essential to practising ethically, collaboratively, and realistically.

CAMHS services frequently experience long waiting lists, high thresholds for acceptance, and limited capacity for urgent intervention. Paramedics may therefore encounter families who have struggled to access assessment or support, or young people whose crises escalate due to unmet needs. Awareness of local pathways, including crisis lines, paediatric liaison services, school safeguarding teams, youth support workers, and voluntary sector organisations, allows paramedics to signpost effectively even when specialist services are overstretched.

Navigating thresholds for referral requires clinical judgement and knowledge of NICE guidance. For example, NICE guideline NG225 (2022) mandates psychosocial assessment following self-harm, while its guideline NG87 (2018) emphasises coordinated MDT management for young people with ADHD experiencing significant impairment. When thresholds are unclear, paramedics can advocate for the young person by clearly communicating concerns to receiving teams, highlighting patterns such as repeated crises, escalating risk, deteriorating school engagement, or social withdrawal.

Advocacy is a core professional skill. Paramedics may need to challenge assumptions, address stigma, and ensure neurodivergent CYP are not dismissed as 'behavioural' or 'non-compliant'. Advocacy also involves supporting families who feel overwhelmed, marginalised, or unheard, particularly those navigating socioeconomic adversity, discrimination, or safeguarding complexities. Compassionate, culturally aware practice enhances equity and helps counter systemic biases that disproportionately affect neurodivergent adolescents.

Finally, working within systems pressures requires recognising the limits of the paramedic role while still striving for holistic care. Effective inter-agency communication, clear documentation, realistic safety planning, and timely referrals all contribute to better outcomes. Paramedics cannot solve structural problems alone, but they can ensure every interaction is grounded in dignity, respect, and evidence-based decision-making.

Conclusion

This chapter has explored neurodiversity as representing natural variation in thinking, communication, and sensory processing, and how neurodevelopmental differences shape how people experience stress, pain, and crisis. For paramedics, recognising these differences helps avoid misinterpretation and promotes safe, respectful care. Small adjustments such as using clear language, offering more processing time, reducing bright lights or noise, and validating alternative communication methods can dramatically improve how neurodivergent individuals engage with assessment and treatment.

Providing good care also means working within the wider multidisciplinary system. Mental health teams, social care, crisis services, and community organisations all play important roles in supporting people beyond the immediate emergency call. Knowing when and how to involve these partners ensures you are delivering genuinely holistic, bio-psycho-social care.

Finally, the chapter emphasises looking after yourself as a clinician. Caring for neurodivergent people during a crisis can be emotionally demanding, so regular reflection, debriefing, and peer support help strengthen confidence, reduce stress, and develop better professional judgement over time. Combining these principles, understanding neurodiversity, adapting communication, working collaboratively, and maintaining wellbeing can all contribute to a safer, more inclusive, and person-centred paramedic practice.

Further learning materials

Multiple-choice questions: Case study 1

MCQ1: Which feature most strongly suggests a sensory-driven autistic meltdown rather than a behavioural crisis?

A. Crying and hyperventilation

B. Lack of verbal communication and shielding ears

C. Refusing to follow parental instructions

D. Running away from the scene

Correct answer: B

Rationale: Sensory overwhelm (covering ears, withdrawal, shutdown) is characteristic of autistic meltdown, not intentional defiance.

MCQ2: According to NICE guideline NG170 (2021a), which communication strategy is recommended when engaging with autistic children in crisis?

A. Use open-ended questions to explore feelings

B. Speak quickly to maintain momentum

C. Use clear, literal, concise language

D. Encourage direct eye contact to build rapport

Correct answer: C

Rationale: NICE emphasises the use of simple, concrete language and avoiding idioms or pressure to maintain eye contact.

MCQ3: A key differential diagnosis in this case is distinguishing meltdown from:

A. ADHD impulsivity

B. Asthma

C. Panic attack

D. Eating disorder

Correct answer: C

Rationale: Panic attacks share acute distress features (hyperventilation, crying) but differ in triggers, trajectory, and sensory overload components.

MCQ4: When determining urgency, which factor increases the need for prompt assessment or onwards referral?

A. The presence of noise and crowds

B. Parent becoming tearful

C. Child repeatedly attempting to self-injure

D. Child refusing to speak

Correct answer: C

Rationale: Active or escalating risk behaviours require immediate assessment and potential CAMHS crisis involvement.

MCQ5: What is the first priority when arriving on scene during a meltdown?

A. Asking detailed questions about medical history

B. Removing bystanders and reducing environmental load

C. Offering the child food or drink

D. Encouraging the child to stand up

Correct answer: B

Rationale: Safety and de-escalation begin with reducing sensory triggers and environmental stressors.

Multiple-choice questions: Case study 2

MCQ1: Which factor best explains Jay's sudden ingestion of medication in the context of ADHD?

A. A planned suicide attempt

B. A desire to attract attention

C. Impulsivity linked to emotional dysregulation

D. Substance dependence

Correct answer: C

Rationale: NICE guideline NG87 (2018) highlights impulsivity and emotional dysregulation as core ADHD features that increase risk-taking behaviours, including sudden ingestion without suicidal planning.

MCQ2: Which communication strategy is most appropriate during assessment of a young person with ADHD in crisis?

A. Rapid questioning to maintain control

B. Long explanations to ensure understanding

C. Minimal, concrete instructions with pauses

D. Avoiding communication until the scene is calm

Correct answer: C

Rationale: *Adolescents with ADHD often benefit from reduced verbal load and clear, simple language to support processing and reduce overwhelm.*

MCQ3: According to NICE guideline NG225 (2022), which of the following indicates the need for hospital conveyance after an impulsive overdose?

A. The adolescent denies wanting to die

B. The quantity of tablets is unknown

C. The adolescent appears embarrassed

D. The adolescent has calmed down

Correct answer: B

Rationale: Any ingestion of unknown or potentially harmful substances in CYP requires ED assessment and observation, regardless of stated intent.

MCQ4: What is the most appropriate MDT referral following this incident?

A. Routine GP appointment only

B. CAMHS crisis team for urgent mental health assessment

C. School to arrange detention

D. Youth offending team for punitive intervention

Correct answer: B

Rationale: CAMHS crisis teams provide urgent psychological assessment and safety planning following self-harm or high-risk behaviour.

MCQ5: Which of the following reflects a neuroaffirming approach for adolescents with ADHD?

A. Highlighting poor choices to reinforce consequences
B. Avoiding family involvement to support autonomy
C. Recognising impulsivity as neurodevelopmental, not intentional
D. Using strict behavioural sanctions during crisis

Correct answer: C

Rationale: Neuroaffirming practice avoids moral judgement and interprets behaviour through developmental and cognitive frameworks.

Guided clinical reasoning questions

Q1: What's most urgent? What life-threatening medical causes must be excluded first (e.g. hypoglycaemia, hypoxia, seizure, head injury, infection, intoxication/overdose)?

Q2: What's driving the behaviour? Is this more consistent with sensory overload, anxiety/panic, pain, trauma response, communication difficulty, neurodevelopmental distress, or deliberate aggression?

Q3: How is the environment affecting risk? What immediate changes can reduce escalation (reduce noise/lights/people, create space, move to quieter area)?

Q4: How will you communicate? What format works best right now (simple literal language, one step at a time, processing time, visual/text, parent as interpreter/support)?

Q5: What's the 'why now?' What has changed recently (school, bullying, routine disruption, service barriers, family stress, sleep, medication, substance use)?

Q6: Risk and safeguarding: Is there self-harm/suicidality, exploitation, neglect, domestic abuse, or carer breakdown? Who is at risk and who is present?

Q7: Consent/capacity and participation: How will you enable assent/consent (adjustments, choices, predictability), and what is your decision-specific capacity view if relevant?

Q8: Disposition: What is the least-restrictive safe next step (ED, CAMHS/crisis pathway, GP/out-of-hours, community support), and what would make non-conveyance unsafe?

Q9: Documentation/handover: What must be recorded and handed over (triggers, effective de-escalation strategies, communication needs, risks/protective factors, rationale)?

Teaching commentary

Neurodivergent children and young people commonly present to paramedics during episodes of escalating distress, often shaped by sensory overload, unmet support needs, and system barriers rather than acute medical pathology alone. The key teaching point is that behaviour is often communication: shutdown, meltdown, avoidance, or agitation may reflect anxiety, pain, trauma responses, or cognitive overload. Safe practice begins with time-critical physiological exclusion, then rapidly shifts to environmental modification, paced communication, and co-regulation with families or trusted adults.

This chapter reinforces that person-centred care in pre-hospital settings is not an 'extra'; it is a safety intervention. Small adjustments, such as, reducing stimulation, simplifying language, offering choices, allowing processing time can prevent escalation, reduce restraint, and support better assessment and decision-making. Finally, learners should recognise the emotional labour involved and use structured reflection and peer support to sustain compassionate, equitable practice.

Reflective practice activity for Case study 1: Autism, sensory overload, and meltdown

This case presents a 13-year-old autistic young person experiencing sensory overload in a public setting. It raises important questions about environmental modification, communication, safeguarding, and trauma-informed decision-making in paramedic practice.

Aligned to the HCPC Standards of Proficiency (2023), this activity invites you to produce a structured reflective account exploring your clinical reasoning, communication approach, and professional responsibilities when supporting neurodivergent CYP in crisis.

Task: Using a recognised reflective model (e.g., What? / So What? / Now What?, Gibbs, or Rolfe), write a 400–600-word reflective account based on Mia's case. Your reflection should demonstrate:

- Understanding of sensory overload and autistic meltdown
- Insight into how environment influences distress
- Adaptation of communication strategies
- Application of trauma-informed and neuroaffirming principles

Link to HCPC Standards of Proficiency. Your reflection should explicitly consider:

- Acting in the best interests of service users
- Adapting communication to individual needs
- Recognising how equality, diversity, and inclusion influence care
- Undertaking effective, compassionate assessment
- Working collaboratively with families and the MDT

Reflection prompts:

- How does recognising sensory overload alter your clinical reasoning?
- What environmental adaptations could reduce escalation?
- How might stigma or bystander judgement influence decision-making?
- How do NICE autism guidelines (2021a) inform your approach?
- How would you balance safeguarding, autonomy, and least-restrictive care?
- What learning will you carry forward into future practice?

Submission guidance: Upload your reflective account to your professional development portfolio as evidence of developing:

- Person-centred crisis care
- Trauma-informed communication
- Inclusive and neuroaffirming practice
- Safe and ethical clinical decision-making

Reflective practice activity for Case study 2: ADHD, impulsivity, and risk

This case presents a 16-year-old young person with ADHD experiencing acute emotional dysregulation and impulsive risk-taking behaviour. The scenario raises important questions about crisis assessment, safeguarding, inter-agency collaboration, and neuroaffirming practice within paramedic care.

Aligned to the HCPC Standards of Proficiency (2023), this activity invites you to produce a structured reflective account exploring your clinical reasoning, communication strategies, and professional responsibilities when supporting neurodivergent adolescents in crisis.

Task: Using a recognised reflective model (e.g., What? / So What? / Now What?, Gibbs, or Rolfe), write a 400–600-word reflective account based on Jay's case. Your reflection should demonstrate:

- Understanding of ADHD-related impulsivity and emotional dysregulation
- Insight into how neurocognitive differences shape crisis behaviour
- Consideration of safeguarding, autonomy, and least-restrictive care
- Awareness of stigma, bias, and diagnostic overshadowing

Link to HCPC Standards of Proficiency. Your reflection should explicitly consider:

- Acting in the best interests of service users
- Adapting communication to individual needs
- Recognising how equality, diversity, and inclusion shape care
- Undertaking effective, compassionate risk assessment
- Working collaboratively with families, police, and the wider MDT

Reflection prompts:

- How did ADHD-related impulsivity influence Jay's presentation and risk profile?
- How would you adapt your communication style to support executive-functioning differences?
- How would you balance safeguarding responsibilities with respect for autonomy?
- How can collaborative working with police reduce escalation?
- How does NICE guidance on ADHD (2018) and self-harm (2022) guide your clinical reasoning?
- What steps can you take to avoid diagnostic overshadowing and challenge stigma?

Submission guidance: Upload your reflective account to your professional development portfolio as evidence of developing:

- Person-centred mental health care
- Neuroaffirming crisis management
- Ethical and legally sound decision-making
- Collaborative, multidisciplinary practice

References

Accardo, A.L., Neely, L.C., Pontes, N.M.H., and Pontes, M.C.F. (2025). Bullying victimization is associated with heightened rates of anxiety and depression among autistic and ADHD youth: National Survey of Children's Health 2016–2020. *Journal of Autism and Developmental Disorders*, *55*(10), 3605–3622. https://doi.org/10.1007/s10803-024-06479-z

Alisic, E., Tyler, M.P., Giummarra, M.J., Kassam-Adams, R., Gouweloos, J., Landolt, M.A., et al. (2017). Trauma-informed care for children in the ambulance: International survey among pre-hospital providers. *European Journal of Psychotraumatology*, *8*(1), 1273587. https://doi.org/10.1080/20008198.2016.1273587

American Psychiatric Association (APA) (2022). *Diagnostic and Statistical Manual of Mental Disorders* (DSM-5-TR). Washington, DC: APA Publishing.

Baron-Cohen, S. (2019). The concept of neurodiversity is dividing the autism community: It remains controversial – but it doesn't have to be. *Scientific American*. https://www.scientificamerican.com/blog/observations/the-concept-of-neurodiversity-is-dividing-the-autism-community/

Betts, D.E., and Patrick, N.J. (2006). *Homespun Remedies: Strategies in the home and community for children with autism spectrum and other disorders*. London: Jessica Kingsley.

Bitsika, V., Heyne, D.A., and Sharpley, C.F. (2022a). The inverse association between psychological resilience and emerging school refusal among bullied autistic youth. *Research in Developmental Disabilities*, *120*, 104121. https://doi.org/10.1016/j.ridd.2021.104121

Bitsika, V., Sharpley, C., and Heyne, D. (2022b). Risk for school refusal among autistic boys bullied at school: Investigating associations with social phobia and separation anxiety. *International Journal of Disability, Development, and Education, 69*(1), 190–203. https://doi.org/10.1080/1034912X.2021.1969544

Black, M.H., Helander, J., Segers, J., Ingard, C., Bervoets, J., de Puget, V.G., et al. (2024). Resilience in the face of neurodivergence: A scoping review of resilience and factors promoting positive outcomes. *Clinical Psychology Review, 113*, 102487. https://doi.org/10.1016/j.cpr.2024.102487

Bloch, C., Burghof, L., Lehnhardt, F., Vogeley, K., and Falter-Wagner, C. (2021). Alexithymia traits outweigh autism traits in the explanation of depression in adults with autism. *Scientific Reports, 11*(1), 2258. https://doi.org/10.1038/s41598-021-81696-5

Bond, L., Frawley, T., Moore, K., Gavin, B., and McNicholas, F. (2025). Challenges for neurodiverse children in acute medical hospitals and opportunities for the new National Children's Hospital to be 'neurodiversity-friendly'. *Irish Journal of Medical Science (1971–), 194*(1), 253–261. https://doi.org/10.1007/s11845-024-03850-y

Botha, M., Dibb, B., and Frost, D.M. (2022). 'It's being a part of a grand tradition, a grand counter-culture which involves communities': A qualitative investigation of autistic community connectedness. *Autism, 26*(8), 2151–2164. https://doi.org/10.1177/13623613221080248

Bowden, S.L.J., and Miller, P.K. (2025). Menstruation among autistic adults: An occupational perspective. *British Journal of Occupational Therapy, 88*(10), 626–634. https://doi.org/10.1177/03080226251341730

Brown, P.C.M., Feldstein Ewing, S.W., and Wilson, A.C. (2025). ADHD (attention-deficit hyperactivity disorder) symptoms are associated with chronic pain interference: Results from a prospective cohort study, *Child: Care, Health and Development, 51*(1), e70016. https://doi.org/10.1111/cch.70016

Carias, K.V., and Wevrick, R. (2019). Clinical and genetic analysis of children with a dual diagnosis of Tourette syndrome and autism spectrum disorder. *Journal of Psychiatric Research, 111*, 145–153. https://doi.org/10.1016/j.jpsychires.2019.01.023

Catts, H.W., Terry, N.P., Lonigan, C.J., Compton, D.L., Wagner, R.K., Steacy, L.M., et al. (2024). Revisiting the definition of dyslexia. *Annals of Dyslexia, 74*(3), 282–302. https://doi.org/10.1007/s11881-023-00295-3

Chapman, R. (2019). Neurodiversity theory and its discontents: Autism, schizophrenia, and the social model of disability, in S. Tekin and R. Bluhm (eds) *The Bloomsbury Companion to Philosophy of Psychiatry* (pp. 371–390). London: Bloomsbury.

Children Act 2004, c.31. London: HMSO.

Children's Commissioner (2023). *The State of Children's Mental Health Services 2023*. London: Children's Commissioner for England.

Chung, P.J., Patel, D.R., and Nizami, I. (2020). Disorder of written expression and dysgraphia: Definition, diagnosis, and management. *Translational Pediatrics, 9*, S46–S54. https://doi.org/10.21037/tp.2019.11.01

Cohn, E.G., and Harrison, M.J. (2025). From principle to practice: Creating neurodiversity-affirming learning environments for students with echolalia. *Research in Autism, 126*, 202628. https://doi.org/10.1016/j.reia.2025.202628

Cohn, E.G., Harrison, M.J., and McVilly, K.R. (2024). 'Let me tell you, I see echolalia as being a part of my son's identity': Exploring echolalia as an expression of neurodiversity from a parental perspective. *Autism: The International Journal of Research and Practice, 28*(5), 1245–1257. https://doi.org/10.1177/13623613231195795

Cortese, S., Bellgrove, M.A., Brikell, I., Franke, B., Goodman, D.W., Hartman, C.A., et al. (2025). Attention-deficit/hyperactivity disorder (ADHD) in adults: Evidence base, uncertainties and controversies. *World Psychiatry, 24*(3), 347–371. https://doi.org/10.1002/wps.21374

Crane, L., Adams, F., Harper, G., Welch, J., and Pellicano, E. (2019). 'Something needs to change': Mental health experiences of young autistic adults in England. *Autism, 23*(2), 477–493. https://doi.org/10.1177/1362361318757048

Dagnan, D., Taylor, L., and Burke, C. (2023). Adapting cognitive behaviour therapy for people with intellectual disabilities: An overview for therapists working in mainstream or specialist services. *The Cognitive Behaviour Therapist, 16*, e3. https://doi.org/10.1017/S1754470X22000587

Department of Health and Social Care (DHSC) (2009). *Reference Guide to Consent for Examination or Treatment* (2nd edition). London: DHSC. https://www.gov.uk/government/publications/reference-guide-to-consent-for-examination-or-treatment-second-edition

Doherty, M., McCowan, S., and Shaw, S.C.K. (2023). Autistic SPACE: A novel framework for meeting the needs of autistic people in healthcare settings. *British Journal of Hospital Medicine, 84*(4), 1–10. https://doi.org/10.12968/hmed.2023.0006

Duinmeijer, I., Peet, S., Janssen, L., Scheper, A., Zwitserlood-Nijenhuis, M., Bliekendaal, W., et al. (2025). Language, communicative participation, and well-being in young children with (presumed) developmental language disorder. *International Journal of Language and Communication Disorders, 60*(3), e70037. https://doi.org/10.1111/1460-6984.70037

Ekström, A., Sandgren, O., Sahlén, B., and Samuelsson, C. (2023). 'It depends on who I'm with': How young people with developmental language disorder describe their experiences of language and communication in school. *International Journal of Language and Communication Disorders, 58*(4), 1168–1181. https://doi.org/10.1111/1460-6984.12850

Elsherif, M.M. (2025). The lived experience of dyspraxia: Challenging ableism and embracing neurodiversity. *Neurodiversity, 3*. https://doi.org/10.1177/27546330251346861

Ergan, S.N. (2025). Exploring epistemic injustice in dyscalculia. *International Journal of Inclusive Education, 29*(14), 2563–2574. https://doi.org/10.1080/13603116.2024.2430538

Faedda, N., Romani, M., Rossetti, S., Vigliante, M., Pezzuti, L., Cardona, F., et al. (2019). Intellectual functioning and executive functions in children and adolescents with attention deficit hyperactivity disorder (ADHD) and specific learning disorder (SLD). *Scandinavian Journal of Psychology, 60*(5), 440–446. https://doi.org/10.1111/sjop.12562

Fielding, C., Streeter, A., Deborah, M.R., and Hanley, M. (2025). Neurodivergent pupils' experiences of school distress and attendance difficulties. *Neurodiversity, 3*. https://doi.org/10.1177/27546330251327056

Garratt, M. (2023). For when you just can't talk to 'normal' people … Exploring the use of informal support structures by supernumerary university paramedic students: Findings from a phenomenological study. *British Paramedic Journal, 7*(4), 1–7. https://doi.org/10.29045/14784726.2023.3.7.4.1

Gill, C.E., and Kompoliti, K. (2020). Clinical features of Tourette syndrome. *Journal of Child Neurology, 35*(2), 166–174. https://doi.org/10.1177/0883073819877335

Goffman, E. (1959). *The Presentation of Self in Everyday Life*. London: Penguin.

Grimwood, T., and Miller, P.K. (2014). How to do things without words, in B. Garvey (ed.) *JL Austin and Language* (pp. 70–85). London: Palgrave Macmillan.

Haft, S.L., Greiner de Magalhães, C., and Hoeft, F. (2022). A systematic review of the consequences of stigma and stereotype threat for individuals with specific learning disabilities. *Journal of Learning Disabilities, 56*, 193–209. https://doi.org/10.1177/00222194221087383

Hatch, B., Kadlaskar, G., and Miller, M. (2023). Diagnosis and treatment of children and adolescents with autism and ADHD. *Psychology in the Schools, 60*(2), 295–311. https://doi.org/10.1002/pits.22808

Health and Care Professions Council (HCPC) (2023). *Standards of Proficiency: Paramedics.* London: HCPC. https://www.hcpc-uk.org/standards/standards-of-proficiency/paramedics/

Isaacs, D., Key, A.P., Cascio, C.J., Conley, A.C., Walker, H.C., Wallace, M.T., et al. (2020). Sensory hypersensitivity severity and association with obsessive-compulsive symptoms in adults with tic disorder. *Neuropsychiatric Disease and Treatment, 16*, 2591–2601. https://doi.org/10.2147/NDT.S274165

Johnson, K.A., Worbe, Y., Foote, K.D., Butson, C.R., Gunduz, A., and Okun, M.S. (2023). Tourette syndrome: Clinical features, pathophysiology, and treatment. *Lancet Neurology, 22*(2), 147–158. https://doi.org/10.1016/S1474-4422(22)00303-9

Joint Royal Colleges Ambulance Liaison Committee (JRCALC) (2025). *JRCALC clinical guidelines update*, July. https://jrcalc.org.uk/publication-date-july-2025/ (accessed 11 December 2025).

Kalisch, L.A., Lawrence, K.A., Baud, J., Spencer-Smith, M., and Ure, A. (2024). Therapeutic supports for neurodiverse children who have experienced interpersonal trauma: A scoping review. *Review Journal of Autism and Developmental Disorders, 11*(4), 733–755. https://doi.org/10.1007/s40489-023-00363-9

Kalokyri, A. (2025). Navigating the interplay of ADHD, social norms, and friendships: Perspectives from secondary school students with ADHD. *Pastoral Care in Education, 43*(3), 415–436. https://doi.org/10.1080/02643944.2025.2495667

Kapp, S.K., Gillespie-Lynch, K., Sherman, L.E., and Hutman, T. (2013). Deficit, difference, or both? Autism and neurodiversity. *Developmental Psychology, 49*(1), 59–71. https://doi.org/10.1037/a0028353

Kazda, L., McGeechan, K., Bell, K., Thomas, R., and Barratt, A. (2022). Association of attention-deficit/hyperactivity disorder diagnosis with adolescent quality of life. *JAMA Network Open, 5*(10), e2236364. https://doi.org/10.1001/jamanetworkopen.2022.36364

Kinnaird, E., Stewart, C., and Tchanturia, K. (2019). Investigating alexithymia in autism: A systematic review and meta-analysis. *European Psychiatry, 55*, 80–89. https://doi.org/10.1016/j.eurpsy.2018.09.004

Kirkpatrick, B., Gilroy, S.P., and Leader, G. (2019). Qualitative study on parents' perspectives of the familial impact of living with a child with autism spectrum disorder who experiences insomnia. *Sleep Medicine, 62*, 59–68. https://doi.org/10.1016/j.sleep.2019.01.032

Lombardi, E., Lepore, F., and Greer, C. (2024). Improving emergency medical services (EMS) care for people with autism in the prehospital setting through sensory and communication aids. *Curēus (Palo Alto, CA), 16*(11), e74702. https://doi.org/10.7759/cureus.74702

Mahoney, W.J., Blaskowitz, M.G., and Johnson, K.R. (2021). Occupational therapy-related assessments for adults with intellectual disability: A scoping review. *American Journal of Occupational Therapy, 75*(3), 7503180100. https://doi.org/10.5014/ajot.2021.046342

Massoni, L. (2025). Imitation and dyspraxia in autism: Clinical and therapeutic implications. *Brain Disorders, 17*, 100191. https://doi.org/10.1016/j.dscb.2025.100191

Mental Capacity Act 2005, c. 9. London: HMSO.

Miller, P.K. (2013). Depression, sense and sensitivity: On pre-diagnostic questioning about self-harm and suicidal inclination in the primary care consultation. *Communication and Medicine, 10*(1), 37–49. https://doi.org/10.1558/cam.v10i1.37

Miller, P.K., Bowden, S.L., Dewison, N., Ingham, B., Thwaites, R., and Dagnan, D. (2025a). 'Sometimes I'm feeling baffled and they're probably feeling baffled': On the experiences of psychological therapists working with autistic people in a structured primary care service for anxiety disorders and depression. *Autism, 29*(10), 2477–2488. https://doi.org/10.1177/13623613251341610

Miller, P.K., Dewison, N., Bowden, S.L.J., Ingham, B., Thwaites, R., and Dagnan, D. (2025b). 'They've almost got, like, a checklist to work down': On the lived experiences of autistic adults who have received a structured therapy service for depression and/or anxiety disorders. *Neurodiversity, 3*. https://doi.org/10.1177/27546330251350037

Moore, H.L., Brice, S., Powell, L., Ingham, B., Freeston, M., Parr, J.R., et al. (2022). The mediating effects of alexithymia, intolerance of uncertainty, and anxiety on the relationship between sensory processing differences and restricted and repetitive behaviours in autistic adults. *Journal of Autism and Developmental Disorders, 52*(10), 4384–4396. https://doi.org/10.1007/s10803-021-05312-1

Morris-Rosendahl, D., and Crocq, M. (2020). Neurodevelopmental disorders: The history and future of a diagnostic concept. *Dialogues in Clinical Neuroscience, 22*(1), 65–72. https://doi.org/10.31887/DCNS.2020.22.1/macrocq

National Institute for Health and Care Excellence (NICE) (2005). *Depression in children and young people: Identification and management* (CG28). London: NICE.

National Institute for Health and Care Excellence (NICE) (2013) *Anxiety disorders: Recognition, assessment and treatment.* London: NICE.

National Institute for Health and Care Excellence (NICE) (2015). *Violence and aggression: Short-term management in mental health, health and community settings* (NG10). London: NICE.

National Institute for Health and Care Excellence (NICE) (2016). *Transition between inpatient mental health settings and community or care settings* (NG53). London: NICE.

National Institute for Health and Care Excellence (NICE) (2018). *Attention deficit hyperactivity disorder: Diagnosis and management* (NG87). London: NICE.

National Institute for Health and Care Excellence (NICE) (2019). *Depression in children and young people: Identification and management* (NG134). London: NICE.

National Institute for Health and Care Excellence (NICE) (2021a). *Autism spectrum disorder in under 19s: Recognition, referral and diagnosis* (NG170). London: NICE.

National Institute for Health and Care Excellence (NICE) (2021b). *Challenging behaviour and learning disabilities* (NG11). London: NICE.

National Institute for Health and Care Excellence (NICE) (2022). *Self-harm: Assessment, management and preventing recurrence* (NG225). London: NICE.

NHS Digital (2023). *Mental health of children and young people in England 2023.* Leeds: NHS Digital.

Nicolaidis, C., Raymaker, D.M., Ashkenazy, E., McDonald, K.E., Dern, S., Baggs, A.E., et al. (2015). 'Respect the way I need to communicate with you': Healthcare experiences of adults on the autism spectrum. *Autism, 19*(7), 824–831. https://doi.org/10.1177/1362361315576221

Nordby, E.S., Guribye, F., Nordgreen, T., and Lundervold, A.J. (2023). Silver linings of ADHD: A thematic analysis of adults' positive experiences with living with ADHD. *BMJ Open, 13*(10), e072052. https://doi.org/10.1136/bmjopen-2023-072052

O'Nions, E., Brown, J., Buckman, J.E.J., Charlton, R., Cooper, C., El Baou, C., et al. (2024). Diagnosis of common health conditions among autistic adults in the UK: Evidence from a matched cohort study. *The Lancet Regional Health – Europe, 41*, 100907. https://doi.org/10.1016/j.lanepe.2024.100907

Paggetti, A., Lazzaro, G., Bacaro, V., Vanacore, N., Vicari, S., and Menghini, D. (2025). Sleep characteristics in children, adolescents, and adults with specific learning disorders: A systematic review and a meta-analysis. *Sleep Medicine, 136*, 106817. https://doi.org/10.1016/j.sleep.2025.106817

Pallisera, M., Vilà, M., Fullana, J., and Valls, M. (2021). Being in control: Choice and control of support received in supported living. A study based on the narratives of people with intellectual disability and support staff. *Journal of Intellectual and Developmental Disability, 46*(2), 164–174. https://doi.org/10.3109/13668250.2020.1802812

Passarello, N., Tarantino, V., Chirico, A., Menghini, D., Costanzo, F., Sorrentino, P., et al. (2022). Sensory processing disorders in children and adolescents: Taking stock of assessment and novel therapeutic tools. *Brain Sciences, 12*(11), 1478. https://doi.org/10.3390/brainsci12111478

Phung, J., Penner, M., Pirlot, C., and Welch, C. (2021). What I wish you knew: Insights on burnout, inertia, meltdown, and shutdown from autistic youth. *Frontiers in Psychology, 12*, 741421. https://doi.org/10.3389/fpsyg.2021.741421

Popit, S., Serod, K., Locatelli, I., and Stuhec, M. (2024). Prevalence of attention-deficit hyperactivity disorder (ADHD): Systematic review and meta-analysis. *European Psychiatry, 67*(1), e68. https://doi.org/10.1192/j.eurpsy.2024.1786

Powell, L., and Bradley, S. (2025). Helping young people find the words: Exploring the impact of psychoeducational materials for neurodivergent young people. *Neurodiversity, 3*. https://doi.org/10.1177/27546330251376508

Pring, K., Malli, M., Hardy, B.W., Rapp, S.R., Storch, E.A., Mink, J.W., et al. (2025). Reframing stigma in Tourette syndrome: An updated scoping review. *European Child and Adolescent Psychiatry, 34*(1), 19–39. https://doi.org/10.1007/s00787-023-02332-3

Quigley, E., and Gallagher, T. (2025). Neurodiversity and higher education: Double masking by neurodivergent students. *European Journal of Special Needs Education*, 1–17. https://doi.org/10.1080/08856257.2025.2511369

Rahman, R., Reid, C., Kloer, P., Henchie, A., Thomas, A., and Zwiggelaar, R. (2024). A systematic review of literature examining the application of a social model of health and wellbeing. *European Journal of Public Health, 34*(3), 467–472. https://doi.org/10.1093/eurpub/ckae008

Rodríguez-Armendariz, E., Vela-Romero, M., and Galiana, A. (2024). Sensory processing challenges in children with neurodevelopmental disorders and genetic conditions: An observational study. *NeuroSci, 5*(3), 339–353. https://doi.org/10.3390/neurosci5030027

Salari, N., Ghasemi, H., Abdoli, N., Rahmani, A., Shiri, M.H., Hashemian, A.H., et al. (2023). The global prevalence of ADHD in children and adolescents: A systematic review and meta-analysis. *Italian Journal of Pediatrics, 49*(1), 48. https://doi.org/10.1186/s13052-023-01456-1

Schneider, M., VanOrmer, J., and Zlomke, K. (2019). Adverse childhood experiences and family resilience among children with autism spectrum disorder and attention-deficit/hyperactivity disorder. *Journal of Developmental and Behavioral Pediatrics, 40*(8), 573–580. https://doi.org/10.1097/DBP.0000000000000703

Silvers, J.A. (2022). Adolescence as a pivotal period for emotion regulation development. *Current Opinion in Psychology, 44*, 258–263. https://doi.org/10.1016/j.copsyc.2021.09.023

Singer, J. (2019). *NeuroDiversity: The birth of an idea*. Self-published Kindle edition.

Tal-Saban, M., Zaguri-Vittenberg, S., and Ivzori, Y. (2025). Enhancing occupational therapists' intervention capabilities with adolescents with neurodevelopmental disorders. *Canadian Journal of Occupational Therapy, 92*(1), 39–49. https://doi.org/10.1177/00084174241272010

Thomas, R., Sanders, S., Doust, J., Beller, E., and Glasziou, P. (2015). Prevalence of attention-deficit/hyperactivity disorder: A systematic review and meta-analysis. *Pediatrics, 135*(4), e994–e1001. https://doi.org/10.1542/peds.2014-3482

Uygur, H. (2025). Unraveling the insomnia puzzle: Sleep reactivity, attention deficit hyperactivity symptoms, and insomnia severity in ADHD patients. *Frontiers in Psychiatry, 15*, 1528979. https://doi.org/10.3389/fpsyt.2024.1528979

Vargas-Salas, O., Alcazar-Gonzales, J., Fernández-Fernández, F.A., Molina-Rodríguez, F.N., Paredes-Velazco, R., and Carcausto-Zea, M. (2025). Neurodivergence and the workplace: A systematic review of the literature, *Journal of Vocational Rehabilitation, 63*(1), 83–94. https://doi.org/10.1177/10522263251337564

Wilson, A.C., and Gullon-Scott, F. (2024). Social anxiety in autistic people: Does the Clark and Wells model fit? *Journal of Autism and Developmental Disorders, 54*(10), 3908–3920. https://doi.org/10.1007/s10803-023-06108-1

World Health Organization (WHO) (2022). *International Statistical Classification of Diseases and Related Health Problems*, 11th revision (ICD-11). Geneva: WHO. https://icd.who.int/en/

YoungMinds (2023). *YoungMinds Annual Report 2023*. London: YoungMinds.

3 Neurocognitive disorders, consent, and critical intervention

Emma Brookes and Paul K. Miller

Introduction

Neurocognitive disorders (NCDs) encompass a range of conditions characterised by a measurably significant decline in cognitive functioning; this decline can affect any or all of memory, attention, language, executive function, perceptual-motor function, and social cognition (APA, 2022). Neurocognitive disorders are acquired, usually progressive, and typically associated with structural or biochemical abnormalities in the brain. Among these, dementia stands out as the most prevalent and extensively studied, representing a significant global health challenge (Nichols et al., 2022).

Dementia is characterised by a chronic and progressive decline in multiple areas of cognitive function, usually related to the disruption of neuronal networks and loss of brain cells, severe enough to interfere with a person's ability to perform everyday activities (APA, 2022; WHO, 2022). It is not a single 'disease', but rather an umbrella term encompassing various aetiologies, the most common of which is Alzheimer's disease, followed by vascular dementia, Lewy body dementia, and frontotemporal dementia (Livingston et al., 2024).

Epidemiology and impact

The global burden of dementia is profound and rising rapidly. As of 2023, more than 55 million people worldwide were living with dementia, and this number is expected to nearly triple by 2050, assuming continued increases in life expectancy and corollary ageing populations (Livingston et al., 2024). In the UK alone, it is estimated that nearly one million people are living with dementia at the time of writing, with costs to the economy now exceeding £40 billion annually, including the costs of all their direct health care and social care, and the labour of more than half a million unpaid carers (McNally, 2025).

Dementia does not occur outside of socioeconomic contexts, and its impacts are complex and interwoven. From an ecological systems perspective (Adkins-Jackson et al., 2023), dementia has effects on the microsystem (e.g. family, friends, immediate caregivers), the mesosystem (e.g. interactions between healthcare services and social support structures), the exosystem (e.g. policy frameworks, economic systems), and finally the macrosystem, which includes societal attitudes towards ageing and mental health. Stigma around cognitive decline can lead to social isolation and under-diagnosis, especially in minority populations (Fazio et al., 2023; Livingston et al., 2024; Mukadam et al., 2011). Families and caregivers often face significant emotional, financial, and psychological burdens, which can only build as increasing levels of care and supervision are required, and burnout is common in this population (Ali et al., 2024; Brites et al., 2025). The increasing prevalence of NCDs also places a significant strain on structural healthcare systems. Emergency and unscheduled care are particularly affected, as people with dementia are more likely to experience adverse events such as falls, infections, and behavioural disturbances that lead to hospital admissions (Courtney-Pratt et al., 2022; Hennah and Miller, 2025; Miller et al., 2019; Parsons et al., 2024). Hospitalisation can, in turn, lead to rapid functional and cognitive decline in this vulnerable group, highlighting the importance of appropriate community-based support and early intervention strategies (Livingston et al., 2024; McNally, 2025).

The role of paramedics

Paramedics are frequently the first point of contact for patients with NCDs during episodes of acute illness or distress. As the landscape of health care evolves towards more integrated and person-centred models, paramedics are increasingly required to adopt a broader clinical scope that includes not only the management of acute medical conditions but also the recognition and support of patients with chronic and complex needs, such as those with dementia (Courtney-Pratt et al., 2022; Han et al., 2024; NICE, 2018).

The role of paramedics in dementia care includes recognising the signs of cognitive impairment during a callout, understanding how neurocognitive decline may influence the patient's presentation and decision-making capacity, and implementing tailored communication strategies to reduce distress and ensure informed consent (Courtney-Pratt et al., 2022; Jones et al., 2023). Moreover, paramedics play a crucial role in safeguarding, particularly where neglect or abuse may be suspected (De Silva et al., 2025; McAtee et al., 2020). Their position within the community also enables them to contribute to continuity of care by signposting to local services and escalating concerns to the appropriate agencies (Choonara and Williams, 2021).

Given their frontline status, paramedics are uniquely placed to influence the patient's journey through the health system, particularly by avoiding unnecessary hospital conveyance where community-based alternatives exist (Han et al., 2024; Parsons et al., 2024). This not only has the potential to improve outcomes for people with dementia, who may become disoriented or agitated in unfamiliar hospital settings, but also reduce pressure on already stretched emergency departments (Jones et al., 2023).

Pathophysiology and types of dementia

Neurocognitive disorders are acquired conditions marked by significant decline in one or more cognitive domains: memory, attention, language, executive function, perceptual-motor function, or social cognition. The DSM-5-TR categorises NCDs as 'mild' or 'major' based on the severity of functional impairment (APA, 2022). Dementia, a 'major' NCD, involves progressive, irreversible neuronal damage affecting synaptic communication and disrupting cognitive function severe enough to interfere with daily activities. While NCDs stem from various causes, including traumatic brain injury, infections, and substance use, most cases arise from neurodegenerative and vascular pathologies (Livingston et al., 2024; McKeith et al., 2017).

Pathophysiology and clinical features by dementia type

Dementia's biological mechanisms vary between subtypes but share common features (Dening and Babu Sandilyan, 2015). Abnormal protein accumulation and neurotransmitter dysfunction cause cortical and subcortical atrophy in regions governing cognition, memory, behaviour, and motor control (Heylen et al., 2025; Lozupone et al., 2026). Neuroinflammation also plays a central role in progression, with microglial activation and oxidative stress driving neuronal damage (Leng and Edison, 2021). Emerging therapeutic strategies target these inflammatory pathways, though none are yet curative.

Alzheimer's disease

Alzheimer's disease accounts for approximately two-thirds of dementia cases globally (Adkins-Jackson et al., 2023). Its pathological hallmarks are aggregates of extracellular beta-amyloid plaques and intracellular neurofibrillary tangles of hyperphosphorylated tau protein, which disrupt neuronal function, inducing inflammation, mitochondrial dysfunction, and cell death (van der Kant et al., 2020). Early involvement of the hippocampus and entorhinal cortex correlates with memory loss, while significant cholinergic dysfunction (i.e. reduced acetylcholine activity in the cortex and hippocampus) impairs attention, learning, and memory (Anderson et al., 2017).

Clinically, Alzheimer's typically initially presents with short-term memory impairment, disorientation, and language difficulties (APA, 2022). Progressive impairments are subsequently likely to develop in visuospatial awareness, reasoning, and social functioning. Later stages bring profound language impairment, mobility loss, and behavioural symptoms including increased agitation or apathy; disease progression typically spans 8–12 years from onset (Livingston et al., 2024).

Vascular dementia

Vascular dementia results from impaired cerebral blood flow due to stroke, small vessel disease, or chronic ischaemia (Yang et al., 2023). While beta-amyloid may be present in some cases of vascular dementia, the primary pathology involves ischaemic and haemorrhagic injury to the periventricular and subcortical regions of the brain, often associated with hypertension, diabetes, and atherosclerosis (Beason-Held et al., 2023).

Clinical presentation is heterogeneous, which is why vascular dementia has particularly high rates of underdiagnosis or misdiagnosis (Huang et al., 2025). Symptoms may appear suddenly, such as in post-stroke, or develop gradually with chronic small vessel disease. Cognitive deficits typically include slowed processing speed, attention difficulties, and executive dysfunction, in contrast with the memory-dominated profile of Alzheimer's disease. Affected individuals may also exhibit motor symptoms, mood disturbances, and/or urinary incontinence depending on the affected brain regions (Yang et al., 2023). Symptom severity often fluctuates, especially immediately following recurrent vascular events.

Lewy body dementia

Lewy body dementia (LBD) involves abnormal alpha-synuclein protein aggregates (Lewy bodies) accumulating in the cortex, brainstem, and limbic regions (Heylen et al., 2025; Lozupone et al., 2026). These deposits disrupt neurotransmitter systems, particularly dopamine and acetylcholine, contributing to both cognitive decline and motor symptoms resembling those in Parkinson's disease (McKeith et al., 2017; Walker et al., 2019). Cholinergic dysfunction is often more pronounced than in Alzheimer's disease, resulting in heightened cognitive fluctuations (Petrova et al., 2020).

The clinical course of LBD varies significantly, combining cognitive and motor features. Affected individuals frequently experience vivid visual hallucinations, disordered REM sleep behaviour, and/or pronounced fluctuations in attention and alertness. Motor symptoms can include bradykinesia and rigidity, and autonomic dysfunction can manifest in postural hypotension and constipation (Camerucci et al., 2024). A critical clinical challenge in the treatment of LBD is marked antipsychotic sensitivity, which can precipitate severe adverse effects including sedation and the prospectively life-threatening neuroleptic malignant syndrome (Seebaluck et al., 2023).

Frontotemporal dementia

Frontotemporal dementia involves progressive frontal and temporal lobe degeneration driven by abnormal tau, TDP-43, or FUS protein accumulations depending on subtype. These proteinopathies disrupt normal cell function, causing selective neuronal loss in regions governing personality, language, and executive function (Takeuchi et al., 2016). Earlier onset than other dementias, and prominent behavioural symptoms, can often lead to misdiagnosis as psychiatric illness (Medina-Rioja et al., 2023; Nicholas et al., 2020).

Clinical presentation shows progressive deterioration in behaviour, personality, or language. The behavioural variant features disinhibition, impulsivity, apathy, and socially inappropriate conduct. Patients often show reduced empathy, with the potential to engender significant distress among family members and carers (Camerucci et al., 2024). Language variants include semantic dementia (loss of word meaning comprehension) and non-fluent primary progressive aphasia (Graviotto et al., 2022). Memory remains relatively preserved early on, potentially further delaying diagnosis.

Other dementia types

Parkinson's disease dementia typically develops in the context of long-standing motor symptoms, usually over one-year post-diagnosis. The clinical profile includes executive dysfunction, attention deficits, and visuospatial impairment (Walker et al., 2019). Mixed dementia, involving both Alzheimer's and vascular pathology, is increasingly recognised as common in older adults, presenting with overlapping memory loss and executive dysfunction symptoms, and may associate with more rapid cognitive decline than either condition alone (Livingston et al., 2024).

Summary

Dementia pathophysiology involves overlapping biological processes which manifest in distinct clinical syndromes, each with characteristic cognitive, behavioural, and motor features. For paramedics and pre-hospital healthcare professionals, understanding the underlying mechanisms and clinical patterns is crucial for early identification, appropriate support, and holistic care planning. Recognition of subtype-specific features, such as memory-dominant decline in Alzheimer's, executive dysfunction in vascular dementia, and fluctuations and antipsychotic sensitivity in LBD, enables tailored pre-hospital responses.

Key points

- Dementia involves progressive neuronal damage through protein aggregation, vascular injury, and neuroinflammation.
- Alzheimer's disease (beta-amyloid plaques, tau tangles) is the most common subtype, presenting with insidious memory loss.
- Vascular dementia results from cerebrovascular damage and affects executive function more than memory.
- Lewy body dementia combines cognitive fluctuations, visual hallucinations, and motor symptoms with high antipsychotic sensitivity.

- Frontotemporal dementia causes early personality and language changes, often mimicking psychiatric illness.
- Understanding dementia subtypes enables paramedics to recognise clinical patterns and tailor pre-hospital responses appropriately.

Clinical presentation and pre-hospital assessment

In emergency and pre-hospital settings, dementia creates distinct assessment challenges. As evidenced above, cognitive decline can substantially alter how individuals interpret their environment, communicate needs, and present with acute illness. Moreover, emergency presentations often differ significantly from those of patients without cognitive impairment, requiring paramedics to adapt assessment approaches while working with limited time and information (Michael et al., 2025; Parsons et al., 2024).

Cognitive deficits in emergency contexts commonly manifest as disorientation to time and place, poor short-term memory, and difficulty understanding instructions (Han et al., 2024). Superficially simple tasks such as unlocking doors may suddenly become impossible, particularly when acute illness and/or environmental stress (such as the arrival of an ambulance) overwhelms limited cognitive reserve. Perhaps more awkwardly for an attending paramedic, the long-term memories of an individual with dementia may remain intact, representing a superficial lucidity that can partially mask the critical issue(s) at hand (Courtney-Pratt et al., 2022; NICE, 2018).

Communication challenges include word-finding difficulties, repeated phrases, and vague or contradictory responses. Affected individuals may struggle with complex or open-ended questions, making history-taking difficult for an attending paramedic. These limitations can be mistaken for hearing loss, language barriers, or non-cooperation unless the underlying cognitive impairment is recognised (Choonara and Williams, 2021; Han et al., 2024). Effective communication in such contexts requires patience, closed questions focused on basic information, and simplified language.

Safety and risk considerations

Safety concerns are paramount in the pre-hospital environment. Individuals with dementia may wander unsupervised, placing themselves at risk of hypothermia or becoming lost, or exhibit poor hazard awareness such as stepping into traffic or touching hot surfaces. This can be a greater issue still where the dementia is yet undiagnosed (Amjad et al., 2022). Signs of self-neglect in the home environment, such as overflowing bins and misplaced medications, require observation and documentation, especially when patients live alone and may be unable to articulate difficulties.

Medical complications frequently prompting emergency response include falls (from poor balance, visual-perceptual deficits, or environmental hazards), incontinence, poor nutrition, dehydration, and medication non-compliance (Han et al., 2024; McNally, 2025; Sampson et al., 2014). Patients are particularly vulnerable to delirium, often the first indicator of underlying infection (e.g. urinary tract infection or pneumonia), constipation, or metabolic disturbance (Dunne and Dunne, 2024). Unlike typical presentations, these conditions may manifest primarily as increased confusion or agitation rather than in terms of physical symptoms.

Environmental cues and routine observations

Scene awareness provides crucial diagnostic and care planning information. Environmental cues such as post-it note reminders, labelled cupboards, pill organisers, and calendars with written schedules can indicate existing cognitive support strategies (Evans and Collier, 2019). Conversely, their absence or evidence of disorganisation inherently highlights unmet needs. These observations should be integrated into clinical assessment and shared with receiving healthcare providers or community services.

Standard observations can be complicated by cognitive impairment and dementia can mask pain perception, thereby preventing effective symptom reporting (Attrill and Schofield, 2024). Chest pain or dyspnoea, for example, may go unrecognised despite significant pathology. Baseline observations may differ from expected norms due to medications (e.g. beta-blockers and anticholinesterases) or autonomic dysfunction common in Lewy body and vascular dementias (as noted above). Vital signs require contextual interpretation, with collateral history regarding baseline status and consideration of subclinical acute illness presentations.

Behavioural and psychological symptoms of dementia

As noted previously, behavioural and psychological symptoms of dementia (BPSD), such as agitation, aggression, hallucinations, depression, anxiety, apathy, and sleep disturbances, occur in the great majority of affected individuals at some point, and can significantly affect pre-hospital assessment and care (Courtney-Pratt et al., 2022; Han et al., 2024).

Agitation and aggression, verbal and/or physical, often represent responses to fear, discomfort, or environmental overstimulation. Loud noises, unfamiliar uniforms, and rushed interactions – all characteristic of emergency response – can escalate such behaviours, particularly when affected individuals struggle to understand what is happening. Wandering, exit-seeking behaviours, and active resistance to care may be misinterpreted as non-compliance rather than manifestations of confusion (Banerjee, 2025; Mast et al., 2022). Visual hallucinations are most common in Lewy body dementia (as discussed earlier) and may cause an individual to significantly misinterpret their surroundings and behave unpredictably. Emotional changes – not least apathy, depression, and anxiety – may be subtle, though lack of engagement, poor eye contact, and/or irritability with a paramedic may indicate psychological distress.

Assessment and non-pharmacological de-escalation strategies

Major assessment barriers to assessment of an individual's state have been largely described above but are typically grounded in an inability and/or reluctance to provide a coherent or accurate medical history (Mast et al., 2022; McNally, 2025; Sampson et al., 2014). Individuals may confuse or minimise symptoms or forget recent events entirely. Carers and family members are often absent during emergency callouts or may be overwhelmed or unaware of recent changes (Brites et al., 2025).

Effective assessment requires simple, closed questions focusing on basic information: name, location, and recent events. Collateral history from carers, neighbours, or care staff is invaluable for understanding baseline function, recent changes, medication compliance, and existing support networks (Choonara and Williams, 2021). Medical documentation, such as hospital discharge summaries, medication administration records, and dementia care plans, should be sought and reviewed (Han et al., 2024; NICE, 2018).

Determining whether a confusion state is acute or chronic is critical to decision-making in an emergency context where dementia is at stake. Sudden mental status change, recent illness or infection, dehydration, missed medications, or recent trauma may indicate delirium requiring urgent investigation and treatment. In the UK, National Institute for Health and Care Excellence (NICE) guidelines recommend non-pharmacological interventions as first-line BPSD management, foregrounding environmental adaptations, carer support, and clear communication (NICE, 2018). In emergency care, this translates to calm, reassuring behaviour, minimal environmental stimulation, and the involvement of carers wherever possible to reduce distress.

Red flags prompting conveyance

Specific clinical red flags that warrant hospital conveyance include sudden deterioration in confusion or consciousness; evidence of acute infection (fever, tachycardia, new incontinence); hypoglycaemia or metabolic derangement; falls with trauma or unexplained injuries; severe agitation unresponsive to de-escalation; safeguarding concerns (neglect, abuse, inadequate supervision); or the lack of a safe discharge plan. Safe non-conveyance, meanwhile, may be considered where confusion is stable and chronic, carer support is available, community pathways are accessible, and no acute medical triggers are identified (Han et al., 2024; Voss et al., 2018). Clear documentation and safety-netting advice are essential in all cases.

Cognitive screening tools can assist assessment in this domain but have pre-hospital limitations. The Abbreviated Mental Test Score (AMTS) is rapid to administrate but may yield unreliable results if patients are distressed or unable to concentrate (Piotrowicz et al., 2019). More intuitive approaches include assessing ability to follow simple commands, orientation to time and place, and response to visual or verbal cues. Communication aids (picture cards, whiteboards) can be helpful. These methods support clinical decision-making and transparently inform handover to hospital staff or community services.

Assessing mental capacity in context

Mental capacity assessment is essential in emergency assessments. Dementia often results in fluctuating capacity; individuals may be able to make some decisions at some times, but not all decisions always (Hinsliff-Smith et al., 2017). In the UK, the 2005 Mental Capacity Act requires the presumption of capacity unless there is unambiguous evidence to conclude otherwise, with any healthcare intervention against an individual's wishes only permissible in their demonstrable best interests (Lepping, 2019; Spacey et al., 2026). If capacity is lacking and there is urgent risk to health or safety, paramedics are authorised to act under necessity and proportionality principles. Key to such capacity assessment is, therefore, distinguishing chronic dementia from acute delirium. While both present with confusion, their underlying causes, courses, and treatments differ significantly. Dementia, as noted throughout, shows progressive, long-term impairment with (relatively) stable patterns over days, months, and years. Delirium has acute onset and fluctuating course, typically triggered by underlying medical issues, not least infection, pain, electrolyte imbalance, or medication side effects (Dunne and Dunne, 2024; Lepping, 2019). Clinical features suggesting delirium include sudden onset of confusion, fluctuating consciousness levels, marked inattention, disorganised thinking, hallucinations, and altered sleep-wake cycles (Dunne and Dunne, 2024). NICE guidance recommends actively seeking and treating underlying delirium causes, which may significantly improve mental state if addressed promptly (NICE, 2023).

Summary

Dementia creates diverse emergency presentation challenges, with cognitive impairment, behavioural symptoms, and physical health complications all contributing to the clinical picture. Paramedics must navigate significant assessment challenges, especially when an individual cannot provide a reliable history or remain engaged. Recognising communication difficulties, behavioural changes, and environmental clues is essential. Distinguishing chronic dementia from acute delirium is critical to safe, effective care. Supported by appropriate training, tools, and interprofessional collaboration, paramedics are well positioned to contribute meaningfully to early identification and management of cognitive impairment.

Key points

- Dementia routinely presents atypically in emergencies. Confusion may mask acute illness, and vital signs may not reflect severity.
- Environmental cues (medication charts, memory aids, disorganisation) provide critical diagnostic and safeguarding information.
- Distinguishing dementia from delirium is essential; delirium has acute onset and requires urgent investigation of underlying causes.
- Red flags for conveyance include sudden confusion worsening, infection, trauma, safeguarding concerns, or lack of carer support.
- Collateral history from carers and environmental observation are vital when individuals with dementia cannot provide reliable accounts.
- Mental capacity assessment must be decision-specific, and paramedics must act in the individual's best interests when capacity is impaired.

Case study: A patient with dementia

Case study: Narrative

At 5:45pm on a cold winter evening, a paramedic crew responded to a category 2 call for a 78-year-old female, Mrs Margaret Turner, reported by a neighbour to be wandering disoriented in the street. The caller stated that Mrs Turner appeared confused, was lightly dressed for the weather, and did not recognise her own home. The incident occurred in a suburban area where Mrs Turner lived alone.

Mrs Turner had a known diagnosis of mixed dementia (Alzheimer's and vascular), with documented progressive cognitive decline over the past five years. Her past medical history included hypertension, Type 2 diabetes, and osteoarthritis. Her daughter, who lived 30 minutes away, was her primary carer and managed her medication and groceries. Mrs Turner had experienced two falls in the last month, one of which led to a minor head injury. According to previous ambulance records, she had become increasingly confused over recent weeks, with multiple calls made by neighbours for welfare concerns. She was under review by a community memory team, and her GP had referred her for increased social support.

The presenting complaint was confusion, exposure to cold, and potential safeguarding concerns due to her wandering behaviour.

Primary survey (ABCDE approach)

Upon arrival, the crew found Mrs Turner approximately 200 metres from her home, standing outside a closed shop. She was underdressed for the conditions, wearing a nightdress and slippers in near-freezing temperatures. Paramedics gently approached and guided her into the ambulance. Based on the ABCDE approach:

Airway was clear and patent.

Breathing was regular, with no signs of respiratory distress or increased effort.

Circulation appeared stable; peripheral pulses were present and skin was cool but perfused.

Disability assessment revealed alertness but notable disorientation, with impaired short-term memory and poor attention. No signs of focal neurological deficit were present.

Exposure, she was noted to be mildly hypothermic, with no visible trauma or injuries.

The crew concluded that there was no immediately life-threatening cause for her confusion and began secondary assessment.

Vital signs

The following observations were recorded:

- Respiratory rate: 18 breaths per minute
- Oxygen saturation: 96% on air
- Pulse: 88 bpm, regular
- Blood pressure: 134/78 mmHg
- Temperature: 35.1°C
- Blood glucose: 7.1 mmol/L
- NEWS2 score: 1

These findings helped exclude hypoxia, hypoglycaemia, and hypotension as immediate causes of altered mental state. The slightly low temperature, combined with her exposure, explained her shivering and some of her agitation. A basic neurological screen revealed no asymmetry, limb weakness, or cranial nerve abnormality, and no evidence of trauma.

Focused mental health assessment

A structured mental state examination (MSE) was conducted to better understand Mrs Turner's psychological and cognitive state.

- *Appearance and behaviour*: She was alert but poorly oriented. Her hygiene appeared adequate, but her clothing was inappropriate for the weather, suggesting a lapse in judgement. She displayed psychomotor agitation, pacing and fidgeting in the ambulance, and was intermittently restless. She attempted to leave several times and expressed a strong desire to return 'home', though could not describe where that was.

- *Speech*: Her speech was coherent but slow. She often repeated herself, and responses were tangential. At times she became frustrated when she could not find the right words, indicating mild aphasia.
- *Mood and affect*: She appeared emotionally flat and anxious. Although she insisted she was 'fine', her affect was incongruent with the situation and her expressed worries about her 'missing mother' were concerning and unrealistic for her age.
- *Thought process and content*: Her thought process was illogical and tangential. She appeared preoccupied with thoughts about household responsibilities, including feeding a pet. There was no clear evidence of active suicidal or homicidal ideation, but her thinking was clearly disorganised.
- *Perception*: She did not appear to be actively hallucinating, though she responded to unseen stimuli and asked questions about people who were not present. Given her known diagnosis of mixed dementia, occasional perceptual disturbances were consistent with her condition.
- *Cognition and insight*: Her orientation was poor. She could not state the time, date, or her location. She misidentified the paramedics as shopkeepers and insisted she needed to return home to carry out 'chores'. Insight into her confusion was absent. She denied that anything was wrong and could not grasp why she was being questioned.

This MSE-informed approach helped guide the clinical impression of cognitive deterioration, likely worsened by delirium, environmental stress, or possible infection.

Capacity assessment

Using the Mental Capacity Act 2005 four-stage framework, the paramedics assessed whether Mrs Turner had the capacity to decide whether to remain at home or attend hospital.

- *Understanding*: She was unable to demonstrate understanding of the current situation. When told she was found wandering in the cold, she dismissed the concern and replied, 'I'm just getting the paper'.
- *Retention*: She could not retain new information beyond a few seconds. When reminded of her location, she quickly forgot and again asked where she was.
- *Use and weighing of information*: She was unable to consider risks, benefits, or alternatives. She could not compare the consequences of staying home alone versus being checked over at hospital.
- *Communication of decision*: Although verbal, her responses were inconsistent and confused. She stated both 'I want to go home' and 'Maybe I live here now' in the space of a few minutes.

Based on this structured assessment, the paramedics concluded that Mrs Turner lacked capacity to make an informed decision about remaining at home. In accordance with the Act, and with her best interests in mind, the team decided to transport her to hospital for further evaluation and safeguarding.

Challenges encountered

- *Communication barriers*: Communication was challenging throughout. Mrs Turner had word-finding difficulties and frequently repeated questions. She showed limited understanding of questions relating to her health or the environment. The crew used short, closed questions, maintained eye contact, and adjusted their tone to be soft and calm. Despite this, information gathering was incomplete without collateral history.
- *Non-compliance and agitation*: Mrs Turner became resistant when asked about her medications or whether she had eaten. At one point, she attempted to leave the ambulance, stating she had 'chores to do'. These behaviours, while not aggressive, indicated increasing anxiety and a potential risk to her safety. The team employed redirection techniques and reassurance, avoiding confrontation or correction.

Ethical and legal considerations

There was a clear need to assess Mrs Turner's capacity. Her disorientation, fluctuating responses, and inability to understand the situation suggested impaired capacity regarding decisions about her immediate care. In line with the Mental Capacity Act 2005, the crew determined she lacked capacity to decide on whether to be assessed further or remain at home. A decision was made in her best interests to convey her to hospital for further evaluation and safeguarding.

Consent was therefore not formal, but action was justified based on clinical necessity and her evident vulnerability. Her property was checked for signs of forced entry or hazards. The crew secured the premises and documented the decision to leave the property temporarily unoccupied.

Management and intervention

Mrs Turner was removed from the cold environment and kept warm in the ambulance. A glucose reading ruled out hypoglycaemia, and her observations were stable. No injuries were noted. Paramedics contacted her daughter, who confirmed she had last seen her mother two days ago and that she was awaiting a reassessment of her care needs.

A review of medications found a blister pack labelled with last Monday's date, with some morning doses skipped. No MAR chart was available. A community dementia diagnosis letter and social work referral were found near the front door.

Collateral history from the daughter indicated a recent urinary tract infection (UTI) treated with antibiotics. She expressed concern about her mother's increased confusion and wandering, stating this was the first time she had left the house at night.

Non-pharmacological and pharmacological interventions

No pharmacological interventions were required at the scene. The focus remained on reducing distress and maintaining comfort. The crew dimmed ambulance lighting, limited noise, and avoided unnecessary handling. Mrs Turner's tremors were attributed to cold and anxiety, not Parkinsonism.

A basic urine dipstick test was not available in the pre-hospital setting, though signs pointed towards possible delirium superimposed on dementia. Differential diagnosis included worsening dementia, possible UTI recurrence, or medication non-compliance.

Transport considerations

Given the circumstances, mild hypothermia, wandering, impaired capacity, lack of supervision, and a recent infection, the decision was made to transport Mrs Turner to hospital. The crew considered community pathways, but out-of-hours services and the absence of an immediate safeguarding plan made this inappropriate.

The crew handed over to the hospital's triage nurse at the local emergency department highlighting: mixed dementia with suspected delirium, mild hypothermia due to environmental exposure, impaired capacity and lack of carer availability, repeat falls, and missed medication concerns.

Patient outcome

Mrs Turner was admitted to the Acute Medical Unit for investigation and monitoring. Blood tests revealed elevated inflammatory markers, and a urine sample confirmed a recurrent UTI. She was started on antibiotics and monitored for signs of delirium. Social services and the safeguarding team were notified.

A capacity assessment performed later determined she lacked capacity to return home safely without supervision. She was referred for an urgent best interests meeting. The outcome, after five days in hospital, was temporary placement in a residential care facility for ongoing support and reablement.

Case study (continued): Applying the Driscoll model of reflection

What?

During the pre-hospital response to Mrs Turner, a patient with known dementia, paramedics faced multiple complex issues. Mrs Turner presented disoriented, hypothermic, and wandering outside her home, with known cognitive decline and recent falls. The paramedic team had to rapidly assess her scene and environment, determine her mental capacity, engage with family for collateral history, and make a decision regarding hospital transport and safeguarding.

They navigated communication difficulties, limited insight from the patient, and legal/ethical challenges related to consent and capacity under the Mental Capacity Act 2005.

So What?

This scenario emphasises several critical principles. First, the need for paramedics to rapidly assess cognitive status and mental capacity in dynamic, pressured pre-hospital environments is increasingly recognised. Recent work shows that paramedics often feel underprepared when responding to people living with dementia, particularly when judgement about capacity, consent, or risk needs to be made on scene (Choonara and Williams, 2021). The ability to adapt to cognitive, communicative, and environmental complexity is therefore a key competency.

Second, collateral history and environmental observation are vital. Without information from Mrs Turner's daughter (regarding recent infection, medication adherence, baseline function), key pieces of her condition and risk profile would have been missed. Evidence supports that incorporating carer/family input improves paramedic assessments of older people with dementia (Jones et al., 2023). Failing to gather such information increases the risk of inappropriate conveyance or missed diagnosis of delirium superimposed on dementia.

Third, the scenario underscores legal and ethical literacy. The paramedics recognised that Mrs Turner lacked capacity to make decisions about her care and conveyed her in her best interests, aligning with statutory frameworks (King et al., 2025; Voss et al., 2018). Misapplication of capacity assessment risks disempowering the patient or exposing practitioners to professional risk.

Finally, inter-agency collaboration proved critical. Liaising with carers, social services, community memory teams, and hospital staff created a continuity of care pathway that extended beyond the callout. Research indicates that paramedics working in isolation often face barriers, whereas integration with dementia and geriatric services leads to better outcomes (Courtney-Pratt et al., 2022).

Now What?

This case supports several actionable recommendations for paramedic services managing similar cases in future.

First, it reinforces the need for training in rapid cognitive and capacity assessment tailored for use in pre-hospital settings. Paramedics should be supported to develop practical skills using simplified tools and scenario-based training to enhance accuracy and confidence. Secondly, services should encourage and facilitate the collection of collateral history as routine practice. This includes structured protocols for contacting next of kin or care providers and prompts to review in-home evidence such as medication administration records (MAR charts), care plans, and environmental safety cues. Thirdly, there should be greater emphasis on documentation of mental capacity assessments and best interests decisions, especially when conveyance is undertaken without consent. Clear documentation protects both the patient and the clinician and ensures transparency in complex care decisions (King et al., 2025; NICE, 2018). Lastly, health systems should continue to invest in community-based alternatives to hospital admission, such as urgent community response teams, crisis intervention, and dementia-specific care pathways. Paramedics, as frontline clinicians, play a critical role in identifying patients who may benefit from these services and facilitating timely referrals (Courtney-Pratt et al., 2022).

This case underscores that effective pre-hospital dementia care is not solely about managing acute medical presentations, it involves recognising vulnerability, applying legal and ethical principles, communicating sensitively, and coordinating care across systems. Enhancing these capabilities within paramedic practice will be essential as dementia prevalence continues to rise globally.

Case study: Lessons

Paramedics play a crucial role in the early identification and management of dementia-related crises. In Mrs Turner's case, the crew's timely response, sensitive communication, and ethical decision-making enabled appropriate safeguarding and treatment. This case reflects the evolving responsibilities of ambulance clinicians in caring for vulnerable populations and demonstrates how high-quality, person-centred care can begin at the front door, or, as in this case, on the pavement!

Best practices for paramedics

Effective pre-hospital care for people living with dementia requires paramedics to deploy specialised communication techniques, behavioural management strategies, ethical reasoning, collaborative practice, and clear understanding of legal responsibilities. This section outlines best practices based on current research, professional guidelines, and statutory frameworks.

Communication techniques for individuals with dementia

As noted throughout the section on 'Clinical presentation and pre-hospital assessment', dementia significantly impairs verbal comprehension, memory, and expressive language, making traditional history-taking methods less effective. Person-centred, simplified approaches are essential (Fazio et al., 2023). Extant research underscores that people with dementia and their carers often experience ambulance encounters as rushed, confusing, and disempowering when communication is not tailored to cognitive ability (Courtney-Pratt et al., 2022; Han et al., 2024; NICE, 2018).

Recommended techniques include speaking slowly and clearly, using short sentences, offering binary choices, and allowing extended processing time (NICE, 2018). Eye-level positioning, non-verbal reinforcement such as smiling or nodding, and avoiding medical jargon are key. Reducing ambient noise, maintaining eye contact, and using visual cues or gestures further support understanding.

Effective communication extends beyond the individual. Engaging early with carers or care home staff helps confirm baseline function, behaviours, and known triggers for distress. It has been well-demonstrated that including family members in care conversations improves paramedic assessment and promotes person-centred care (Brites et al., 2025; Han et al., 2024; McNally, 2025).

De-escalation and behavioural management strategies

Behavioural and psychological symptoms of dementia (BPSD), including agitation, anxiety, delusions, hallucinations, and wandering, can be exacerbated during ambulance callouts. As discussed above, these behaviours often reflect unmet needs, discomfort, or confusion rather than intentional resistance. Best practice involves reducing environmental stressors, speaking calmly, validating emotions, and avoiding confrontation (Fazio et al., 2023; Molony et al., 2025).

Where possible, paramedics should use distraction, redirection, and reassurance rather than correction or restraint. Validation techniques, originally developed in therapeutic settings, have been shown to reduce agitation and distress in crisis response situations (Choonara and Williams, 2021; Courtney-Pratt et al., 2022). Paramedics should also assess for physical or clinical causes behind behavioural changes. Pain, infection, hunger, constipation, or missed medication may all contribute. NICE guidelines in the UK emphasise that non-pharmacological approaches should always be first-line responses to BPSD, with medications such as antipsychotics reserved for extreme risk scenarios and after senior review (NICE, 2018).

Ethical considerations: Capacity, consent, and best interests

Working with individuals who have impaired cognition raises complex ethical considerations around consent, autonomy, and decision-making. The Mental Capacity Act 2005 provides a legal framework for assessing capacity and making best interests decisions when individuals cannot do so themselves (Spacey et al., 2026). As outlined above, paramedics must assess whether the person understands, retains, weighs, and communicates a decision. If not, they are permitted to act in the person's best interests, considering the least restrictive option and involving carers where possible.

There is strong evidence to suggest, however, that paramedics at all levels of experience often express uncertainty about applying the Mental Capacity Act in practice, particularly in time-pressured situations (Courtney-Pratt et al., 2022; Han et al., 2024; Jones et al., 2023). Training on mental capacity and consent should therefore be embedded into continuing professional development. In situations where an individual refuses care but lacks capacity, paramedics must clearly document their rationale for overriding this refusal, ensuring decisions align with necessity and proportionality principles (NICE, 2018).

Involving family or legal advocates in care decisions not only helps establish best interests but also improves outcomes and supports relational ethics (Choonara and Williams, 2021; Voss et al., 2018), and a paramedic's willingness to involve carers in decisions can be reflexively influenced by their confidence, empathy, and knowledge of the legal framework (Jones et al., 2023).

Interdisciplinary collaboration

Delivering safe and effective care to people with dementia cannot be achieved by paramedics in isolation. Interdisciplinary collaboration is vital, particularly with GPs, memory clinics, community mental health teams, adult social care, and hospital frailty teams. Working together improves continuity of care and avoids unnecessary hospital admissions (King et al., 2025; Lofthouse-Jones et al., 2021), and early contact with a known GP, keyworker, or informal carer can help establish a plan aligning with the person's existing care preferences and reduces emergency conveyance needs (Han et al., 2024; McNally, 2025).

Whether conveying to hospital or referring to community care, paramedics should ensure that dementia status, observed behaviours, known risks, and safeguarding concerns are communicated clearly to the next provider (NICE, 2018).

Legal and professional responsibilities

Paramedics in the UK are bound by professional standards set by the Health and Care Professions Council (HCPC), including duties to respect service users, communicate effectively, make informed decisions, and safeguard vulnerable individuals. In the context of dementia, these responsibilities mean recognising cognitive impairment, adapting communication, acting lawfully around capacity, and involving others appropriately (HCPC, 2024). Documentation is a core legal responsibility therein. Paramedics are expected to accurately record findings, including indicators of cognitive impairment, the results of any mental capacity assessments, consent decisions, safeguarding actions, and the rationale for treatment or conveyance. Clear records protect both the individual and practitioner, particularly when decisions deviate from standard expectations due to ethical or capacity issues.

Paramedics must also maintain their competence. Dementia education is not yet universally standardised in paramedic programmes, though research indicates it improves attitudes, communication skills, and clinical confidence (Jones et al., 2023). Ongoing professional development in dementia care, capacity law, and ethical decision-making is essential as the population ages and pre-hospital dementia presentations increase.

Best practice: Summary

Paramedics are frequently first responders to people living with dementia during moments of crisis. Best practice in this context relies on five key domains: clear and adapted communication, effective de-escalation of behavioural symptoms, legally sound and ethical decision-making, collaborative working with carers and professionals, and adherence to legal and regulatory responsibilities. As the UK population ages and dementia rates continue to rise, paramedics will play an increasingly important role in identifying, managing, and advocating for people living with dementia within and beyond the emergency care system.

Future directions and challenges

Evolving role of paramedics in dementia care

The paramedic role in dementia care is undergoing significant transformation. Having traditionally responded to acute medical emergencies, paramedics now encounter increasing numbers of people with dementia, yet many report feeling underprepared and unclear about their role in dementia-specific care (Han et al., 2024). This gap indicates a need for clearer role definitions, protocols, and pathways that position paramedics as integral actors in the dementia care continuum rather than simply conveyance agents.

Paramedics may increasingly act as community dementia first responders: recognising cognitive impairment early, working with care networks, facilitating non-conveyance or alternative care pathways, and advocating for safety in out-of-hospital settings. Paramedic referrals to community memory services, falls teams, and rapid community response teams may become standard. This shift demands that paramedics incorporate knowledge of dementia trajectories, communication strategies, and safeguarding frameworks into their skillset. As current literature highlights, the lack of a defined paramedic role in dementia care remains a systemic hindrance (De Silva et al., 2025). Ambulance services and policymakers must actively reconfigure job descriptions, training frameworks, and performance metrics to reflect this evolving paradigm.

Advancements in pre-hospital dementia screening and management

Screening, assessment, and management of dementia in the pre-hospital context continue to develop. Although recognised screening tools are widely used in hospital settings, their adaptation for paramedic use remains limited. Recent studies advocate for tailored, rapid tools that paramedics can deploy reliably in the field (Jones et al., 2023). Mobile electronic patient records with embedded dementia flags, decision-support prompts, and home-environment risk checklists hold promise for streamlining on-scene assessment and safe decision-making (Han et al., 2024).

Another promising direction is integration of paramedics into community paramedicine models focused on home-based care and non-conveyance pathways (McCann, 2022; Parsons et al., 2024). Home-based paramedicine services, when aligned with geriatric and memory services input, can reduce hospital admissions and improve satisfaction in older, cognitively impaired individuals. Furthermore, assistive technologies and remote monitoring, including wearable sensors, GPS location monitoring, and cognitive-support applications, are gaining traction (Cullen et al., 2022). While not yet mainstream in ambulance services, these trends suggest paramedics will need to become familiar with interpreting remote-monitor data and liaising with technology-enabled care teams.

However, challenges persist. Evidence of validated screening tools for paramedic use remains limited, and competing on-scene priorities may hinder implementation. Non-conveyance decisions must be backed by robust community pathways, clear documentation, and inter-agency collaboration. The literature notes that paramedics work best when supported by dementia-inclusive systems rather than working in isolation (Han et al., 2024).

Training and education needs

Training and education represent a central pillar of the future agenda. Recent research evaluating the impact of dementia-specific education on student paramedics found significant improvements in knowledge and confidence even after brief educational modules (Jones et al., 2023). Nonetheless, such training is rarely mandatory. To deliver high-quality dementia care, curricula for undergraduate and continuing professional development must include modules on cognitive impairment recognition, communication strategies, behavioural management, legal and ethical issues, and safe decision-making for non-conveyance.

Simulation-based training, case studies, interprofessional learning (with geriatrics, memory teams, and social care), and exposure to dementia-friendly environments should be developed. Leadership and policy experts recommend that ambulance services institute formal competencies in dementia care for paramedics, aligned with national dementia strategies and regulatory frameworks (De Silva et al., 2025). Ongoing audit, feedback, and research into paramedic-led dementia care initiatives can further refine training and integration.

Policy and healthcare system changes

Policy and health system changes will play a decisive role in shaping future paramedic involvement in dementia care. National dementia strategies increasingly emphasise early detection, community-based care, and hospital-avoidance models. The 2024 Lancet Commission update on dementia prevention and care emphasised community resilience, integrated care models, and new workforce roles including paramedics (Livingston et al., 2024).

These high-level policy drivers provide a mandate for ambulance services to align with dementia-friendly systems, develop alternative pathways, and invest in workforce adaptation.

System-level enablers include electronic health record sharing between ambulance, primary care, and memory services; community risk registers highlighting people with dementia; and funding models rewarding appropriate non-conveyance. Conversely, obstacles include fragmented commissioning, variable local dementia services capacity, and a risk-averse conveyance culture in some ambulance services. Policy frameworks must therefore incentivise collaboration, support paramedic triage models, and define outcome metrics beyond simple conveyance rates (De Silva et al., 2025).

Additionally, the professional regulatory environment is evolving. Bodies such as the Health and Care Professions Council and the Royal College of Paramedics emphasise safeguarding, interprofessional collaboration, and lifelong learning. Integrated system policy requires paramedics to function not just as clinicians responding to immediate crises but as connectors in multidisciplinary dementia care networks.

Future directions: Summary

The future of paramedic involvement in dementia care is defined by four interwoven strands: redefining the paramedic role, implementing robust pre-hospital screening and management tools, building workforce capabilities through focused education, and aligning with health system policy shifts. As dementia prevalence grows globally and healthcare delivery increasingly occurs outside hospital settings, paramedics are well positioned to lead change. Realising this potential requires investment in training, research into field-adapted screening and referral pathways, and strong system-wide integration. Paramedics, often first responders in moments of crisis, are uniquely positioned to advocate for safer alternatives and initiate early interventions that may prevent further deterioration. The shift towards community-based care and expanding roles such as advanced paramedics, urgent care responders, and community paramedics offer promising pathways to more responsive, preventative, and person-centred dementia care. However, this evolution depends on system-wide collaboration, adequate resourcing, and dementia-specific training.

Conclusion

Neurocognitive disorders, and in particular dementia, continue to present significant clinical, ethical, and societal challenges that demand a nuanced and compassionate response from across the healthcare system. Throughout this chapter, several key themes have emerged, reinforcing the complex interplay between biology, behaviour, systems of care, and frontline clinical practice, especially within the domain of paramedicine.

A recurring theme herein has been the progressive and multifaceted nature of dementia, which disrupts not only memory and cognition, but also behaviour, communication, and physical health. This complexity necessitates that paramedics move beyond traditional, time-pressured models of acute care to provide more person-centred, contextually aware, and relationally sensitive interventions. The unpredictable presentations of dementia, particularly during crises or acute illness, require heightened clinical vigilance, flexible communication strategies, and an ability to recognise both typical symptoms and subtle deviations from baseline (Han et al., 2024). Another central theme is the importance of integrated assessment and decision-making, particularly in differentiating dementia from delirium, identifying behavioural and psychological symptoms of dementia, and determining whether hospital conveyance is necessary. This involves gathering collateral histories, using observational skills to interpret environment and behaviour, and balancing clinical risk with the patient's known wishes and routines (Livingston et al., 2024).

Ethical and legal considerations are woven throughout pre-hospital dementia care. Paramedics must navigate fluctuating capacity, consent, safeguarding concerns, and best interests decisions often with limited information and time. This highlights the need for clear legal understanding, ethical frameworks, and confidence in multi-agency referral processes. The evolving role of paramedics as autonomous clinicians in community settings demands sustained training in these areas, along with competence in engaging families, carers, social care, and other health professionals (Parsons et al., 2024).

Finally, systemic and educational gaps remain in preparing paramedics for the rising demand and complexity of dementia care. There is a clear need for enhanced dementia-specific training in undergraduate and postgraduate programmes. At policy level, investment is required in community care alternatives, clearer escalation pathways, and digital tools for information-sharing and care continuity (Han et al., 2024).

Implications for paramedic practice

For paramedics, dementia care is no longer peripheral, it is becoming a routine and expanding aspect of practice. The implications are broad: clinical pathways must be adapted to account for cognitive impairment; communication strategies must be flexible and individualised; paramedics must feel equipped to assess risk, support autonomy, and involve families in decision-making. Person-centred dementia care means understanding the person behind the diagnosis, their preferences, fears, routines, and social environment. It means managing behavioural symptoms with empathy, avoiding unnecessary pharmacological interventions, and recognising hospital environments themselves may cause harm for people with dementia.

Paramedics, often first responders in moments of crisis, are uniquely positioned to advocate for safer alternatives and initiate early interventions that may prevent further deterioration (Han et al., 2024; Parsons et al., 2024). The shift towards community-based care and expanding roles such as advanced paramedics, urgent care responders, and community paramedics offer promising pathways to more responsive, preventative, and person-centred dementia care. However, this evolution depends on system-wide collaboration, adequate resourcing, and dementia-specific training.

Final thoughts on improving pre-hospital dementia care

Improving pre-hospital care for people living with dementia is not simply about clinical competence, it is about compassion, respect, and adaptability. It involves recognising each patient as more than a diagnosis, understanding the pressures on families and carers, and working within systems that may be fragmented or under strain. To move forward, the practice must continue to challenge outdated assumptions about cognitive impairment and emergency care. It must build evidence-based models that encourage autonomy, avoid institutional harm, and ensure paramedics are equipped with the tools, knowledge, and confidence to deliver excellent care in any setting. Ultimately, excellence in dementia care begins with understanding, is sustained by teamwork, and is measured not only in clinical outcomes but in the dignity and comfort of our patients.

Further learning materials

Multiple-choice questions

MCQ1: Which statement best describes dementia in clinical terms?

A. A single disease with a fixed course
B. A chronic, progressive decline in cognition severe enough to impair daily functioning
C. An acute confusional state that resolves with treatment
D. A psychiatric disorder defined by hallucinations and delusions

Correct answer: B

Rationale: Dementia is an umbrella syndrome of progressive cognitive decline that interferes with everyday functioning.

MCQ2: Which feature most strongly suggests delirium rather than dementia?

A. Gradual decline over years
B. Stable confusion day-to-day
C. Acute onset with fluctuating attention and consciousness
D. Early memory-dominant impairment

Correct answer: C

Rationale: Delirium is characterised by acute onset and fluctuating attention/level of awareness.

MCQ3: A 'memory-dominant' early presentation is most typical of:

A. Vascular dementia
B. Alzheimer's disease
C. Frontotemporal dementia
D. Lewy body dementia

Correct answer: B

Rationale: Alzheimer's disease typically begins with prominent short-term memory impairment.

MCQ4: Which cognitive domain is often disproportionately affected in vascular dementia compared with Alzheimer's disease?

A. Executive function/processing speed
B. Immediate recall only
C. Long-term autobiographical memory
D. Procedural memory only

Correct answer: A

Rationale: Vascular dementia commonly presents with slowed processing and executive dysfunction due to cerebrovascular injury.

MCQ5: A patient with dementia has vivid visual hallucinations and marked fluctuations in attention. This most suggests:

A. Frontotemporal dementia
B. Lewy body dementia
C. Alzheimer's disease
D. Normal ageing

Correct answer: B

Rationale: Visual hallucinations and cognitive fluctuations are core features of Lewy body dementia.

MCQ6: A key pre-hospital safety risk that is especially relevant in dementia is:

A. Medication intolerance due to allergies
B. Wandering with poor hazard awareness and exposure risk
C. Primary hallucinations causing violence in all cases
D. Hyperglycaemia as the most common cause of confusion

Correct answer: B

Rationale: Dementia increases risk of wandering, exposure, falls, and poor hazard awareness in the community.

MCQ7: Which approach is most consistent with best practice communication with a person with dementia?

A. Open-ended questioning to encourage narrative detail
B. Rapid questioning to save time
C. Short sentences, closed questions, and extra processing time
D. Correcting inaccuracies immediately to 'reorient' the patient

Correct answer: C

Rationale: Simplified language, closed questions, and extra processing time reduce cognitive load and distress.

MCQ8: Under the Mental Capacity Act 2005, capacity is best described as:

A. Global and fixed once dementia is diagnosed
B. Decision-specific and may fluctuate
C. Determined solely by age and diagnosis
D. Absent whenever a person refuses care

Correct answer: B

Rationale: Capacity is assessed for a specific decision at a specific time and can fluctuate in dementia/delirium.

MCQ9: Which is a red flag prompting conveyance for a person with dementia in the pre-hospital setting?

A. Stable chronic confusion with reliable carer support
B. Sudden deterioration in confusion or consciousness
C. Mildly repetitive speech
D. Known dementia with normal observations and safe supervision

Correct answer: B

Rationale: Sudden cognitive change may indicate delirium or acute illness requiring urgent investigation.

MCQ10: In Lewy body dementia, why should clinicians be cautious with anti-psychotics?

A. They have no effect on agitation

B. They can cause marked sensitivity reactions including severe adverse effects

C. They worsen memory only, without other risks

D. They are always contraindicated in all dementias

Correct answer: B

Rationale: People with LBD can have severe antipsychotic sensitivity, including potentially life-threatening reactions.

MCQ11: Which environmental cue most strongly suggests existing cognitive support needs at home?

A. A TV on in the background

B. Post-it note reminders, labelled cupboards, pill organisers

C. A tidy living room

D. A pet bed

Correct answer: B

Rationale: Memory aids and medication organisers often indicate known cognitive impairment and compensatory strategies.

MCQ12: Which assessment principle is most important when a person with dementia gives an unreliable history?

A. Rely on patient report only to respect autonomy

B. Avoid speaking to carers to preserve confidentiality

C. Seek collateral history and integrate environmental observations

D. Treat all confusion as dementia progression

Correct answer: C

Rationale: Collateral history and scene cues are often essential to identify baseline function, acute change, and risk.

Guided clinical reasoning questions

Q1: Is this dementia, delirium, or both? What is the time course (acute/fluctuating vs. gradual/stable)?

Q2: What reversible causes must I exclude first? Hypoglycaemia, hypoxia, infection, trauma, medication effects, dehydration, pain, constipation.

Q3: What is the immediate risk? Wandering/exposure, falls risk, unsafe home environment, aggression/distress, safeguarding concerns.

Q4: What does the environment tell me? Medication packs, missed doses, food/fluids, hazards, neglect, cognitive aids, heating, locked doors.

Q5: What collateral history is essential? Baseline cognition/function, recent change, recent infection, falls, medication adherence, support network.

Q6: How will I adapt communication? Simple phrases, closed questions, one speaker, calm tone, reduce stimulation, validation and reassurance.

Q7: Capacity – what decision is being made right now? Can the patient understand / retain / weigh / communicate about *this* decision?

Q8: What is the least restrictive safe plan? Conveyance vs. supported stay at home with urgent community response / carers / safeguarding.

Q9: What red flags override non-conveyance? Acute deterioration, infection signs, head injury/trauma, unsafe supervision, severe agitation, safeguarding.

Q10: What must be documented and handed over? Baseline vs. acute change, capacity reasoning, risks observed, collateral sources, environment cues, safety netting.

Reflective questions for learners

Q1: When did I last risk diagnostic overshadowing, assuming 'it's just dementia' and what would I do differently?

Q2: How did my communication style change, or not, when the patient was confused, repetitive, or distressed?

Q3: What cues did I notice in the environment, and what did I miss because I was task-focused?

Q4: How confident am I applying the Mental Capacity Act 2005 under time pressure, and what support/tools would help?

Q5: Did I choose the least restrictive option that was still safe? What influenced that decision (risk, time, system pressures)?

Q6: How did I involve carers/family appropriately, and how did I manage confidentiality and safeguarding duties?

Q7: What emotional responses did this type of call evoke (frustration, anxiety, protectiveness), and how might that affect decisions?

Q8: What is one concrete change I will make next shift when attending a person with suspected dementia/delirium?

Teaching commentary

Dementia presentations in pre-hospital care are rarely 'just confusion'. Paramedics must balance time-critical exclusion of reversible causes, especially delirium triggers with person-centred communication and safeguarding awareness. Environmental cues and collateral history often carry the diagnostic weight when the patient cannot provide a reliable history. Decision-making should be anchored in capacity as decision-specific, best interests, and the least restrictive safe plan while recognising clear red flags that necessitate conveyance. Good practice is measured not only by clinical accuracy, but also by maintaining dignity, reducing distress, and ensuring continuity through high-quality documentation and handover.

References

Adkins-Jackson, P.B., George, K.M., Besser, L.M., Hyun, J., Lamar, M., Hill-Jarrett, T.G., et al. (2023). The structural and social determinants of Alzheimer's disease related dementias. *Alzheimer's and Dementia, 19*(7), 3171–3185. https://doi.org/10.1002/alz.13027

Ali, A.M., Alkhamees, A.A., Hallit, S., Al-Dwaikat, T., Khatatbeh, H., and Al-Dossary, S. (2024). The Depression Anxiety Stress Scale 8: Investigating its cutoff scores in relevance to loneliness and burnout among dementia family caregivers. *Scientific Reports, 14*(1), 13075–13012. https://doi.org/10.1038/s41598-024-60127-1

American Psychiatric Association (APA) (2022). *Diagnostic and Statistical Manual of Mental Disorders* (DSM-5-TR). Washington, DC: APA Publishing.

Amjad, H., Samus, Q.M., Huang, J., Gundavarpu, S., Bynum, J.P.W., Wolff, J.L., et al. (2022). Acute care utilization risk among older adults living undiagnosed or unaware of dementia. *Journal of the American Geriatrics Society, 70*(2), 470–480. https://doi.org/10.1111/jgs.17550

Anderson, R.M., Hadjichrysanthou, C., Evans, S., and Wong, M.M. (2017). Why do so many clinical trials of therapies for Alzheimer's disease fail? *The Lancet, 390*(10110), 2327–2329. https://doi.org/10.1016/S0140-6736(17)32399-1

Attrill, L., and Schofield, P. (2024). Perspectives on approaching pain management in patients with dementia. *Pain Management, 14*(3), 153–161. https://doi.org/10.2217/pmt-2023-0095

Banerjee, S. (2025). Systematic literature review of wandering prevention technologies for dementia care. *Journal of Technology in Human Services, 43*(3), 234–245. https://doi.org/10.1080/15228835.2025.2528781

Beason-Held, L.L., Kerley, C.I., Chaganti, S., Moghekar, A., Thambisetty, M., Ferrucci, L., et al. (2023). Health conditions associated with Alzheimer's disease and vascular dementia. *Annals of Neurology, 93*(4), 805–818. https://doi.org/10.1002/ana.26584

Brites, R., Brandão, T., Nunes, O., Hipólito, J., and Pires, C.T. (2025). The impact of caregiving on informal caregivers of people with dementia: Family functioning, burden, and burnout. *Journal of Clinical Psychology in Medical Settings, 32*(2), 325–335. https://doi.org/10.1007/s10880-024-10052-2

Camerucci, E., Mullan, A.F., Turcano, P., Stang, C.D., Bower, J., Benarroch, E.E., et al. (2024). A population-based approach to the argument on brain-first and body-first pathogenesis of Lewy body disease. *Annals of Neurology*, *96*(3), 551–559. https://doi.org/10.1002/ana.27006

Choonara, E., and Williams, J. (2021). What factors affect paramedics' involvement of people with dementia in decisions about their care? A qualitative study. *British Paramedic Journal*, *5*(4), 1–8. https://doi.org/10.29045/14784726.2021.3.5.4.1

Courtney-Pratt, H., Eccleston, C., Lucas, P., Tierney, L., Harris, W., Campbell, B., et al. (2022). Experience of paramedics providing care to people living with dementia: The working with uncertainty. *Australasian Journal of Paramedicine*, *19*, 1–6. https://doi.org/10.33151/ajp.19.929

Cullen, A., Mazhar, M.K.A., Smith, M.D., Lithander, F.E., Ó Breasail, M., and Henderson, E.J. (2022). Wearable and portable GPS solutions for monitoring mobility in dementia: A systematic review. *Sensors*, *22*(9), 3336. https://doi.org/10.3390/s22093336

Dening, T., and Babu Sandilyan, M. (2015). Dementia: Definitions and types. *Nursing Standard*, *29*(37), 37–42.

De Silva, M., Peters, A., De Waal, B., Christopher, L., and Naidoo, N. (2025). Paramedic roles, purpose, and practices when responding to older adults in abusive contexts: A systematic review. *Journal of Applied Gerontology*, *45*(1), 110–121. https://doi.org/10.1177/07334648251330347

Dunne, C.P., and Dunne, S.S. (2024). Casting light on the links between delirium, infection, and dementia risk. *The Lancet Healthy Longevity*, *5*(2), e90–e91. https://doi.org/10.1016/S2666-7568(24)00003-5

Evans, N., and Collier, L. (2019). An exploration of the experience of using calendar reminders for people with dementia and family carers. *Dementia*, *18*(5), 1912–1933. https://doi.org/10.1177/1471301217734916

Fazio, S., Stratton, L., Kline, C., and Molony, S. (2023). Providing 'just enough' support for individuals to live well with dementia. *Generations*, *47*(1), 1–12. https://generations.asaging.org/just-enough-support-live-well-dementia/

Graviotto, H.G., Sorbara, M.G., Rodriguez, C.M.T., and Serrano, C. (2022). 12-item version of Boston Naming Test: Usefulness in the diagnosis of primary progressive aphasia, frontotemporal dementia, and Alzheimer's disease. *Dementia and Neuropsychologia*, *16*(2), 181–186. https://doi.org/10.1590/1980-5764-dn-2021-0043

Han, M.X., Ross, L., Hemingway, L., Anderson, D., and Gosling, C. (2024). Out-of-hospital paramedic interactions with people living with dementia: A scoping review. *Age and Ageing*, *53*(7), afae143. https://doi.org/10.1093/ageing/afae143

Health and Care Professions Council (HCPC) (2024). *Standards of Conduct, Performance and Ethics*. London: HCPC. https://www.hcpc-uk.org/standards/standards-of-conduct-performance-and-ethics/

Hennah, M., and Miller, P.K. (2025). Early-career physiotherapists' experiences of working with people with dementia: An exploratory phenomenological study. *Physiotherapy Practice and Research*, *47*(1), 113–121. https://doi.org/10.1177/22130683251409085

Heylen, A., Vermeiren, Y., Engelborghs, S., Van Acker, F., De Deyn, P.P., and Debby, V.D. (2025). Correlation analyses between MIBG myocardial scintigraphy and monoamine levels in dementia with Lewy bodies show potential link with the serotonergic system. *Clinical Parkinsonism and Related Disorders*, *12*, 100346. https://doi.org/10.1016/j.prdoa.2025.100346

Hinsliff-Smith, K., Feakes, R., Whitworth, G., Seymour, J., Moghaddam, N., Dening, T., et al. (2017). What do we know about the application of the Mental Capacity Act (2005) in healthcare practice regarding decision-making for frail and older people? A systematic literature review. *Health and Social Care in the Community*, *25*(2), 295–308. https://doi.org/10.1111/hsc.12310

Huang, W., Zeng, R., Li, Y., Hua, Y., Liu, L., Chen, M., et al. (2025). Identification of Alzheimer's disease and vascular dementia based on a Deep Forest and near-infrared spectroscopy analysis method. *Spectrochimica Acta A: Molecular and Biomolecular Spectroscopy, 326*, 125209. https://doi.org/10.1016/j.saa.2024.125209

Jones, D., Capstick, A., Faisal, M., and Frankland, J. (2023). The impact of dementia education on student paramedics' preparedness to care, knowledge, confidence and attitudes towards dementia: An analytic survey. *British Paramedic Journal, 8*(1), 9–17. https://doi.org/10.29045/14784726.2023.6.8.1.9

King, R., Downer, T., Lord, B., Flanagan, B., and Oprescu, F. (2025). A practical example of how to apply constructivist grounded theory methodology: Exploring patient experiences during paramedic-led healthcare. *Research in Nursing and Health, 48*(4), 508–521. https://doi.org/10.1002/nur.22468

Leng, F., and Edison, P. (2021). Neuroinflammation and microglial activation in Alzheimer disease: Where do we go from here? *Nature Reviews Neurology, 17*(3), 157–172. https://doi.org/10.1038/s41582-020-00435-y

Lepping, P. (2019). Capacity issues at the front door. *British Journal of Hospital Medicine, 80*(9), 513–516. https://doi.org/10.12968/hmed.2019.80.9.513

Livingston, G.H., Huntley, J., Liu, K.Y., Costafreda, S.G., Selbæk, G., Alladi, S., et al. (2024). Dementia prevention, intervention, and care: 2024 report of the Lancet Standing Commission. *The Lancet, 404*(10452), 572–628. https://doi.org/10.1016/S0140-6736(24)01296-0

Lofthouse-Jones, C., King, P., Pocock, H., Ramsay, M., Jadzinski, P., England, E., et al. (2021). Reducing ambulance conveyance for older people with and without dementia: Evidence of the role of social care from a regional, year-long service evaluation using retrospective routine data. *British Paramedic Journal, 6*(3), 58–69. https://doi.org/10.29045/14784726.2021.12.6.3.58

Lozupone, M., Leccisotti, I., Mollica, A., Berardino, G., Moretti, M.C., Altamura, M., et al. (2026). Neuropsychiatric symptoms and apolipoprotein E genotypes in neurocognitive disorders. *Neural Regeneration Research, 21*(4), 1528–1541. https://doi.org/10.4103/NRR.NRR-D-24-01274

Mast, B.T., Ertle, E.M., Kolanowski, A., Mountain, G., Moniz-Cook, E., and Halek, M. (2022). Person-centered assessment of apathy and resistance to care in people living with dementia: Review of existing measures. *Alzheimer's and Dementia: Translational Research and Clinical Interventions, 8*(1), e12316. https://doi.org/10.1002/trc2.12316

McAtee, R., Claar, V., Spradley, L., and Thomasson, W. (2020). Elder abuse and neglect: Training first responders in rural Arkansas to recognize, respond, and report. *Innovation in Aging, 4*(suppl. 1), 46–47. https://doi.org/10.1093/geroni/igaa057.151

McCann, L. (2022). *The Paramedic at Work: A sociology of a new profession.* Oxford: Oxford University Press.

McKeith, I.G., Boeve, B.F., Dickson, D.W., Halliday, G., Taylor, J., Weintraub, D., et al. (2017). Diagnosis and management of dementia with Lewy bodies: Fourth consensus report of the DLB Consortium. *Neurology, 89*(1), 88–100. https://doi.org/10.1212/WNL.0000000000004058

McNally, S. (2025). Healthier environments and prevention can help us manage dementia better. *British Medical Journal, 389*, r1163. https://doi.org/10.1136/bmj.r1163

Medina-Rioja, R., Gonzalez-Calderon, G., and Masellis, M. (2023). Frontotemporal dementia. *Canadian Medical Association Journal, 195*(48), e1660. https://doi.org/10.1503/cmaj.230407

Mental Capacity Act 2005, c. 9. London: HMSO.

Michael, T., Chapin, L.A., and Quitoriano, C.D. (2025). Paramedicine students' experiences on placement: Preparedness for the emotional impacts of witnessing trauma. *BMC Medical Education, 25*(1), 951–913. https://doi.org/10.1186/s12909-025-07277-6

Miller, P.K., Booth, L., and Spacey, A. (2019). Dementia and clinical interaction in frontline radiography: Mapping the practical experiences of junior clinicians in the UK. *Dementia, 18*(3), 1010–1024. https://doi.org/10.1177/1471301217700742

Molony, S., Fazio, S., Barrere, C., Zimmerman, S., Sanchez, R., Montminy, J., et al. (2025). Perspectives on living well with dementia. *Journal of Applied Gerontology.* https://doi.org/10.1177/07334648251338307

Mukadam, N., Cooper, C., and Livingston, G.H. (2011). A systematic review of ethnicity and pathways to care in dementia. *International Journal of Geriatric Psychiatry, 26*(1), 12–20. https://doi.org/10.1002/gps.2484

National Institute for Health and Care Excellence (NICE) (2018) *Dementia: Assessment, management and support for people living with dementia and their carers* (NG97). London: NICE. https://www.nice.org.uk/guidance/ng97

National Institute for Health and Care Excellence (NICE) (2023). *Delirium: Prevention, diagnosis and management in hospital and long-term care* (CG103). London: NICE. https://www.nice.org.uk/Guidance/CG103

Nicholas, J., Grossman, M., McMillan, C.T., Massimo, L., Van Deerlin, V.M., Warren, J.D., et al. (2020). Age at symptom onset and death and disease duration in genetic frontotemporal dementia: An international retrospective cohort study. *The Lancet Neurology, 19*(2), 145–156. https://doi.org/10.1016/S1474-4422(19)30394-1

Nichols, E., Steinmetz, J.D., Vollset, S.E., Abd-Allah, F., Abdoli, A., Abu-Gharbieh, E., et al. (2022). Estimation of the global prevalence of dementia in 2019 and forecasted prevalence in 2050: An analysis for the Global Burden of Disease Study 2019. *The Lancet Public Health, 7*(2), e105–e125. https://doi.org/10.1016/S2468-2667(21)00249-8

Parsons, C., Escobar, C., Jasani, A., Zhao, D., Gliatto, P., Blutinger, E., et al. (2024). Community paramedicine in dementia care. *Journal of the American Geriatrics Society, 72*(7), 2167–2173. https://doi.org/10.1111/jgs.18872

Petrova, T., Orellana, C., Jelic, V., Oeksengaard, A., Snaedal, J., Hógh, P., et al. (2020). Cholinergic dysfunction, neurodegeneration, and amyloid-beta pathology in neurodegenerative diseases. *Psychiatry Research: Neuroimaging, 302*, 111099. https://doi.org/10.1016/j.pscychresns.2020.111099

Piotrowicz, K., Romanik, W., Skalska, A., Gryglewska, B., Szczerbińska, K., Derejczyk, J., et al. (2019). The comparison of the 1972 Hodkinson's Abbreviated Mental Test Score (AMTS) and its variants in screening for cognitive impairment. *Aging Clinical and Experimental Research, 31*(4), 561–566. https://doi.org/10.1007/s40520-018-1009-7

Sampson, E.L., White, N., Leurent, B., Scott, S., Lord, K., Round, J., et al. (2014). Behavioural and psychiatric symptoms in people with dementia admitted to the acute hospital: Prospective cohort study. *British Journal of Psychiatry, 205*(3), 113. https://doi.org/10.1192/bjp.bp.113.130948

Seebaluck, J., Colebatch, J.G., and Chan, B.S. (2023). Butyrophenone-induced neuroleptic malignant syndrome in Lewy body dementia: A cautionary tale. *Emergency Medicine Australasia, 35*(1), 183–184. https://doi.org/10.1111/1742-6723.14113

Spacey, A., Booth, L., Bowden, S.L.J., and Miller, P.K. (2026). Exploring diagnostic radiographers' experiences and understandings of informed consent and capacity assessment during general radiography imaging examinations of persons living with dementia: A qualitative interview study of UK practice. *Radiography, 32*(2), 103309. https://doi.org/10.1016/j.radi.2025.103309

Takeuchi, R., Toyoshima, Y., Tada, M., Tanaka, H., Shimizu, H., Shiga, A., et al. (2016). Globular glial mixed four repeat tau and TDP-43 proteinopathy with motor neuron disease and frontotemporal dementia. *Brain Pathology, 26*(1), 82–94. https://doi.org/10.1111/bpa.12262

van der Kant, R., Goldstein, L.S.B., and Ossenkoppele, R. (2020). Amyloid-β-independent regulators of tau pathology in Alzheimer disease. *Nature Reviews Neuroscience, 21*(1), 21–35. https://doi.org/10.1038/s41583-019-0240-3

Voss, S., Brandling, J., Taylor, H., Black, S., Buswell, M., Cheston, R., et al. (2018). How do people with dementia use the ambulance service? A retrospective study in England: The HOMEWARD project. *BMJ Open, 8*(7), e022549. https://doi.org/10.1136/bmjopen-2018-022549

Walker, L., Stefanis, L., and Attems, J. (2019). Clinical and neuropathological differences between Parkinson's disease, Parkinson's disease dementia and dementia with Lewy bodies – current issues and future directions. *Journal of Neurochemistry, 150*(5), 467–474. https://doi.org/10.1111/jnc.14698

World Health Organization (WHO) (2022). *International Statistical Classification of Diseases and Related Health Problems*, 11th revision (ICD-11). Geneva: WHO. https://icd.who.int/en/

Yang, X., Chen, C., Wang, A., Li, C., and Cheng, G. (2023). Imaging, genetic, and pathological features of vascular dementia. *European Neurology, 86*(4), 277–284. https://doi.org/10.1159/000531088

4 Mental health and long-term conditions: Chronic illness, complexity, and social isolation

Emily Holland, Gemma Goadsby, Yuet Wah Patrick, and Jo Augustus

Introduction

Long-term conditions are illnesses that last a year or more and affect multiple aspects of a person's life (NICE, 2023; NHS England, 2019). They are usually incurable and require ongoing symptom management. Such conditions include non-communicable diseases (e.g. diabetes and cancer), long-duration communicable diseases (e.g. HIV), and long-term mental health conditions, particularly severe and enduring mental illnesses.

With rising prevalence and an ageing population, multimorbidity has become a major healthcare challenge (Academy of Medical Sciences, 2018; Ho et al., 2022; NIHR, 2021). People with multiple long-term conditions experience poorer outcomes across all measures. Outcomes worsen further when mental and physical health conditions co-exist (Naylor et al., 2012; Firth et al., 2019; NHS England, 2024b). This is especially evident in people with a severe and enduring mental illness, for whom life expectancy is 15–20 years less than the general population due to preventable physical diseases and difficulties accessing high-quality health care (Firth et al., 2019; NHS England, 2024b).

Mental health can impact physical health and vice versa. People with long-term conditions experience higher rates of anxiety, depression, stress, and PTSD (Naylor et al., 2012), often linked to the burden of self-management, uncertainty, and social isolation. Conversely, those with mental health conditions may struggle to maintain physical health due to social inequalities and reduced capacity for health-promoting behaviours.

Paramedics are frequently called to the aid of people with a long-term condition. A holistic understanding of how long-term illness affects psychological wellbeing, daily functioning, and social circumstances will help paramedics tailor their approach. It is important to acknowledge that patients managing a long-term condition are usually experts in their own experience. Because people with multimorbidity often present with overlapping issues, paramedics' skills in rapid differentiation and whole-person assessment are particularly valuable.

This chapter explores common long-term conditions encountered in pre-hospital care, their psychological impacts, clinical presentation, assessment approaches, and best practices for paramedic management.

Common long-term conditions encountered in pre-hospital care

Diabetes mellitus

Diabetes mellitus is a condition that causes dysregulation of blood sugar levels. This can be due to a lack of insulin production in the body (Type 1) or a resistance to insulin that develops over time (Type 2). In the UK, it is estimated that approximately 5.8 million people have diabetes, accounting for estimated undiagnosed cases, and this number is rising (NHS England, 2024a).

Diabetes requires complex management that is demanding and pervasive across all aspects of an individual's life. Some people with Type 2 diabetes do not need to monitor their blood glucose levels on a daily basis. Others, however, and all people with Type 1 diabetes, do need to monitor their blood glucose levels on a daily basis, which involves either regular finger-prick blood testing or the wearing of a continuous glucose monitoring device. Management can involve taking daily oral medications, regular insulin injections, or using a pump. Fear of hypoglycaemic episodes is also common. Diet and lifestyle choices impact on blood glucose management, requiring adequate education and understanding, as well as discipline to adhere to recommendations. There are constant calculations, risk assessments, and problem-solving that the individual or their carers need to manage on a day-to-day basis. This places a significant mental burden on those living with the condition, which can negatively impact their mental wellbeing. This is sometimes referred to as 'diabetes distress', where the emotional burden of self-management becomes overwhelming (Dennick et al., 2017; Fisher et al., 2010; Poole and Hackett, 2024).

The mental health conditions that are common amongst people with diabetes include depression (two to three times more likely than the general population), anxiety, and disordered eating behaviours such as binge eating and insulin restriction/omission (Farooqi et al., 2019; Horsbøl et al., 2024; Grigsby et al., 2002). These are associated with poor management, disengagement from services, increased risk of diabetes distress, increased risk of complications, and impaired quality of life.

Chronic respiratory diseases

Chronic respiratory diseases include conditions such as chronic obstructive pulmonary disease (COPD) and asthma. COPD is an umbrella term for progressive, largely irreversible, lung conditions that can limit daily function. COPD mainly affects middle-aged or older adults who smoke, or who have been exposed to environmental irritants. Asthma is usually diagnosed in childhood but can develop at any age. Both conditions are characterised by difficulty breathing (dyspnoea) (Hinson-Enslin et al., 2025; Yohannes and Alexopoulos, 2014).

The relationship between chronic respiratory disease and mental health is multifaceted. Dyspnoea can have significant psychological impact, such as anxiety around feeling unable to breathe or fear of another exacerbation. This can manifest in avoidance behaviours and hypervigilance to try and avert another acute episode, or denial around the severity of symptoms and not seeking medical assistance. Acute episodes can also be a source of trauma, particularly if this has led to time in intensive care. The symptoms can impact on daily functions as well and limit the person's ability to do what they used to do. This decrease in independence can lead to feeling out of control, becoming socially isolated, and decreased mood overall.

The link between respiratory disease and mental health is also seen in the increased prevalence of respiratory disease amongst people with a severe and enduring mental illness (SMI). The prevalence of smoking amongst people with SMI is higher than in the general population, attributed to a range of factors such as self-medicating, increased exposure through social circles, and cessation programmes not being accessible to this population (Royal College of Physicians, 2018; NHS England, 2024b). People with SMI also tend to be more socially disadvantaged and can be affected by environmental factors such as poor housing, high levels of pollution in their neighbourhood, and occupational hazards.

Cardiovascular diseases

Cardiovascular diseases (CVD) are a group of disorders of the heart and blood vessels. These include coronary heart disease (angina, myocardial infarction, heart failure), cerebrovascular disease (stroke and transient ischaemic attacks), peripheral artery disease, and aortic atherosclerosis (including aneurysms). The causes of these conditions usually stem from atherosclerosis (the build-up of plaque on arterial walls), which narrows the arteries and increases the risk of an embolism forming.

Lifestyle factors are a major contributor to CVD. Smoking, poor diet, drug and alcohol misuse, and a sedentary lifestyle all predispose to the development of CVD. Mental health conditions, particularly depression, anxiety, and post-traumatic stress disorder (PTSD), are also recognised as an independent risk factor for developing CVD (Coughlin, 2011; Gilsanz et al., 2017). Someone with depression, for example, may be more inclined to make poor lifestyle choices as a result of their symptoms. Low energy and poor self-esteem can also reduce an individual's motivation to engage in health improvement behaviours. However, it is acknowledged that there is a more complex, interrelated connection between mental health and cardiovascular health. Medication used when treating SMI has side effects that are risk factors for developing CVD, such as weight gain and arrhythmias. Major adverse cardiac events, such as a myocardial infarction, can trigger onset of PTSD or worsen pre-existing mental health conditions. Mental health conditions can also result in pathophysiological changes. PTSD impacts on nervous system activity, which can lead to blood pressure dysregulation. Hormone dysregulation, such as prolonged release of cortisol, and elevated inflammation markers have also been associated with mental health conditions, both of which can accelerate the progression of CVD (Civieri et al., 2024).

Cerebrovascular disease impacts in other ways on mental health, including emotional dysregulation and an increase in depression and anxiety after stroke. This has been linked to the pathology of stroke causing physical damage to the regions of the brain responsible for mood and emotion but can also be due to identity change that may occur. Depending on the severity of the stroke, the individual may have a sudden change in support needs and communication abilities, which can be isolating and frustrating.

Neurological conditions

Neurological conditions encompass disorders of the brain, spinal cord, and nerves. The most common conditions are Parkinson's disease, multiple sclerosis, and epilepsy. These can be acquired through injury or infection, or passed on genetically. Most often, they are degenerative and gradually progressive, although some are intermittent and unpredictable such as epilepsy.

Given that neurological conditions affect the brain and nerves, they can affect a range of different bodily functions and impact how an individual engages with the world. Symptoms are classified as motor, sensory, cognitive, or communicative in nature. Motor symptoms impact movement, balance, and coordination, or can cause a loss of function altogether. Sensory symptoms include numbness, tingling, and pain. Cognitive changes may impact memory, personality, and mood, or cause confusion. Communicative symptoms negatively affect speech and word-finding abilities. Other symptoms include fatigue, dizziness, and visual or hearing deficits. Even amongst individuals who have the same condition, not only will the severity of their symptoms differ but also which aspects of their functioning are most impacted. Due to the complexity of these disorders, multidisciplinary input is imperative but can be difficult to coordinate (Brauckmann et al., 2024; Wang et al., 2018; Jones et al., 2008; Firth et al., 2019).

Autoimmune and inflammatory conditions

Autoimmune and inflammatory conditions, such as lupus and rheumatoid arthritis, result from the immune system's abnormal response. When the immune system recognises a foreign substance, immune cells and signalling molecules trigger an inflammatory response, allowing immune cells to travel through the bloodstream to the affected area and eliminate the threat. In inflammatory conditions, this is usually an overreaction of inflammation in response to non-harmful stimuli such as the body's own cells. Autoimmunity is a process in which the immune system begins to fight the body's own cells, such as with rheumatoid arthritis and lupus.

Autoimmune and inflammatory conditions are often systemic. Common features of most of these conditions include pain, fatigue, and malaise. Whilst different conditions have unique features, their symptoms are non-specific. There are often diagnostic delays in identifying and treating these conditions. Sometimes, diagnosis is conducted via a process of exclusion, which can require many tests and be frustrating for the individual (Squance et al., 2014; McWilliams et al., 2019; Harwood et al., 2025).

Chronic kidney disease and dialysis patients

Chronic kidney disease (CKD) is a progressive condition where there is a decline in kidney function, thus impairing the body's ability to filter waste and regulate fluid and electrolytes. It is a common condition, with prevalence increasing with age. Severity ranges from no symptoms in the early stages to requiring renal replacement therapy, such as dialysis or transplants, in the later stages. Dialysis, typically undertaken several times per week, is life-sustaining but requires a significant time commitment.

Amongst people with CKD, the rates of depression and anxiety are higher than in the general population (Kommer et al., 2025). As with the previous conditions discussed, the relationship between kidney disease and mental health is bidirectional. Depression and anxiety can reduce adherence to dialysis schedules, medication, and dietary guidelines, which can subsequently increase the risk of complications and accelerate disease progression. In people requiring dialysis, the frequent hospital visits, invasive procedures, and fear of complications can have a toll on mental health. Dialysis can also have a financial and social impact, with difficulties working and engaging with social life.

Cancer and palliative care considerations

Cancer encompasses a group of diseases characterised by uncontrolled cell growth, often requiring complex treatments such as surgery, chemotherapy, and radiotherapy. These interventions can be physically taxing and emotionally overwhelming. A cancer diagnosis is a profound psychological stressor. Depression and anxiety are highly prevalent in this population, and individuals often experience loneliness, guilt, and existential concerns (Grassi et al., 2023; Ikhile et al., 2024; Mitchell et al., 2013). Treatment burden is also significant, with the side effects of treatment including fatigue, pain, and cognitive changes. Poor mental health can negatively affect cancer prognosis by reducing adherence to treatment and impairing immune function (Paslaru et al., 2025).

Clinical presentation and pre-hospital assessment

Individuals living with a long-term condition often present with complex care needs that extend beyond the assessment of a single disease process. Historically, health was viewed as the absence of disease; however, a complex interplay exists between the biological, psychological, and social factors that shape health outcomes: the biological condition (long-term condition) exists within the individual's social context and shapes psychological experiences, all of which significantly affect health behaviours and outcomes. Understanding this complexity and far-reaching impact of long-term conditions enables paramedics to carry out comprehensive assessments and tailored care based on an individual's circumstances.

Several theoretical frameworks and models exist to support the assessment of people living with long-term conditions, and which can be applied in the pre-hospital environment. For reasons of brevity, only a few are mentioned here. The bio-psycho-social model (Engel, 1977) recognises the complex nature of assessment, supporting paramedics to explore all the domains that impact health and wellbeing. Signs and symptoms are not assessed in isolation – they are considered in the broader context of the patients' unique circumstances. Enquiring about the patient's ideas, concerns, and expectations (ICE) offers insight into their individual experiences and hopes.

The chronic care model (Wagner, 1998) can also be applied outside traditional healthcare settings, helping empower individuals with long-term conditions. It provides a framework for proactive person-centred assessment and management, identifying the elements required for high-quality care of long-term conditions: the community, the health system, self-management support, delivery system design, decision support, and clinical information. In 2003, the model was expanded to include population health promotion components, accounting for the complexity of long-term conditions, recognising social determinants and inequities as crucial factors in health outcomes. Viewing pre-hospital assessment through the lens of these models encourages paramedics to consider not only an acute presentation but also the complex interplay between chronic disease and the social and the psychological systems.

It is important to recognise that patients may have had different experiences throughout their healthcare journey. Diagnostic overshadowing, originally linked to intellectual disability, is gaining recognition in the context of physical long-term conditions, particularly those with complex care needs (Jones et al., 2008; Hallyburton, 2022). It occurs when new symptoms are misattributed to an existing diagnosis, 'overshadowing' consideration of exacerbations or new conditions, potentially delaying diagnosis or treatment.

The risk of diagnostic overshadowing further increases when a patient has multiple long-term conditions owing to the complexity involved. Though outside the scope of this chapter, it is thought-provoking to note that diagnostic overshadowing is linked to diagnostic delay for some long-term conditions, due to the complex overlap of symptoms that are commonly seen in other conditions. For example, fatigue and joint pain may be attributed to depression, rather than originating from the autoimmune disease systemic lupus erythematosus (SLE). Harwood et al. (2025) reported the average diagnostic delay for SLE to be 7.5 years, but it could be up to 40 years. The overlap of symptoms and variation from patient to patient can make it easy to err towards a more comfortable and better understood condition, with devastating consequences for the patient's physical and mental health.

Bias in pre-hospital assessment can lead to substandard care and the erosion of trust, with individuals left feeling frustrated or dismissed if their concerns are misattributed without comprehensive assessment. Such experiences can contribute to disengagement from services and the development of negative health behaviours. This could be perceived as an individual being 'non-compliant', but with empathy and understanding, paramedics can explore the influencing factors within the bio-psycho-social model, such as practical barriers, fear, or mistrust. Goode et al. (2022) note how previous adverse experiences significantly influence the way older adults make decisions on current and future care needs.

Experiences of diagnostic overshadowing can themselves be traumatic. Trauma-informed care, first described in mental health services by Harris and Fallot (2001), recognises this impact, aiming to understand and mitigate negative health consequences based on six guiding principles: safety, trust, choice, collaboration, empowerment, and cultural consideration. Trauma-informed care requires a cultural shift that recognises the sensitive nature of mental health problems, viewing social or behavioural issues as potential indicators of trauma. Trauma-informed care is *not* treatment of trauma. Instead, it encourages patients to safely express their feelings and experiences by asking, 'What happened to you?' instead of 'What is wrong with you?' (Berring et al., 2024). Integrating trauma-informed care into pre-hospital assessment helps paramedics to recognise how trauma interacts with physical, psychological, and social factors to influence health outcomes.

Recognising the multifaceted complexity and influences of long-term conditions in pre-hospital assessment can be profoundly meaningful for patients, enabling psychological safety and trust. The person-centred approach encourages patients to be active participants in their care, rather than passive recipients of it (Brown et al., 2022; Wagner, 1998).

Exacerbation, vital signs, and monitoring

The nature of long-term conditions means that patients may experience symptoms that fluctuate in severity or overlap with those of new conditions, which can complicate pre-hospital assessment. Some abnormalities may reflect the patient's documented 'normal' parameters, while others may indicate short- or long-term complications such as a change in the long-term condition requiring intervention, or a new pathology unrelated to the long-term condition.

Metacognition, or thinking about thinking, is useful to mitigate the cognitive pitfall of diagnostic overshadowing. With clinical curiosity, paramedics can consider if the presentation represents a known fluctuation in the individual's long-term condition, an exacerbation or relapse requiring management, or something new. Incorporating the patient's lived experiences and awareness of condition-specific markers of complication can guide recognition. There are often overlapping symptoms such as pain and reduced mobility across long-term conditions, but each one has specific markers and symptoms associated with it. A vast array of condition-specific markers is shown in Table 4.1. This list is far from exhaustive and is designed to encourage further reading on the concepts listed.

As discussed earlier, some abnormalities may be known and documented; physiological parameters may differ from typical clinical ranges yet still be normal for the patient. To differentiate chronic from acute abnormalities, vital signs and symptoms need to be interpreted in the context of the patient's condition and baseline, using trend recognition to identify any deviation. A common example is a patient living with chronic Type 2 respiratory failure – their baseline peripheral oxygen saturation (SpO_2) may be 88–92% in the context of chronic hypoxaemia. This differs from the values expected in patients without the condition, yet unnecessary oxygen administration can cause worsening hypercapnia. The NEWS2 score is used to identify clinical deterioration in patients with acute illness. It contains a second SpO_2 scale to reflect the baseline deviation for patients with documented hypercapnic respiratory failure, allowing the physiological abnormality to be interpreted in the context of the patient's condition. Patients who live with other long-term conditions are not always accounted for in the same way, requiring paramedics to compare the findings with documented baseline values to ensure a safe assessment that does not over-diagnose or, more importantly, under-diagnose a patient's presentation.

These overarching principles also apply to patients presenting with mental health conditions. A common misconception is that vital signs are unnecessary in these patients. As social determinants and psychosocial factors can significantly influence health behaviours, pre-hospital assessment may be the only opportunity to monitor physical health. It is an opportunity to identify underlying organic causes, reveal potential unknown comorbidities, or declining health, serving as a platform for health promotion.

Functional status and disability assessment

Functional independence is the ability to safely and autonomously carry out activities of daily living (ADLs) and instrumental activities of daily living (IADLs). The potential for shifting baselines in some long-term conditions highlights the dynamic nature of functional independence, where observations during assessment only represent that moment in time. An acute event can significantly limit the degree of functional independence. Equally, an individual may have relatively good function one day but experience a decline the next

Table 4.1: Specific markers of long-term conditions

Long-term condition	Preferred term	Condition-specific markers (***exemplary, not exhaustive***)
Diabetes mellitus (Type 1 and Type 2)	Exacerbation	Hypoglycaemia, hyperosmolar hyperglycaemic state, diabetic ketoacidosis (Poole and Hackett, 2024)
Chronic respiratory diseases (COPD, asthma)	Exacerbation	Increased work of breathing, adventitious lung sounds, altered mental status, hypoxia, fatigue, sputum changes, right-sided heart failure, hypercapnia, inability to complete sentences, sputum changes (Sneath et al., 2019)
Cardiovascular diseases (heart failure, hypertension)	Exacerbation	*Heart failure*: respiratory distress, peripheral and pulmonary oedema, tachycardia, arrythmia, fatigue, weakness, hypotension (Bounds et al., 2024) *Hypertensive emergency*: altered mental state, seizures, visual disturbances, stroke, aortic dissection, haematuria, acute coronary syndrome (Alhasan and Yaseen, 2021)
Neurological conditions (Parkinson's, multiple sclerosis, epilepsy)	Relapse (multiple sclerosis, epilepsy) Exacerbation (Parkinson's)	*Parkinson's*: akinesia, delirium, hypotension, infection, aspiration pneumonia *Multiple sclerosis*: dysphagia, respiratory failure, heat sensitivity, severe fatigue, weakness (Wang et al., 2018) *Epilepsy*: status epilepticus, injury, postictal state (Brauckmann et al., 2024)
Mental health disorders (schizophrenia, bipolar disorder)	Relapse	Neuroleptic malignant syndrome, suicidality, serotonin syndrome, acute psychosis, self-neglect, catatonia, acute behavioural disturbance (Briggs et al., 2024)

(*continued*)

Table 4.1: *(continued)*

Long-term condition	**Preferred term**	**Condition-specific markers (*exemplary, not exhaustive*)**
Autoimmune and inflammatory diseases (lupus, rheumatoid arthritis)	Exacerbation or Flare	*Lupus*: Butterfly rash, neuropsychiatric symptoms, lupus nephritis, thrombosis, sepsis (Squance et al., 2014) *Rheumatoid arthritis*: extreme pain, swelling, stiffness in multiple joints, sepsis, rapid weight loss, fever, night sweats, atlantoaxial subluxation (McWilliams et al., 2019)
Chronic kidney disease and dialysis patients	Exacerbation (acute-on-chronic kidney disease)	Dialysis disequilibrium syndrome, access site complications, hypotension, air embolism, hyperkalaemia, uraemic encephalopathy, pulmonary oedema (Lau et al., 2024)
Cancer and palliative care considerations	Relapse used when cancer returns after remission; progression if disease continues to worsen; oncological emergency	*Neurological emergencies*: increased intracranial pressure, spinal cord compression *Metabolic and endocrine emergencies*: tumour lysis syndrome, hyponatraemia, syndrome of inappropriate antidiuretic hormone secretion (SIADH), hypercalcaemia, hypomagnesaemia, adrenal insufficiency *Vascular emergency*: superior vena cava obstruction *Infectious emergency*: neutropenic sepsis or fever (Gri et al., 2023)

Table 4.2: Functional independence

ADLs/IADLs	Examples	Relevance
ADLs: Basic self-care tasks	Bathing, dressing, feeding oneself, toileting, grooming, mobility, transferring	These are fundamental to independent living. Altered capability indicates more severe functional decline
IADLs: More complex, independent living tasks	Using communication devices and technology, preparing meals, managing finances, taking medications, doing laundry and housework, shopping, managing transportation	These reflect the higher-level functioning required for independent living, with changes in ability often the first sign of functional decline

due day to fluctuations in the symptoms experienced. For an accurate picture, an individual's baseline is compared to their current ability, exploring recent changes (Table 4.2).

As with other elements of pre-hospital assessment, the patient's functional status extends beyond the physical challenges of a condition; it is significantly influenced by social determinants and psychosocial factors, with depression noted to be the strongest determinant of function in older adults (Goodarzi et al., 2024; NICE, 2022). The context-specific nature of the patient must be considered to ensure management plans are accessible and tailored to the individual; patients may experience increased levels of independence in their adapted home but encounter considerable difficulty in other environments.

A loss of independence can lead to feelings of decreased autonomy and control, with feelings of psychological burden becoming heightened if reliance on others subsequently increases. A negative feedback loop may develop, where declining functional independence exacerbates mental health challenges, which then further reduces functional independence.

Living with a long-term condition or experiencing limitations with ADLs and IADLs does not necessarily constitute frailty. However, a two-way relationship exists with ADLs being predictors of IADLs and vice versa. Frailty, defined as decreased physiological reserves, which increases an individual's vulnerability to health stressors, is typically assessed in older adults. Several tools exist to measure frailty in this population, including the Clinical Frailty Scale (Rockwood, 2005), which is recommended for use in individuals aged 65 and over. Nonetheless, frailty can occur in younger populations, manifesting in different ways across the life course. There is a lack of clarity surrounding the validity and impact of frailty measures across age groups; indeed, Spiers et al. (2021) highlight the need for further research to address this gap.

Paramedics can discuss the underlying drivers of health with patients, incorporating their support network of family, friends, and caregivers where appropriate. A conversation can be the first step in highlighting the many factors that can influence functional independence, building an insightful picture incorporating patients' lived experiences and the paramedic's environmental observations. Health promotion and education promote self-management where appropriate, validating experiences and encouraging individuals to be active participants in their care.

Medication review and compliance issues

It is likely that patients living with a long-term condition will be prescribed medications for management of the condition. Regular medication reviews are key to optimising their use, thus reducing adverse events which could be challenging to identify in complex conditions.

Compliance is multifactorial – non-adherence may be intentional or unintentional. Treatment regimens can be complex and overwhelming, compounded by the physical symptoms of some conditions which challenge cognition or dexterity, for example, leading to unintentional non-adherence. Some medications also have a direct impact on functional independence. It is beyond the scope of this chapter to discuss all medication interactions, but an example is antipsychotic medications prescribed for schizophrenia. Antipsychotics can have significant, yet common extrapyramidal side effects, causing involuntary, drug-induced movement disorders (Table 4.3). Extrapyramidal side effects directly impact an individual's quality of life and functional independence, affecting social function, communication, and movement. This can cause negative treatment responses from patients leading to treatment failure.

Reeve et al. (2022) report that many people taking five or more medicines per day (polypharmacy) feel overburdened by their treatment. Additionally, polypharmacy increases the risk of prescribing cascades. This occurs when a

Table 4.3: Summary of common extrapyramidal side effects

Extrapyramidal side effects	Description
Acute dystonia	*Hypokinetic*: Involuntary muscle contractions that may affect any skeletal muscle. Leads to abnormal postures or repetitive movements which may be painful
Parkinsonism	*Hypokinetic*: Slowed motor functions (bradykinesia), cogwheel rigidity, and resting tremor. Characteristics include a slow shuffling gait and imbalance, stooped posture, and reduced facial expression
Akathisia	*Hyperkinetic*: A feeling of restlessness with a strong, uncontrollable need to move
Tardive dyskinesia	*Hyperkinetic*: Involuntary, jerky, and twisting movements that mainly involve the face and tongue but may also spread to the trunk and limbs

side effect from a medication is mistaken for a new medical condition, resulting in the potentially unnecessary prescribing of another medication. Paramedics can encourage individuals to undertake a medication review in primary care, leading to the safe reduction, replacement, or de-prescription of medications that are either no longer effective or causing harm. Engaging patients and caregivers in educational conversations can empower them to instigate and have meaningful discussions with the appropriate healthcare professionals.

Presentation and assessment: Summary

Individuals living with a long-term condition usually have to navigate complex and fluctuating health experiences; however, with the appropriate support, many maintain a good quality of life. For paramedics, recognising the interplay between physical, psychological, and social factors is fundamental to delivering holistic, person-centred care. A comprehensive and empathetic assessment encourages paramedics to see the person beyond the illness, allowing the person to feel heard and supported.

Case study: Chronic illness and social isolation

Case study: Narrative

A paramedic working alone on a rapid response vehicle attends a welfare concern for a 34-year-old woman, Amara. A friend has raised concerns after being unable to contact her and receiving no response at Amara's home address. The friend reports that Amara has missed several medical appointments recently and has appeared increasingly withdrawn and low in mood. She describes Amara's health as 'varying from day to day', but notes that in recent weeks Amara has required more support with everyday tasks due to increased brain fog, fatigue, and joint pain.

Amara has a diagnosis of systemic lupus erythematosus (SLE) and experiences fluctuating symptoms that include fatigue, joint and muscle pain, photosensitivity, shortness of breath, brain fog, anxiety, and depression. She is prescribed hydroxychloroquine and has recently started prednisolone. She reports adherence to her medication regimen but struggles to remember doses without prompting. Her depression is currently managed through active monitoring.

Amara lives alone in a ground-floor flat that has been adapted to meet her needs. She is the only member of her family living in the UK and has a limited social network. She finds it difficult to maintain friendships because she often has to cancel plans due to unpredictable lupus flares. Her friend provides informal caregiving support, although both find this challenging because Amara's needs fluctuate and a fixed schedule of support is not always effective. Amara previously worked part-time as a shop assistant but has been unable to sustain employment due to the unpredictability of her lupus flares, which makes planning and maintaining work responsibilities difficult.

Amara smokes five cigarettes a day and does not drink alcohol. When her health permits, she enjoys creating crafts at home, which supports her well-being; however, she has been unable to do so recently due to a combination of apathy, fatigue, and joint pain. When asked about the loss of interest in a previously enjoyed activity, Amara explains that not being able to work has affected her sense of identity and increased her stress levels, which she believes have exacerbated her physical symptoms. She also describes noticing signs of burnout in her caregiver due to increased reliance on her friend. Amara states, 'I often feel like a burden, so I have shut myself away.' She acknowledges feeling more depressed recently and demonstrates rumination, repeatedly questioning, 'Why did this happen to me?'

To monitor the severity of depressive symptoms, the paramedic completes a PHQ-9 assessment with Amara. Amara scores 10, indicating moderate depression.

During the consultation, Amara gestures to unopened hospital letters on a nearby surface and explains that she has missed several appointments and does not intend to attend further because she no longer trusts healthcare professionals. She describes feeling overwhelmed by the volume of appointments and reports difficulty concentrating and retaining information due to brain fog. She states that she often feels unheard during consultations and that her experiences are dismissed as 'just part of your lupus diagnosis', without further follow-up. Amara expresses significant frustration, explaining that it took years to obtain an SLE diagnosis after periods of misdiagnosis and being told she had 'health anxiety'. She now feels that her concerns are routinely attributed to lupus without thorough investigation. She also reports feeling rushed during appointments after overcoming practical barriers to attend, with limited opportunity to process information or ask questions. Over time, these experiences have intensified her distress and contributed to increasing withdrawal, social isolation, and disengagement from care.

Amara apologises for requiring an ambulance response and states that she feels misunderstood in relation to her long-term condition, and feels alone and unsupported.

Primary survey

No abnormalities identified. All vital signs within range. Review of systems reveals no deviation from Amara's baseline.

Capacity assessment

Based on the Mental Capacity Act 2005, it is recognised that Amara's emotional state, fatigue, and pain levels may influence the ability to complete some elements of CURE; however, she is assessed to have capacity.

Critical questions

- What are the implications of not comprehensively exploring Amara's presentation, when the symptoms are consistent with those she experiences from lupus?

Table 4.4: Focused mental health assessment (MSE-informed)

Appearance and behaviour	Unkempt, wearing loungewear. Appears subdued but is making appropriate eye contact as rapport builds. Movements are consistent with pain
Speech	Coherent but reduced rate of speech. No slurring. Appropriate responses followed by long pauses
Mood and affect	Reports feeling extremely tired. Still has the motivation to engage but feels people have a lack of understanding of her condition due to its fluctuating nature, so finds it easier to socially isolate. This aligns with the observed mood, flat but reactive to conversation
Thought process and content	Denies suicidal ideation or intent. Expresses guilt about being a burden to her friend. Feels dismissed by healthcare professionals and overwhelmed by the task of remembering and keeping up with appointments
Perception	No perceptual disturbances observed or reported
Cognition and insight	Orientated to person, place, and time. Reports frequent brain fog and forgetfulness, particularly when fatigued but does demonstrate insight of the situation. Able to acknowledge independently that she has withdrawn from care and support due to feeling dismissed and overwhelmed

Table 4.5: Functional assessment

ADLs/IADLs	Assessment
ADLs: Basic self-care tasks	Able to manage ADLs independently in adapted home, though it can take a significant amount of time on days with increased symptoms, such as fatigue and joint pain. Requires support with ADLs in unfamiliar environments
IADLs: More complex, independent living tasks	Difficulty managing IADLs consistently due to fluctuating nature of her condition. Often requires support from caregiver

- What factors are contributing to a negative feedback loop?
- How can the paramedic contribute to improving Amara's health, wellbeing, and engagement with services?

Key learning points from Amara's case

- Long-term conditions like lupus can fluctuate, with symptoms overlapping those of mental health problems.
- Past negative healthcare experiences can damage trust and reduce engagement with services.
- Trauma-informed care helps patients feel safe, heard, and respected.
- Diagnostic overshadowing can occur when all symptoms are attributed to a known diagnosis.
- Depression may arise from the condition itself, the emotional impact of living with it, or the side effects of her medication.
- Psychosocial stressors can create a negative feedback loop that worsens physical and mental health.
- A bio-psycho-social approach supports holistic assessment and person-centred care.

Table 4.6: Examples of potential interventions for Amara

Referrals + Interventions (*exemplary, not exhaustive*)	**Rationale**
Primary care review	*Medication review*: Potential antidepressant therapy and possible adverse effect from steroids. Review and follow-up of depression and lupus management. Possible antidepressant therapy
Cognitive behavioural therapy (CBT)	*Online CBT*: The online nature increases accessibility, covering processes including avoidance, rumination, and interpersonal difficulties
Social prescribing	Connect to a link worker, providing support that includes: • personalised care and support planning with shared decision-making • connect to community groups to reduce isolation and increase support networks • supported self-management • aid attendance at medical appointments • support to navigate the referrals that have been made

(*continued*)

Table 4.6: *(continued)*

Referrals + Interventions (*exemplary, not exhaustive*)	Rationale
Carer support	With consent, the informal caregiver can be signposted to local support services
Social care needs assessment	A formal review of care needs
Specialist lupus nurse	Provides support to people with lupus and their families
Health promotion	Make every contact count approach: • supporting Amara to recognise triggers, manage stress, smoking cessation, and coping strategies • encourages sustainable behaviour changes that improve overall wellbeing
Health education	Providing information and increasing understanding about health, illness, and behaviours, supporting informed decisions. For example, understanding lupus, the relationship between steroids and depression, and how wider factors affect physical health

Best practices for paramedics in managing long-term conditions

Effective communication with patients and caregivers

Whilst paramedics may encounter the same individual repeatedly, they are unlikely to know the full journey the person has been on regarding their experience with their long-term condition. People with a long-term condition live with it on a daily basis and are the experts in their own experience. To harness this expertise, listening should be the paramedic's main priority. This is the first step in adopting a person-centred approach.

Taking a structured approach to history-taking and asking open questions allow paramedics to start 'data gathering'. Whilst paramedics will often be attending for a physical concern, it is important to be professionally curious about the other aspects of the person's life by incorporating questions about their psychological and social wellbeing. Whilst the individual may not think this is relevant to their assessment, it can be useful information when adapting management plans to their specific needs.

Another aspect of communication that should be considered is how paramedics deliver education and advice. Individuals with a long-term condition may be well versed in their condition but will perhaps not be able to retain information provided to them when they are unwell. Health literacy should also be considered. Providing written advice can be useful for patients to refer to if they forget what was said. Setting clear worsening care advice with time frames and expectations can also help with building confidence in self-management and avoiding re-contact.

Recognising and managing acute exacerbations of chronic illnesses

Chronic illnesses do not follow a clear and predictable path and progression is often non-linear and can fluctuate. How these developments present will be unique to each person and rely on recognising changes from the individual's baseline. Establishing a baseline of the patient's experiences can support recognition of an exacerbation of a chronic illness. For example, an individual with rheumatoid arthritis may live with significant levels pain each day; however, today it is unmanageable and is seriously affecting their ability to function.

A phenomenon all clinicians must consider during assessment is diagnostic overshadowing, the attribution of a person's symptoms to their existing mental health condition. This can overlook underlying medical causes, potentially causing a delayed or missed diagnosis and negative health outcomes. Difficult communication (the 'poor historian') can also further exacerbate this issue, together with impaired insight into recognising and interpreting their own physical symptoms (Squance et al., 2014; Harwood et al., 2025; Lupus UK, 2025).

Viewed through a bio-psycho-social lens, paramedics should start with managing the physical manifestations of the disease. Then, paramedics should consider psychological and social support for the patient. Social support can also have positive protective effects on an individual with mental health concerns secondary to chronic health conditions.

Enhancing patient education and self-management support

Starting with prevention, addressing lifestyle risk factors such as smoking, physical activity, and diet can be a way to empower individuals. Supporting patients to recognise the benefits that small changes can make can help improve their physical health as well as boost their self-esteem through achieving small goals. Goal-setting is recognised as a beneficial way of enhancing a feeling of control over one's situation. Long-term conditions can feel overwhelming and never-ending, so supporting patients to gain clarity on a challenge can help them to move towards an action- and solution-focused mindset. Most importantly, this allows for recognition of success when goals are achieved as little wins that combine to achieve greater change.

For some, the only encounter with emergency services they have may be with the paramedics. When attending someone for mental health support, whilst it may not be clinically relevant to their current presentation, taking their blood pressure, checking their blood sugars, or asking a brief health history may identify early signs of treatable long-term conditions such as hypertension or diabetes. If this is accompanied with brief advice about what these conditions are and how they can be managed, this may help improve long-term outcomes for this patient group.

Multi-agency collaboration (GPs, community nurses, social services)

Managing long-term conditions requires a 'whole team approach', drawing on the expertise of a variety of disciplines. An individual with a long-term condition will likely already be receiving care from GPs in primary care, specialists, community nurses, pharmacists, and mental health professionals. Each will have a role in managing the care of various aspects of a condition. Together, they can combine to care holistically for the individual and understand the impact the condition may have on various aspects of living. Studies have shown that multidisciplinary team working in the care of chronic conditions improves overall patient satisfaction, knowledge, and health behaviours (Shi et al., 2025).

Multidisciplinary team working can also improve staff job satisfaction through enhanced skill development, knowledge-building, and greater autonomy. However, multi-agency collaboration is not without its challenges. Role definition and understanding are important to establish, both for the benefit of staff and for patients. Clearly defined roles enhance coordination of care and improve accountability and autonomy.

Ethical considerations: Patient autonomy

The patient-led approach may seem counterintuitive. However, a clinician-centred approach can create a divide between patient and clinician and can result in a paternalistic approach. The paternalistic model of health care creates a dynamic where the clinician tells the patient what to do, and the 'good patient' complies with the advice, whereas the 'difficult patient' is non-compliant. In this model, the clinician is the expert, whose authority must be adhered to. Whilst this expert advice may follow the ethical principles of beneficence and non-maleficence, with the clinician aiming to do what is best for the patient, this can be at the cost of patient autonomy. The inherent power dynamic that can occur with this approach may result in the patient's wishes being overridden or the full understanding of what would be in their best interests not being considered.

Prioritising patient autonomy in the management of long-term conditions is essential to maintaining a person-centred approach. Paramedics can achieve this by centring all decision-making on the patient and considering their wishes, concerns, and preferences. Explaining your rationale for your differentials and management plan can encourage questions from the patient and improves their overall knowledge of their condition. Throughout the consultation, asking the patient what their preferences are and whether they have any hesitations can allow for joint decision-making and troubleshooting early on. Overall, this approach results in greater 'buy-in' and improves compliance with management plans.

Future directions and challenges

The paramedic role is changing, driven by evolving patterns of community utilisation of emergency services, and the expansion of the role into new workplaces, such as urgent care settings and primary care. This shift reflects broadened healthcare priorities outlined in the Fit for the Future: 10 year Health Plan for England and the development of integrated care systems, which emphasise prevention, early intervention, and integrated care pathways. As a result, paramedics will increasingly support patients in the management of chronic diseases, not only to deliver emergency care but also focusing on prevention and proactive management (Department of Health and Social Care, 2025; Briggs et al., 2024).

From emergency care to prevention

Historically, paramedics have operated within a reactive model, responding to crises and transporting patients to hospital. However, the growing burden of chronic disease and multimorbidity demands a proactive approach. Prevention is now central to healthcare policy, aiming to reduce hospital admissions and improve quality of life. If patients are empowered to improve their health through brief interventions, education, screening, and referrals, outcomes are significantly better than waiting until emergency care is required.

The Make Every Contact Count (MECC) initiative aims to deliver health promotion interventions through routine interactions with health and social care staff. This can be in the form of brief interventions to provide advice, support, or signposting to other services, as a way of improving health outcomes. MECC provides a practical tool for paramedics to incorporate preventive strategies into routine encounters. By using every patient interaction as an opportunity for health promotion, such as smoking cessation advice or signposting to mental health support, paramedics can contribute meaningfully to population health (NHS England, 2016; Public Health England, 2020; NICE, 2023).

Empowering patients to manage their conditions independently is a cornerstone of modern health care. Paramedics can reinforce self-care strategies during home visits, provide tailored education, and encourage adherence to treatment plans. Community-based care supports patients to remain in their homes, where social support may be stronger and risks associated with hospitalisation are minimised. However, effective self-management depends on better connectivity between primary care, social services, and mental health so that patients receive consistent messages and support across all services.

Effective signposting and community integration

Paramedics frequently encounter patients whose needs extend beyond the immediate clinical presentation, such as social isolation, poor medication adherence, or mental health crises. Effective signposting to community resources, mental health services, and social care can prevent escalation and improve outcomes. Integration into community-based care models and primary care networks enables paramedics to collaborate with GPs, nurses, physiotherapists, and occupational therapists, ensuring holistic care.

Models of care such as 'Hospital at Home' are being rolled out across the UK, supporting active treatment for chronic and complex conditions in the home setting rather than in hospital. These models reduce risks associated with hospital admissions, such as infections, muscle deterioration, and social isolation, while allowing patients to remain in familiar environments with better social support (British Geriatrics Society, 2022; NIHR, 2025; NHS England, 2024b).

Although healthcare reforms, including integrated care pathways and implementation of the Fit for the Future: 10 year Health Plan for England, aim to integrate services and prioritise prevention, challenges remain. Currently, systems are fragmented with poor interoperability between providers, often limited by poor communication between electronic health records. Recruitment and retention issues within the workforce impact on patient experience and reduce the therapeutic relationship that can support long-term change in individuals. Funding constraints also limit investment in digital infrastructure and training that would be required to address these challenges. Policy must support paramedics' expanded scope and provide clear frameworks for community-based practice and ensure equitable access to resources.

Advances in remote monitoring and telemedicine

Digital health technologies, including remote monitoring and teleconsultations, are reshaping chronic disease management. Paramedics can play a pivotal role in deploying and interpreting these tools, particularly during home visits or community clinics. Wearable devices that track vital signs, such as blood pressure or oxygen saturation, enable early detection of deterioration and timely intervention. Telemedicine allows remote specialist input, expanding the scope of what can be managed in the home environment. However, barriers persist amongst persons with severe and enduring mental illness, older adults, people living in rural locations, and members of poorer socioeconomic groups (Badr et al., 2024). These inequities risk widening health disparities unless addressed through targeted policies, funding, and inclusive design.

Training and education needs

The evolving scope of paramedic practice demands advanced training in chronic disease management, mental health, and digital health literacy. Education must also address the complexity of multimorbidity, where physical and psychological conditions intersect. Physical illnesses often co-exist with mental health disorders, creating a cycle of poor adherence, increased hospitalisations, and reduced quality of life. Paramedics must navigate these complexities, balancing clinical priorities with psychosocial needs. This requires time, training, and access to multidisciplinary support. Skills in motivational interviewing, cultural competence, and health coaching will become increasingly important. Furthermore, as paramedics become increasingly involved with primary care and multidisciplinary team working, they need a better understanding of community resources, care pathways, and collaborative working.

Conclusion

Living with a long-term conditions is a complex experience shaped by the interaction of physical illness, mental health, and social context. This chapter has shown how these factors intertwine, influencing a person's wellbeing, confidence, and engagement with care. For paramedics, recognising this interplay is essential when assessing and supporting individuals living with chronic illness.

As practice evolves, paramedics are increasingly involved in prevention, early intervention, and community-based care. Approaches such as Make Every Contact Count, trauma-informed care, and effective multidisciplinary working help address the wider influences on health and promote more personalised support. New models of care, including Hospital at Home and remote monitoring, offer opportunities for improved patient experience, though digital exclusion and health inequalities remain challenges (NHS England, 2023).

Clinical curiosity, metacognition, and awareness of diagnostic overshadowing are crucial when mental and physical health needs co-exist. Ultimately, supporting people with long-term conditions requires seeing the person beyond the diagnosis, promoting autonomy, and building trust. By adopting holistic, compassionate practice, paramedics can play a meaningful role in helping individuals live well with long-term conditions.

Further learning materials

Multiple-choice questions

MCQ1: Which statement best reflects the relationship between mental and physical health in people with long-term conditions?

A. Mental health problems usually develop after physical deterioration

B. Mental health affects physical health and vice versa

C. Mental health concerns are secondary to physical illness

D. Psychological distress only occurs in severe disease

Correct answer: B

Rationale: Mental health both affects and is affected by long-term physical illness, influencing outcomes and engagement.

MCQ2: Which feature is most characteristic of diabetes distress?

A. Acute psychotic symptoms
B. Emotional burden related to ongoing self-management
C. Intentional non-adherence to treatment
D. Cognitive impairment due to hypoglycaemia

Correct answer: B

Rationale: Diabetes distress reflects the emotional load of continuous monitoring and decision-making.

MCQ3: Diagnostic overshadowing occurs when:

A. Symptoms worsen despite treatment
B. New symptoms are attributed to an existing diagnosis without adequate assessment
C. A patient refuses investigation
D. A diagnosis is delayed due to service access issues

Correct answer: B

Rationale: Overshadowing risks missed or delayed diagnoses, particularly in multimorbidity.

MCQ4: Which paramedic approach best reflects trauma-informed care?

A. Focusing on efficiency to reduce on-scene time
B. Prioritising symptom checklists
C. Asking 'What happened to you?' rather than 'What's wrong with you?'
D. Avoiding discussion of past healthcare experiences

Correct answer: C

Rationale: Trauma-informed care emphasises safety, trust, and understanding lived experience.

MCQ5: Which change is most likely to indicate early functional decline?

A. Difficulty with bathing
B. Inability to transfer independently
C. Difficulty managing medications and appointments
D. Incontinence

Correct answer: C

Rationale: IADL changes often precede deterioration in basic self-care.

Guided clinical reasoning questions

Q1: *Assessment*: Which aspects of Amara's presentation could be mistakenly attributed solely to lupus?

Q2: *Assessment*: What cues suggest depression related to social isolation rather than disease progression?

Q3: *Assessment*: How does knowledge of Amara's baseline function shape your assessment?

Q4: *Risk and complexity*: What factors contribute to a negative feedback loop between Amara's physical and mental health?

Q5: *Risk and complexity*: How does missed follow-up increase long-term risk, even when vital signs are normal?

Q6: *Capacity and autonomy*: Why does Amara retain capacity despite fatigue, pain, and low mood?

Q7: *Capacity and autonomy*: How can paramedics support autonomy while addressing disengagement from care?

Q8: *Management*: What immediate paramedic actions could help rebuild trust in healthcare services?

Q9: *Management*: How might brief intervention or signposting alter Amara's longer-term trajectory?

Reflective questions for learners

Q1: How might previous experiences of dismissal influence a patient's willingness to engage with you?

Q2: When symptoms overlap with a known diagnosis, how do you guard against diagnostic overshadowing?

Q3: What assumptions might clinicians make about 'non-attendance' or 'non-compliance'?

Q4: How can paramedics balance efficiency with relational, person-centred care?

Teaching commentary

This chapter has highlighted the complexity of caring for people living with long-term conditions, where physical illness, mental health, and social context interact dynamically. The case of Amara illustrates how fluctuating symptoms, diagnostic overshadowing, and past negative healthcare experiences can erode trust and engagement, even in the absence of acute physiological deterioration. Teaching should emphasise bio-psycho-social assessment, trauma-informed communication, functional evaluation, and the importance of understanding baseline status. Also of importance are discussion of autonomy, capacity, and shared decision-making, reinforcing the paramedic role in prevention, early intervention, and re-engagement with community-based care.

References

Academy of Medical Sciences (2018). *Multimorbidity: A priority for global health research.* https://acmedsci.ac.uk/file-download/82222577 (accessed 25 November 2025).

Alhasan, D., and Yaseen, A. (2021). Hypertensive emergencies in the ambulance: Characteristics, clinical presentations and complications – a prospective cohort study. *Open Access Emergency Medicine, 13*, 75–81. https://doi.org/10.2147/oaem.s293413

Badr, J., Motulsky, A., and Denis, J-L. (2024). Digital health technologies and inequalities: A scoping review of potential impacts and policy recommendations. *Health Policy, 146*, 105122. https://doi.org/10.1016/j.healthpol.2024.105122

Berring, L.L., Holm, T., Hansen, J.P., Delcomyn, C.L., Sondergaard, R., and Hvidhjelm, J. (2024). Implementing trauma-informed care – Settings, definitions, interventions, measures, and implementation across settings: A scoping review. *Healthcare, 12*(9), 908. https://doi.org/10.3390/healthcare12090908

Bounds, C.G., Campos, A., Bains, G.S., and Goldstein, S. (2024). *EMS field identification of heart failure.* https://www.ncbi.nlm.nih.gov/books/NBK442029/ (accessed 25 November 2025).

Brauckmann, V., Hudasch, D., Gräff, P., Riecke, T., Aktas, G., Mayor, J., et al. (2024). Prehospital neurological emergencies – a survey on the state of prehospital neurological assessment by emergency medical professionals. *BMC Emergency Medicine, 24*, 164. https://doi.org/10.1186/s12873-024-01076-w

Briggs, H., Clarke, S., and Rees, N. (2021). Mental health assessment and triage in an ambulance clinical contact centre. *Journal of Paramedic Practice, 13*(5), 196–203. https://doi.org/10.12968/jpar.2021.13.5.196.

British Geriatrics Society (2022). *Bringing hospital care home: Virtual wards and Hospital at Home for older people.* https://www.bgs.org.uk/virtualwards (accessed 10 December 2025).

Brown, T., Ashworth, H., Bass, M., Rittenberg, E., Levy-Carrick, N., Grossman, S., et al. (2022). Trauma-informed care interventions in emergency medicine: A systematic review. *Western Journal of Emergency Medicine, 23*(3), 334–344. https://doi.org/10.5811/westjem.2022.1.53674

Civieri, G., Abohashem, S., Grewal, S.S., Aldosoky, W., Qamar, I., Hanlon, E., et al. (2024). Anxiety and depression associated with increased cardiovascular disease risk through accelerated development of risk factors. *JACC Advances, 3*(9), 101208. https://doi.org/10.1016/j.jacadv.2024.101208

Coughlin, S.S. (2011). Post-traumatic stress disorder and cardiovascular disease. *Open Cardiovascular Medicine Journal, 5*, 164–170. https://doi.org/10.2174/1874192401105010164

Dennick, K., Sturt, J., and Speight, J. (2017). What is diabetes distress and how can we measure it? A narrative review. *Journal of Diabetes Complications, 31*(5), 898–911. https:doi.org/10.1016/j.jdiacomp.2016.12.018

Department of Health and Social Care (2025). *Fit for the Future: 10 Year Health Plan for England.* https://www.gov.uk/government/publications/10-year-health-plan-for-england-fit-for-the-future/fit-for-the-future-10-year-health-plan-for-england-executive-summary (accessed 20 May 2025)

Engel, G.L. (1977). The need for a new medical model: A challenge for biomedicine. *Science, 196*(4286), 129–136. https://doi.org/10.1126/science.847460

Farooqi, A., Khunti, K., Abner, S., Gillies, C., Morriss, R., and Seidu, S. (2019). Comorbid depression and risk of cardiac events and cardiac mortality in people with diabetes: A systematic review and meta-analysis. *Diabetes Research and Clinical Practice, 156*, 107816. https://doi.org/10.1016/j.diabres.2019.107816

Firth, J., Siddiqi, N., Koyanagi, A., Siskind, D., Rosenbaum, S., Galletly, C., et al. (2019). The Lancet Psychiatry Commission: A blueprint for protecting physical health in people with mental illness. *The Lancet Psychiatry, 6*(8), 675–712. https://doi.org/10.1016/S2215-0366(19)30132-4

Fisher, L., Mullan, J.T., Arean, P., Glasgow, R.E., Hessler, D., and Masharani, U. (2010). Diabetes distress but not clinical depression or depressive symptoms is associated with glycemic control in both cross-sectional and longitudinal analyses. *Diabetes Care, 33*(1), 23–28. https://doi.org/10.2337/dc09-1238

Gilsanz, P., Winning, A., Koenen, K.C., Roberts, A.L., Sumner, J.A., Chen, Q., et al. (2017). Post-traumatic stress disorder symptom duration and remission in relation to cardiovascular disease risk among a large cohort of women. *Psychological Medicine, 47*(8), 1370–1378. https://doi.org/10.1017/S0033291716003378

Goodarzi, F., Khoshravesh, S., Ayubi, E., Bashirian, S., and Barati, M. (2024). Psychosocial determinants of functional independence among older adults: A systematic review and meta-analysis. *Health Promotion Perspectives, 14*(1), 32–43. https://doi.org/10.34172/hpp.42354

Goode, D., Ryan, A., Melby, V., and Slater, P. (2022). Care experiences of older people with mental health needs and their families in emergency medical services settings. *International Journal of Older People Nursing, 18*(1), e12500. https://doi.org/10.1111/opn.12500

Grassi, L., Caruso, R., Riba, M.B., Lloyd-Williams, M., Kissane, D., Rodin, G., et al. (2023). Anxiety and depression in adult cancer patients: ESMO Clinical Practice Guideline. *ESMO Open, 8*(2), 101155. https://doi.org/10.1016/j.esmoop.2023.101155

Gri, N., Longhitano, Y., Zanza, C., Monticone, V., Fuschi, D., Piccioni, A., et al. (2023). Acute oncologic complications: Clinical-therapeutic management in critical care and emergency departments. *Current Oncology, 30*(8), 7315–7334. https://doi.org/10.3390/curroncol30080531

Grigsby, A.B., Anderson, R.J., Freedland, K.E., Clouse, R.E., and Lustman, P.J. (2002). Prevalence of anxiety in adults with diabetes: A systematic review. *Journal of Psychosomatic Research, 53*(6), 1053–1060. https://doi.org/10.1016/s0022-3999(02)00417-8

Hallyburton, A. (2022). Diagnostic overshadowing: An evolutionary concept analysis on the misattribution of physical symptoms to pre-existing psychological illnesses. *International Journal of Mental Health Nursing, 31*(6), 1360–1372. https://doi.org/10.1111/inm.13034

Harris, M., and Fallot, R.D. (2001). Envisioning a trauma-informed service system: A vital paradigm shift. *New Directions for Mental Health Services, 2001*(89), 3–22. https://doi.org/10.1002/yd.23320018903

Harwood, R., Wincup, C., D'Cruz, D., and Sloan, M. (2025). Diagnostic overshadowing in systemic lupus erythematosus (SLE): A qualitative study. *Lupus, 34*(8), 819–831. https://doi.org/10.1177/09612033251345184

Hinson-Enslin, A.M., Espinoza, L.E., and Talleff, J.L. (2025). Mental health conditions of adults with chronic obstructive pulmonary disease and comorbidities. *Journal of Social, Behavioral and Health Sciences, 19*(1). https://doi.org/10.5590/JSBHS.2025.19.1660

Ho, I.S.S., Azcoaga-Lorenzo, A., Akbari, A., Davies, J., Hodgins, P., Khunti, K., et al. (2022). Variation in the estimated prevalence of multimorbidity: Systematic review and meta-analysis of 193 international studies. *BMJ Open, 12*(4). https://doi.org/10.1136/bmjopen-2021-057017

Horsbøl, T.A., Hoffmann, S.H., Thorsted, A.B., Rosenkilde, S., Lehn, S.F., Kofoed-Enevoldsen, A., et al. (2024). Diabetic complications and risk of depression and anxiety among adults with type 2 diabetes. *Diabetic Medicine*, *41*(4), e15272. https://doi.org/10.1111/dme.15272

Ikhile, D., Ford, E., Glass, D., Gremesty, G., and van Marwijk, H. (2024). A systematic review of risk factors associated with depression and anxiety in cancer patients. *PLoS One*, *19*(3), e0296892. https://doi.org/10.1371/journal.pone.0296892

Jones, S., Howard, L., and Thornicroft, G. (2008). 'Diagnostic overshadowing': Worse physical health care for people with mental illness. *Acta Psychiatrica Scandinavica*, *118*(3), 169–171. https://doi.org/10.1111/j.1600-0447.2008.01211.x

Kommer, A., Claßen, P.C., Schleicher, E.M., Weinmann-Menke, J., Kostev, K., and Labenz, C. (2025). Chronic kidney disease is associated with incident depression and anxiety: A cohort study. *Clinical Kidney Journal*, *18*(7), 1234–1243. https://doi.org/10.1093/ckj/sfaf186

Lau, D.C.W., Shaw, E., McMullen, S., Cowling, T., Witges, K., Amitay, E.L., et al. (2024). Acute and chronic complication profiles among patients with chronic kidney disease in Alberta, Canada: A retrospective observational study. *BMC Nephrology*, *25*(1), 244. https://doi.org/10.1186/s12882-024-03682-z

Lupus UK (2025). *What is lupus?* https://lupusuk.org.uk/what-is-lupus/ (accessed 25 November 2025).

McWilliams, D.F., Rahman, S., James, R.J.E., Ferguson, E., Kiely, P.D.W., Young, A., et al. (2019). Disease activity flares and pain flares in an early rheumatoid arthritis inception cohort: Characteristics, antecedents and sequelae. *BMC Rheumatology*, *3*(1), 49. https://doi.org/10.1186/s41927-019-0100-9

Mental Capacity Act 2005, c. 9. https://www.legislation.gov.uk/ukpga/2005/9/contents (accessed 11 December 2025).

Mitchell, A.J., Ferguson, D.W., Gill, J., Paul, J., and Symonds, P. (2013). Depression and anxiety in long-term cancer survivors compared with spouses and healthy controls: A systematic review and meta-analysis. *The Lancet Oncology*, *14*(8), 721–732. https://doi.org/10.1016/S1470-2045(13)70244-4

National Institute for Health and Care Excellence (NICE) (2022). *Depression in adults: Treatment and management* (NG222). London: NICE. https://www.nice.org.uk/guidance/ng222/chapter/recommendations (accessed 25 November 2025).

National Institute for Health and Care Excellence (NICE) (2023). *Multimorbidity.* https://cks.nice.org.uk/topics/multimorbidity/ (accessed 25 November 2025).

National Institute for Health and Care Research (NIHR) (2021). *Multiple long-term conditions (multimorbidity): Making sense of the evidence.* https://doi.org/10.3310/collection_45881

National Institute for Health and Care Research (NIHR) (2025). *Hospital at Home and virtual wards: what works?* NIHR Evidence Collection. https://evidence.nihr.ac.uk/collection/hospital-at-home-and-virtual-wards-what-works/ (accessed 10 December 2025).

Naylor, C., Galea, A., Parsonage, M., McDaid, D., Knapp, M., and Fossey, M. (2012). *Long-term conditions and mental health.* London: The King's Fund. https://www.kingsfund.org.uk/insight-and-analysis/reports/long-term-conditions-mental-health (accessed 25 November 2025).

NHS England (2016). *Making Every Contact Count (MECC): Consensus statement.* https://www.england.nhs.uk/publication/making-every-contact-count-mecc-consensus-statement/ (accessed 10 December 2025).

NHS England (2023). *Inclusive digital healthcare: A framework for NHS action on digital inclusion.* https://www.england.nhs.uk/long-read/inclusive-digital-healthcare-a-framework-for-nhs-action-on-digital-inclusion/ (accessed 10 December 2025).

NHS England (2024a). *News: NHS identifies over half a million more people at risk of type 2 diabetes in a year.* https://www.england.nhs.uk/2024/06/nhs-identifies-over-half-a-million-more-people-at-risk-of-type-2-diabetes-in-a-year/ (accessed 10 December 2025).

NHS England (2024b). *Improving the physical health of people living with severe mental illness.* https://www.england.nhs.uk/long-read/improving-the-physical-health-of-people-living-with-severe-mental-illness/ (accessed 10 December 2025).

Paslaru, A.M., Plesea-Condratovici, A., Moroianu, L-A., Isailă, O-M., Rebegea, L.F., Pavel, L.L., et al (2025). Mind over malignancy: A systematic review and meta-analysis of psychological distress, coping and therapeutic interventions in oncology. *Medicina, 61*(6), 1086. https://doi.org/10.3390/medicina61061086

Poole, L., and Hackett, R.A. (2024). Diabetes distress: The psychological burden of living with diabetes. *The Lancet Diabetes and Endocrinology, 12*(7), 439–441. https://doi.org/10.1016/S2213-8587(24)00126-8

Public Health England (PHE) (2020). *Making Every Contact Count (MECC): Evaluation guide.* https://www.gov.uk/government/publications/making-every-contact-count-mecc-practical-resources/mecc-evaluation-guide-2020 (accessed 10 December 2025).

Reeve, J., Maden, M., Hill, R., Turk, A., Mahtani, K., Wong, G., et al. (2022). Deprescribing medicines in older people living with multimorbidity and polypharmacy: The TAILOR evidence synthesis. *Health Technology Assessment, 26*(32), 1–148. https://doi.org/10.3310/aafo2475

Rockwood, K. (2005). A global clinical measure of fitness and frailty in elderly people. *Canadian Medical Association Journal, 173*(5), 489–495. https://doi.org/10.1503/cmaj.050051

Royal College of Physicians (2018). *Hiding in plain sight: Treating tobacco dependency in the NHS.* https://www.rcp.ac.uk/media/bdnj2ykk/hiding-in-plain-sight.pdf (accessed 10 December 2025).

Shi, Y., Li, H., Yuan, B., and Wang, X. (2025). Effects of multidisciplinary teamwork in non-hospital settings on healthcare and patients with chronic conditions: A systematic review and meta-analysis. *BMC Primary Care, 26*, 110. https://doi.org/10.1186/s12875-025-02814-0

Sneath, E., Bunting, D., Hazell, W., Tippett, V., and Yang, I.A. (2019). Pre-hospital and emergency department pathways of care for exacerbations of chronic obstructive pulmonary disease (COPD). *Journal of Thoracic Disease, 11*(suppl. 17), S2221–S2229. https://doi.org/10.21037/jtd.2019.10.37

Spiers, G.F., Kunonga, T.P., Hall, A., Beyer, F., Boulton, E., Parker, S., et al. (2021). Measuring frailty in younger populations: A rapid review of evidence. *BMJ Open, 11*(3), e047051. https://doi.org/10.1136/bmjopen-2020-047051

Squance, M.L., Reeves, G.E.M., and Bridgman, H. (2014). The lived experience of lupus flares: Features, triggers, and management in an Australian female cohort. *International Journal of Chronic Diseases, 2014*, 816729. https://doi.org/10.1155/2014/816729

Wagner, E.H. (1998). Chronic disease management: What will it take to improve care for chronic illness? *Effective Clinical Practice, 1*(1), 2–4. PMID: 10345255. https://pubmed.ncbi.nlm.nih.gov/10345255/ (Accessed: 25 November 2025).

Wang, C., Ruiz, A., and Mao-Draayer, Y. (2018). Assessment and treatment strategies for a multiple sclerosis relapse. *Journal of Immunology and Clinical Research, 5*(1), 1032. https://pmc.ncbi.nlm.nih.gov/articles/PMC6223639/

Yohannes, A.M., and Alexopoulos, G.S. (2014). Depression and anxiety in patients with COPD. *European Respiratory Review, 23*(133), 345–349. https://doi.org/10.1183/09059180.00007813

5 Women's mental health: Maternity

Susan Rhind, Sarah Hilton, Yuet Wah Patrick, and Jo Augustus

Introduction

Ambulance services play a vital role in providing unscheduled maternity care in the UK, despite maternity and newborn presentations comprising less than 1% of ambulance calls. Variability in maternity education among paramedics and the complexity of unscheduled care create challenges for safe decision-making, particularly when gestation is unknown or antenatal records are inaccessible. For many women, especially those living in socioeconomic deprivation, paramedics may be the first or only healthcare professionals they encounter during pregnancy, reflecting wider inequalities in access to antenatal care and increased reliance on emergency services (Jardine et al., 2021). Persistent racial and socioeconomic disparities contribute to stark variations in maternal outcomes. Women from the global majority remain at significantly higher risk of illness and death during pregnancy and labour, driven not by biological factors but by structural inequalities, racism, and poor access to culturally responsive care (Linton, 2025). Migrant women, including those seeking asylum, face additional barriers such as language difficulties, fear of NHS charging regulations, and frequent relocations, all of which can delay or prevent antenatal engagement.

Understanding maternity care in the pre-hospital environment requires recognising that perinatal health is shaped not only by physiological processes but also by profound psychological, emotional, and social determinants. Negative or traumatic birth experiences influence long-term psychological wellbeing. Mental health intersects with every stage of pregnancy, from the neuroendocrine changes that influence mood and anxiety, to the psychological impact of complications, pain, loss of control, and the trauma associated with emergency or unplanned births (Henriksen et al., 2017; Baptie et al., 2020). Inequalities, language barriers, stigma, and previous negative maternity experiences further compound vulnerability, influencing how women seek help and how they engage with clinicians during emergencies. Women frequently report feeling excluded from decision-making, poorly informed, or unsupported during labour, which can contribute to heightened anxiety, fear, and loss of autonomy (Flanagan et al., 2019; Findlay et al., 2024; Hill et al., 2025). Such experiences are consistently linked to postnatal depression, post-traumatic stress disorder (PTSD), anxiety disorders, and impaired parent–infant bonding (Henriksen et al., 2017; Baptie et al., 2020). Psychological factors now account for a substantial proportion of maternal deaths between six weeks and one year postpartum, including 34% of suicides recorded between 2020 and 2022 (Benton et al., 2024; Felker et al., 2024). This chapter, therefore, integrates mental health considerations throughout its discussion of perinatal physiology, emergency clinical presentations, birth trauma, and communication, highlighting the need for trauma-informed, culturally safe, and psychologically aware paramedic practice focused on both immediate safety and long-term wellbeing.

Key physiological differences during pregnancy

During pregnancy, women may experience various symptoms due to physiological, metabolic, and psychological changes. The types of symptoms, and their duration and severity, can vary among pregnant women and may differ across trimesters. Fatigue, urinary frequency, upper/lower back pain, and poor sleep quality are the most common symptoms reported by pregnant women that limit daily activities and can cause distress and impact on their mental wellbeing (Kiyak, 2024). Sleep disruption is common in both early and late pregnancy due to hormonal shifts, discomfort, and nocturia, further elevating the risk of anxiety and depressive symptoms, affecting concentration, coping capacity, and help-seeking behaviours.

Nausea and vomiting and changes in physical appearance such as body shape, weight gain, and stretch marks, can be a cause of concern for some women, triggering stress and anxiety. Increased blood volume and metabolic demands can lead to light-headedness, breathlessness, and weakness, which can contribute to feeling overwhelmed and anxious. Cognitive changes which can result in forgetfulness or 'brain fog' often make it more challenging for women to continue to perform to the same standards in their working or personal lives.

Alongside the physical adaptations of pregnancy, significant neuroendocrine changes occur that influence maternal mood, cognition, and emotional regulation. Rising levels of progesterone and oestrogen have well-documented sedative and anxiolytic effects, yet in some women they contribute to heightened emotional sensitivity, irritability, or low mood due to their interaction with γ-aminobutyric acid (GABA) and serotonergic pathways (Marx et al., 2023). Cortisol levels increase progressively throughout gestation as part of normal foetal development, but this physiological hypercortisolism can amplify stress responses and vulnerability to anxiety, especially when compounded by socioeconomic stressors or previous trauma (Henriksen et al., 2017; Felker et al., 2024). These neuroendocrine and physiological factors mean that psychological distress may present subtly or overlap with somatic symptoms, underscoring the importance of paramedics adopting a sensitive, holistic, and trauma-informed approach when assessing women in the perinatal period.

Overview of maternity presentations relevant to the pre-hospital setting

This section provides an overview of some maternity presentations from UK ambulance services.

Miscarriage and still births

A miscarriage is the loss of a pregnancy within 23 weeks and 6 days of gestation. Any loss from 24 weeks is called a stillbirth. If the baby is born alive, even before 24 weeks, and lives even for a matter of minutes, it is considered a live birth and a neonatal death. Approximately 15% of confirmed pregnancies end in miscarriage, although the actual number is higher as many women miscarry without knowing they are pregnant (Ghosh et al., 2021).

Perinatal loss can trigger intense short- and long-term psychological distress because a moment expected to bring joy instead results in profound grief. This grief is often complicated by a lack of memories of the baby, feelings of biological failure (especially for mothers), limited social validation, and uncertainty about future pregnancies (Human et al., 2014). A woman who has miscarried or experiences a stillbirth is at risk of PTSD, depression, and complicated grief (Henriksen et al., 2017), with 20% of women developing anxiety and/or depression (NICE, 2023a). The impact extends beyond the parents to the wider family and social environment and because society often minimises these losses, parents may feel isolated. As grief affects the whole family, support should be given to the family as a unified system rather than as individuals.

Ectopic pregnancies

An ectopic pregnancy is when the fertilised ovum implants itself outside of the uterus. The most common site of implantation is in the fallopian tube (97%) but other sites include interstitial tissue, the ovaries, abdomen, and cervix. In the UK, approximately 1% of pregnancies are ectopic, or around 12,000 each year, of which approximately 0.2 per 1,000 ectopic pregnancies result in maternal death (MBRRACE, 2024). Nearly two-thirds of these deaths are associated with substandard clinical care. Vulnerability to adverse outcomes is heightened among women who face barriers accessing timely medical attention, including recent migrants, asylum seekers, refugees, and individuals with limited English language proficiency or literacy skills. These groups may experience delays in help-seeking, reduced engagement with healthcare services, and challenges in navigating the healthcare system, thereby increasing the risk of severe complications (NICE, 2023a).

Risk factors include a previous ectopic pregnancy, pelvic inflammatory disease, tubal damage, previous pelvic surgery, smoking, age over 35, infertility and fertility treatment including in vitro fertilisation (IVF), having multiple sexual partners, and black ethnicity (Hendricks et al., 2020; NICE, 2023). However, about a third of women who have an ectopic pregnancy will have no discernible risk factors (RCOG, 2016). Many of the signs and symptoms of ectopic pregnancy are atypical and resemble other common conditions, making recognition of an ectopic pregnancy challenging in the pre-hospital setting. It is, therefore, imperative to suspect ectopic pregnancy in women of childbearing age to allow for prompt intervention and prevent complications including tubal rupture and death from hypovolaemic shock.

Unexpected out-of-hospital birth and imminent birth in the pre-hospital setting

Unexpected birth that has occurred in an unplanned location such as the home or public space without the support of a healthcare professional is often referred to as a birth before arrival (Hill et al., 2025). Imminent birth is the clinical stage of labour where birth is occurring or about to occur; an imminent birth can happen within any setting and is assessed on key physical signs and maternal behaviour, such as the urge to push or bear down, bulging perineum, parting of the labia, or a visible presenting part (Marshall and Raynor, 2020; JRCALC, 2025). Births before arrival and imminent birth can include associated risks for the mother such as increased risk of postpartum haemorrhage, shoulder dystocia, and perineal tears. The newborn is at increased risk of hypothermia, hypoxia, injury, prematurity, low birthweight, and hypoglycaemia, leading to unfavourable neonatal outcomes, including increased perinatal and neonatal mortality.

An unplanned out-of-hospital birth can be an anxious and stressful experience for the mother and her partner. They may have concerns about potential complications and may feel guilty about not reaching hospital in time. These factors can lead to a negative birth experience that may have a lasting effect on all involved. A confident and reassuring paramedic presence can reduce any psychological complications, allowing the mother and her partner to focus on the experience of the birth (Hill et al., 2025).

Venous thromboembolism

Venous thromboembolism (VTE) is considered the leading cause of maternal mortality in the UK and pulmonary embolism represents the most life-threatening complication of VTE (RCOG, 2015; Felker et al., 2024; Linton, 2025). Black women continue to experience maternal deaths from thrombosis, thromboembolism, and cardiac disease at nearly three times the rate of white women, and this is attributed to systemic inequalities, racial bias in health care, and social determinants of health, rather than biological factors alone (Felker et al., 2024; Linton, 2025). Risk factors for VTE include a history of previous VTE or thrombophilia, acquired heart disease, advanced maternal age (over 35 years), immobility or long-distance travel, and co-morbidities such as hypertension, urinary tract infections, pre-eclampsia, and obesity. The Royal College of Obstetricians and Gynaecologists (2015) associates obesity with an increased risk of pulmonary embolism. Felker et al. (2024) note that mental health comorbidities may influence physical health or the quality of care for women with heart disease. Cardiovascular complications are often accompanied with dyspnoea as a symptom which can be misinterpreted as panic or anxiety. It is important to assess any breathing difficulties for an underlying clinical cause to avoid misdiagnosis.

Pre-eclampsia and eclampsia

Pre-eclampsia is challenging to define because its signs and symptoms vary widely, making this pregnancy complication unpredictable. It can progress to severe within days and can lead to multi-organ dysfunction, affecting both the mother and the newborn. Guidance defines pre-eclampsia as a pregnancy complication that presents after 20 weeks' gestation with new-onset hypertension of at least 140/90mmHg and either proteinuria or liver and kidney dysfunction; pre-eclampsia can vary in severity with 'severe' categorised as hypertension over 160/110mmHg associated with ongoing or recurrent headaches, nausea, vomiting, epigastric pain, and visual disturbances (Li et al., 2016; NICE, 2023b; Boyle, 2024). Eclampsia can develop during the antenatal, intrapartum, or postnatal stages of pregnancy and is commonly defined as new onset, unexplained seizures that are associated with the signs and symptoms of pre-eclampsia. Although eclamptic seizures are closely associated with cardiac arrest and intracerebral haemorrhage, many seizures resolve in a short period of time.

There are numerous risk factors for pre-eclampsia; however, like its unpredictability, pre-eclampsia can present with no identifiable risk factors (Li et al., 2016; NICE, 2023b; Di Martino et al., 2025; Nakimuli et al., 2025). One risk factor is previous episodes of pre-eclampsia, eclampsia, or hypertension during pregnancy, which suggests that some women are more prone to the condition with each pregnancy. This can instil anxiety if the woman becomes pregnant again as they are at higher risk.

Antepartum haemorrhage

Antepartum haemorrhage (APH) is bleeding that originates from or into the genital tract within 24 weeks of pregnancy until prior to the birth of the baby (RCOG, 2011). The causes of APH include placenta praevia where the placenta covers the cervix, placental abruption where the placenta separates from the uterus prematurely, vasia praevia where foetal blood vessels cross or are close to the cervix, increasing risk of rupture, uterine rupture, and local causation such as bleeding from the vagina, vulva, or cervix (RCOG, 2011; Acosta, 2024). Antepartum haemorrhage is difficult to assess in the pre-hospital setting due to possible concealed blood loss or where the underlying cause is unclear; a history of trauma may increase clinical suspicion but timely recognition and prompt conveyance to definitive care remain crucial. The condition is associated with serious risk, including preterm birth, intrauterine growth restriction, hypoxia-induced cerebral palsy, and neonatal death (Acosta, 2024).

Postpartum haemorrhage

Primary PPH (postpartum haemorrhage) is blood loss of more than 500mL from the genital tract within 24 hours of childbirth (WHO, 2012; Mavrides et al., 2016; Escobar et al., 2022). The Royal College of Obstetricians and Gynaecologists (2016) further classifies PPH based on the volume of blood lost, with a loss of 500 to 1000 mL classified as 'minor'. Major classification is further divided into 'moderate' (1000–2000mL) and 'severe' (>2000mL). Predisposing risk factors for primary PPH include previous PPH, previous caesarean delivery, placenta praevia, advanced maternal age, ethnic origin, racial group, and socioeconomic status (Kramer et al., 2011; Bryant et al., 2012). Guidelines outline common causes of PPH; Tone, Trauma, Tissue, and Thrombin, colloquially known as 'The 4 Ts', which provides a simple and memorable guide for assessment and management. Uterine atony (tone) is considered the most common cause of primary PPH; delayed medical support or unassisted births can further increase the risk of trauma such as perineal tears.

Where there is evidence of hypovolaemia and blood loss with palpated uterine tone, internal tears should be suspected and PPH management should be undertaken with time-critical conveyance expedited for further care (Kramer et al., 2011; Bryant et al., 2012; Elser et al., 2025). Tissue-related causes of PPH such as a retained placenta or membranes can prevent effective uterine contractions contributing to primary PPH.

In cases of secondary PPH, which occurs from 24 hours up to 6 weeks postpartum, retained products disrupt the uterus returning to its normal size and recovering; if products remain within the uterus, there is an increased risk of infection, endometritis, and ongoing bleeding (Chainarong et al., 2022; Elser et al., 2025; Ubom et al., 2025).

Postpartum haemorrhage is an extremely distressing event and is associated with acute stress for all those involved. Clear and calm communication regarding interventions is paramount.

Clinical assessment

Ambulance service providers are familiar with early warning scores to detect deterioration, but the physiology of pregnancy and the perinatal period requires a different approach. Maternity Early Warning Scores (MEWS) used in hospital settings are designed around pregnancy physiology and trigger escalation when parameters move outside safe ranges (Gerry et al., 2024). However, they do not fully align with the scope of practice or diagnostic capacity of ambulance clinicians. For this reason, the Prehospital Maternity Decision Tool (PMDT) has been developed within JRCALC guidance to support recognition of deterioration in women who are pregnant, suspected to be pregnant, or recently pregnant (JRCALC, 2024).

National Early Warning Score 2 (NEWS2), commonly used in adult prehospital care, is not appropriate for pregnant or postnatal women because it does not account for the normal physiological changes of pregnancy. It is, therefore, essential that paramedics proactively establish pregnancy status in all girls and women of childbearing potential. The PMDT uses pregnancy-specific parameters and a clear red–amber–green flagging system to highlight when urgent or time-critical transfer is required. Subtle changes such as a slight rise in respiratory rate, new-onset tachycardia, or borderline hypotension may indicate significant pathology in the perinatal context and should not be dismissed as 'normal' if they deviate from expected pregnancy physiology.

Psychological assessment considerations

Although the PMDT provides a structured framework for recognising physiological deterioration, psychological assessment is an equally critical component of safe perinatal care. Mental health presentations in pregnancy and the postpartum period can be rapid in onset and may initially be mistaken for distress or fatigue. Paramedics should remain alert to mental health 'red flags', including marked agitation, confusion, disorientation, severe anxiety, withdrawal, hallucinations, delusional beliefs, or sudden changes in behaviour. These may indicate acute mental illness, substance use, hypoxia, sepsis, or metabolic disturbance, and should always prompt urgent escalation.

Simple, compassionate screening questions can help identify emerging psychological or emotional risk:

'How are you feeling emotionally right now?'
'Does anything feel frightening or overwhelming?'
'Have you noticed any thoughts or experiences that feel unusual for you?'
'Is there anything worrying you that we haven't talked about yet?'

Such questions allow women to express fear or distress while enabling clinicians to distinguish between expected psychological responses and symptoms suggesting more serious pathology.

Recognition of postpartum psychosis is especially important, as it is a rare but life-threatening psychiatric emergency typically presenting within the first two weeks after birth. Symptoms may include hallucinations, delusional thinking, severe mood swings, insomnia, disorganised behaviour, or an abrupt loss of insight. Early identification and rapid conveyance to specialist care are crucial, as postpartum psychosis is associated with high risks of suicide and harm if not addressed promptly (Benton et al., 2024).

Importantly, psychological distress may mask or mimic clinical deterioration. Fear, panic, past trauma, and pain can all influence breathing patterns, heart rate, and communication, leading to misattribution of physiological changes. Conversely, women experiencing shock, hypovolaemia, or sepsis may appear withdrawn, flat, or unusually calm, which can be misinterpreted as coping or emotional shutdown. A trauma-informed, culturally sensitive approach acknowledging how fear, discrimination, and previous maternity experiences shape help-seeking supports more accurate assessment and promotes safety for both mother and baby.

The PMDT aligns with MEWS thresholds but is streamlined for pre-hospital use, focusing on key markers of deterioration, symptom clusters, and 'red flag' presentations such as suspected ectopic pregnancy, pre-eclampsia/eclampsia, acute haemorrhage (APH/PPH), and sepsis (JRCALC, 2024). It reinforces structured assessment, including brief obstetric history (gestation, parity, antenatal complications), presenting symptoms (e.g. pain, bleeding, headache, visual disturbance, reduced foetal movements), and targeted examination. Applying the PMDT alongside clinical judgement supports earlier recognition of time-critical conditions and promotes appropriate pre-alert and conveyance to the correct receiving unit.

Newborn transition and initial assessment

Unplanned out-of-hospital births, particularly births before arrival, are often perceived as challenging and high-risk incidents by ambulance personnel. Babies born in uncontrolled environments are at increased risk of hypothermia, hypoglycaemia, jaundice, low birthweight, and admission to the neonatal intensive care unit (Loughney et al., 2006; Ford and Pett, 2008; McLelland et al., 2014, 2018; Thornton and Dahlen, 2018; Smith et al., 2025). Newborn transition refers to the complex physiological changes that occur in the minutes and hours after birth, including the initiation of breathing, conversion of fluid-filled lungs to aerated lungs, and redirection of circulatory flow away from the placenta (Graves and Haley, 2013; Chakkarapani et al., 2024).

Closure of foetal shunts, including the ductus arteriosus, occurs gradually. During this time, oxygen-rich and oxygen-poor blood may mix, so post-ductal oxygen saturations in the feet can be lower than pre-ductal values. For this reason, right-hand or right-wrist pulse oximetry is recommended as the most accurate site for monitoring newborn oxygen saturations in the first minutes after birth (Backes et al., 2022; Chakkarapani et al., 2024). Rather than expecting immediate 'normal adult' values, paramedics should anticipate a gradual rise over the first 10 minutes of life and interpret saturations in that context (RCUK, 2025).

Thermoregulation and skin-to-skin contact

Newborns lose heat rapidly after birth, with an estimated temperature drop of 0.1–0.3°C per minute if not adequately protected (Graves and Haley, 2013; Widström et al., 2019; Goodwin et al., 2022). Limited subcutaneous fat, wet skin, and a high surface area-to-mass ratio, combined with immature thermoregulatory mechanisms, increase the risk of hypothermia. To maintain temperature, newborns rely on non-shivering thermogenesis, which increases oxygen and glucose consumption and can contribute to hypoxia and hypoglycaemia if environmental warmth is not optimised.

In pre-hospital settings, it is not always possible to achieve ideal thermal conditions, but simple measures can significantly reduce heat loss. These include closing doors and windows, minimising drafts, turning up the heating where possible, drying the newborn thoroughly, placing a hat on the head, and promoting skin-to-skin contact on the mother's chest, covered with a clean, dry towel, or blanket (Graves and Haley, 2013; Widström et al., 2019). Temperature should be among the first recorded observations and reassessed regularly, aiming to maintain a range of 36.5–37.5°C (JRCALC, 2025; RCUK, 2025). However, studies show that pre-hospital clinicians frequently omit temperature assessment or record temperatures below 36.5°C following a birth before arrival, citing lack of neonatal equipment, low confidence, or the baby 'appearing well' (McClelland et al., 2019; Donnellan et al., 2020; Goodwin et al., 2022).

Skin-to-skin contact confers benefits beyond thermoregulation. It is associated with improved respiratory and heart rate stability, reduced crying, and lower risk of hypoglycaemia. For mothers, skin-to-skin contact can reduce stress and anxiety, support maternal–infant bonding, and promote early initiation of breastfeeding, which in turn enhances oxytocin release, uterine contraction, and lactation (Carfoot et al., 2005; Marin et al., 2010; Ruiz et al., 2023). Initial newborn assessment can usually be completed while the baby remains in skin-to-skin contact, alongside drying, stimulation, and delayed cord clamping, provided there are no immediate resuscitation concerns.

Continuous assessment

Newborn assessment should be continuous and documented, focusing on breathing, heart rate, and muscle tone rather than skin colour alone. Colour can be difficult to interpret reliably, particularly in a diverse population with a wide range of skin tones (Dumas et al., 2013; RCUK, 2025). Research has demonstrated significant variability between clinicians' assessments of cyanosis and pallor, suggesting that colour alone is a poor indicator of wellbeing (O'Donnell et al., 2007; Sotiropoulos et al., 2022). Paramedics should therefore prioritise objective measures of respiratory effort, heart rate, tone, and temperature over subjective impressions of colour when judging newborn stability.

Case study: A maternity-related emergency

Case study: Narrative

At 11:30am you are dispatched to 22-year-old Zara, reported to be in labour with abdominal pain. A transporting ambulance is 20 minutes away. You arrive at a small, terraced house where family members crowd the hallway, anxious and distressed. In the bedroom, Zara is seated on a towel on the floor, holding a newborn wrapped in a blanket. There is visible blood loss estimated at around 400 mL.

Through initial conversation and use of professional interpretation support, Zara confirms she is 19+3 weeks gestation, a singleton pregnancy, and that she attended only an early dating scan. She has since struggled to access antenatal care due to digital barriers, limited English literacy, and the socioeconomic constraints of her household. Her 12-year-old brother who speaks English attempts to interpret, but it is clear he cannot safely or ethically fulfil this role. You arrange professional interpretation immediately.

Primary survey and baby assessment

Using RCUK newborn assessment guidance (2025), findings are:

- *Colour*: dark red with purple extremities
- *Tone:* floppy
- *Breathing:* absent
- *Heart rate:* none detected

The baby is extremely small, consistent with 19-week gestation; eyelids and digits remain fused, and the umbilical cord is intact with placenta in situ. At this gestation, survival-focused care is not appropriate, and guidance from the British Association of Perinatal Medicine (2026) and JRCALC (2025) directs clinicians to provide comfort-focused care.

You gently support Zara in holding the baby while ensuring privacy and dignity. Comfort-focused care aims to avoid any interventions that may cause discomfort or medically futile attempts at resuscitation, instead prioritising warmth, closeness, and family time.

Maternal assessment

Zara is alert, orientated, and able to express her needs clearly with interpreter support. She shows understanding that the baby has died, demonstrating capacity for decision-making. Vital signs are within normal ranges, and bleeding has slowed. She reports no abdominal pain and is haemodynamically stable, but the placenta remains in situ, placing her at increasing risk of postpartum haemorrhage (PPH) and infection.

Ongoing maternal assessment is required, using the Prehospital Maternity Decision Tool (PMDT) to interpret clinical observations within pregnancy-specific parameters (JRCALC, 2024). Even subtle deterioration can signal early haemorrhage or sepsis in perinatal patients.

Pregnancy loss

Pregnancy loss at any gestation can trigger acute psychological responses, and Zara's presentation should be assessed with this in mind. Women may experience acute stress reactions, including emotional numbness, dissociation, tearfulness, panic, or difficulty processing information. Shock may manifest as slowed speech, flat affect, or an apparently calm demeanour, which can be misinterpreted as coping. These reactions are normal but require sensitive handling, clear communication, and awareness that psychological distress may interact with physiological symptoms. Paramedics should remain attentive to signs of escalating anxiety, confusion, or withdrawal, which may indicate acute mental health need alongside the physical considerations of preterm birth.

Management priorities

For the baby:

- Support Zara and her family in providing comfort-focused care.
- Maintain warmth and dignity, swaddling the baby carefully.
- Encourage bonding if desired; avoid assumptions, recognising culturally influenced preferences.
- If the family wishes, the baby's name – Aarav – may be used, reinforcing personhood and validating the family's grief (BAPM, 2026).

For Zara:

- Perform frequent observations at 5-minute intervals (JRCALC, 2024).
- Prioritise timely conveyance to an obstetric-led unit, as the retained placenta increases risk of PPH.
- Prepare to manage potential blood loss during transport. Estimating and documenting visible blood loss are essential for receiving clinicians.
- Consider maternal analgesia such as Entonox if contractions resume but avoid manipulating the cord or applying traction to deliver the placenta.

Alongside physical assessment, Zara's emotional wellbeing requires active support. Validating her reactions acknowledging the grief, fear, and shock she may be experiencing can reduce feelings of isolation and distress. Paramedics should remain vigilant for acute mental health red flags, such as agitation, disorientation, intrusive thoughts, expressions of guilt, or detachment, which may signal early trauma responses or severe distress. Trauma-informed language is essential: avoiding euphemisms, offering choices wherever possible, and explaining each action can help restore a sense of control. Given Zara's cultural background and the involvement of her family, bereavement care must also be culturally safe, ensuring her beliefs, rituals, and communication preferences are respected while avoiding assumptions. Sensitive, culturally attuned practice supports both immediate psychological stabilisation and longer-term emotional recovery.

After birth, accurately assessing uterine tone is critical. A firm, 'cricket ball' uterus suggests lower PPH risk; a soft or high uterus warrants urgent reassessment. If the placenta is not delivered within 20 minutes, guidelines recommend time-critical transfer due to rising PPH risk.

Communication and cultural safety

Communication is central to trauma-informed care, particularly in pre-hospital pregnancy loss (Berry et al., 2023). Professional interpretation must be used instead of family members (especially children) both to ensure clarity and to protect the emotional wellbeing of young relatives (Heath et al., 2023).

Clear, direct language is recommended; euphemisms can create damaging misunderstandings and false hope. In this case, it is vital to explain compassionately that Aarav was born too early for survival, even with medical intervention.

Cultural considerations should be explored sensitively. Many families draw upon specific rituals or customs following pregnancy loss and offering options rather than making assumptions helps support autonomy and dignity. Where appropriate, taking photographs or offering memory-making items such as 'cuddle pockets' may support grief and long-term coping (SANDS, 2021; BAPM, 2026).

Communication plays a central role in shaping psychological outcomes after perinatal loss. Poor or unclear communication has been strongly associated with increased trauma symptoms and heightened risk of long-term psychological distress, including PTSD (Berry, 2022; Flanagan et al., 2019). For Zara, whose first language is not English, the potential for misinterpretation or misunderstanding further increases vulnerability. Ensuring accurate, compassionate, and unambiguous communication supported by professional interpretation services is therefore essential to prevent additional harm. Transparent explanations about the baby's condition, what has happened, and what will happen next can reduce confusion, minimise traumatic processing, and support a more dignified and emotionally safe experience for the patient and her family.

Documentation

Accurate, detailed documentation is essential because maternal deaths and neonatal deaths (from 22 weeks to 28 days) are reviewed under national governance structures such as the Maternity and Newborn Safety Investigations (MNSI) and the Perinatal Mortality Review Tool (PMRT). Records must:

- outline the sequence of events
- document clinical findings and decision-making
- include any barriers to antenatal care
- record communication using interpretation services
- summarise handover information clearly

Zara's limited access to antenatal care linked to language, digital exclusion, and socioeconomic constraints should be documented, as these factors contribute to systemic inequalities in maternal health outcomes (Goodwin et al., 2018).

Psychological needs and trauma-informed care

Pregnancy loss carries immediate and long-term psychological risks including PTSD, anxiety, depression, nightmares, panic attacks, and intrusive thoughts (Berry, 2022). Zara's emotional response is shaped by her cultural background, support networks, and the unexpected nature of the loss. Paramedics should monitor for acute distress, dissociation, or expressions of guilt or self-blame, and should signpost appropriately for early mental health support. Red flags requiring urgent escalation include suicidal ideation, severe withdrawal, inability to care for self, and overwhelming grief that impairs functioning.

Trauma-informed practice emphasises compassion, predictability, choice, and empowerment. Small actions asking permission before examinations, explaining each step, and validating feelings can profoundly influence long-term psychological outcomes.

Case study: Lessons

Maternity emergencies not only involve significant physiological risk but also carry profound psychological implications that can shape a woman's wellbeing long after the acute event has passed. Evidence demonstrates that women who experience unexpected or traumatic perinatal events, including unplanned out-of-hospital birth, severe maternal illness, and pregnancy loss, have a heightened likelihood of developing PTSD, postnatal depression, and anxiety disorders (Henriksen et al., 2017; Arnold et al., 2025). These risks are further amplified by factors such as fear, pain, loss of control, poor communication, cultural misunderstanding, or a lack of emotional support at the time of the incident. For many, the pre-hospital encounter is a pivotal moment that shapes both their immediate coping and their long-term emotional recovery. Paramedics therefore play a critical role in delivering psychological first aid: offering calm, validating communication; reducing uncertainty; supporting dignity; and ensuring culturally sensitive, trauma-informed care. Such approaches not only improve patient experience but may also reduce the likelihood of enduring psychological harm.

Key learning points

- Pre-hospital maternity emergencies require balancing clinical priorities with psychological and bereavement needs, demanding confidence, structured assessment, and sensitive communication.
- Effective care must integrate cultural humility, acknowledging the patient's social background, beliefs, and preferences when providing support.
- Language barriers, limited health literacy, and wider structural inequities can significantly shape antenatal access, risk profiles, and emergency presentations.
- The Prehospital Maternity Decision Tool (PMDT) provides essential guidance for recognising clinical deterioration in pregnant or recently pregnant patients.
- Trauma-informed, culturally safe, and person-centred practice is crucial for supporting positive experiences, reducing long-term psychological distress, and enhancing overall safety in maternity care.

Psychological safety for paramedics in maternity care

Paramedics attending maternity emergencies often work in unfamiliar, high-pressure, and emotionally charged environments, where outcomes can change rapidly and may involve traumatic events such as perinatal loss or severe maternal complications. These situations can trigger feelings of anxiety, self-doubt, or moral distress, particularly as maternity accounts for a small proportion of routine paramedic work, limiting confidence and experience. Psychological safety means that clinicians feel able to express uncertainty, seek help, and discuss difficult emotions without fear of judgement or blame. A psychologically safe workplace promotes reflective practice, structured debriefs, and access to professional and peer support, helping to reduce burnout and enhance resilience. Fostering psychological safety is not optional: it is crucial for protecting clinician wellbeing and sustaining compassionate, high-quality maternity care in the pre-hospital environment.

Future directions

Future pre-hospital maternity care must prioritise both physical safety and mental wellbeing. NHS England highlights maternal mental health as a key national focus, recognising that mental illness remains a leading cause of death in the year after birth. Paramedics will need stronger training in recognising perinatal mental health red flags such as severe anxiety, trauma responses, or postpartum psychosis and in using trauma-informed, culturally sensitive communication. More research is needed to understand how mental health crises present in the pre-hospital setting and how psychological first aid affects long-term outcomes. Closer integration with perinatal mental health teams and clearer referral pathways will help ensure women receive timely, holistic support. Treating physical and mental health as inseparable will be central to improving outcomes.

Conclusion

This chapter has explored the unique challenges involved in providing safe, effective, and compassionate pre-hospital maternity care. Paramedics must navigate rapid physiological changes, unpredictable clinical presentations, and the complex social and cultural factors that shape women's experiences during pregnancy and birth. Unscheduled or emergency maternity events are not only clinically demanding but can carry profound emotional and psychological consequences for women and families. It is, therefore, essential that paramedics recognise their role not only in managing physical risk but also in preventing trauma, supporting emotional safety, and responding to distress with sensitivity. Awareness of the long-term psychological impact of events such as pregnancy loss, severe illness, or unplanned birth underscores the importance of clear communication, reassurance, and validation. Embedding culturally safe, trauma-informed practice into everyday care will help ensure that women feel respected and understood, reduce the risk of lasting harm, and promote positive outcomes across diverse communities.

Further learning materials

Multiple-choice questions

MCQ1: *Inequalities and access*: Which statement best reflects why some women rely on ambulance services for maternity care?

A. Maternity calls are common in ambulance practice

B. Paramedics routinely access full antenatal records

C. Structural barriers can limit antenatal access, increasing emergency reliance

D. Antenatal care is equally accessible across populations

Correct answer: C

Rationale: Socioeconomic barriers, language, and system factors can reduce antenatal engagement.

MCQ2: *Gestation and terminology*: In the UK, a pregnancy loss at 19+6 weeks is classified as?

A. Stillbirth

B. Miscarriage

C. Neonatal death

D. Maternal death

Correct answer: B

Rationale: Loss before 24 weeks is classified as miscarriage.

MCQ3: *Escalation tool*: Why is NEWS2 not appropriate for pregnant/postnatal women?

A. It is only validated in hospital settings

B. It does not account for pregnancy physiology

C. It cannot be used for mental health presentations

D. It requires laboratory tests

Correct answer: B

Rationale: Pregnancy alters baseline physiology; PMDT/MEWS-style parameters are more appropriate.

MCQ4: *Red flags – postpartum psychosis*: Which presentation most strongly suggests postpartum psychosis?

A. Tearfulness and worry about feeding
B. Low mood and fatigue at 3 months postpartum
C. Hallucinations, delusional beliefs, and disorganised behaviour within 2 weeks of birth
D. Anxiety during labour with hyperventilation

Correct answer: C

Rationale: Rapid-onset psychotic symptoms early postpartum is a psychiatric emergency.

MCQ5: *Interpretation and safeguarding*: In Zara's case, the most appropriate approach to communication is?

A. Use the 12-year-old brother to interpret as he is present
B. Use family interpretation if the scene is time-critical
C. Use professional interpretation and avoid child interpreters
D. Communicate only with the family spokesperson

Correct answer: C

Rationale: Professional interpretation supports accuracy, consent, and safeguards children.

MCQ6: *Baby care at 19 weeks*: At 19+6 weeks with no signs of life, the correct care priority for the baby is?

A. Full neonatal resuscitation per RCUK algorithm
B. Comfort-focused care with warmth, dignity, and family time
C. Immediate transport to NICU without assessment
D. Oxygen via mask and chest compressions

Correct answer: B

Rationale: At this gestation, survival-focused interventions are not appropriate; comfort care is indicated.

Guided clinical reasoning questions

Q1: *Assessment*: What history is essential when antenatal records are unavailable (gestation, parity, complications, bleeding, pain, reduced movements)?

Q2: *Assessment*: Using PMDT, what physiological changes would trigger urgent escalation in a perinatal patient?

Q3: *Clinical risk*: In Zara's scenario, what are the immediate maternal risks associated with placenta in situ?

Q4: *Clinical risk*: What findings would increase suspicion of evolving haemorrhage or sepsis despite initially 'normal' observations?

Q5: *Communication and cultural safety*: What trauma-informed language would you use to explain the baby's death clearly and compassionately (avoiding euphemism)?

Q6: *Communication and cultural safety*: What culturally safe options could you offer the family (rituals, naming, memory-making) without assumptions?

Q7: *Psychological considerations*: What signs might indicate acute stress responses (dissociation, numbness, panic), and how might they affect consent and recall?

Q8: *Psychological considerations*: What perinatal mental health red flags would require urgent escalation (e.g. psychosis, suicidal ideation, severe withdrawal)?

Q9: *Professional practice*: What must be documented in this case to support continuity of care and governance review (clinical findings, interpretation use, barriers to antenatal access, decision-making)?

Q10: *Professional practice*: What debrief/support would you access after a perinatal loss call to protect clinician wellbeing?

Reflective questions for learners

Q1: How might language barriers and digital exclusion shape risk, help-seeking, and trust during maternity emergencies?

Q2: What could unintentionally increase trauma during pre-hospital care (rushed explanations, euphemisms, lack of choice), and how would you avoid this?

Q3: How do you balance time-critical clinical actions with dignity, privacy, and family needs following pregnancy loss?

Q4: What helps you stay compassionate and grounded in emotionally intense maternity calls?

Teaching commentary

This chapter supports learners to manage pre-hospital maternity emergencies using structured assessment (PMDT) while maintaining trauma-informed, culturally safe practice. Zara's case highlights pregnancy loss, communication barriers, and the clinical risks of retained placenta, requiring clinicians to balance time-critical maternal safety with bereavement care and dignity. Teaching should emphasise avoiding NEWS2 in perinatal patients, recognising subtle deterioration, using professional interpretation (not children), and documenting clinical and contextual factors including barriers to antenatal access. The chapter also reinforces awareness of perinatal mental health emergencies (including postpartum psychosis) and the importance of debriefing and psychological safety for clinicians following traumatic events.

References

Acosta, L. (2024). Antepartum haemorrhage, in M. Boyle (ed.) *Emergencies Around Childbirth: A handbook for midwives* (pp. 57–70). London: Routledge.

Arnold, L., Völkel, M., Rosendahl, J., and Rost, M. (2025). A multi-level meta-analysis of the relationship between decision-making during birth and postpartum mental health. *Health Psychology and Behavioral Medicine, 13*(1), 2456032. https://doi.org/10.1080/21642850.2025.2456032

Backes, C.H., Hill, K.D., Shelton, E.L., Slaughter, J.L., Lewis, T.R., Weisz, D.E., et al. (2022). Patent ductus arteriosus: A contemporary perspective for the pediatric and adult cardiac care provider. *Journal of the American Heart Association, 11*, e025784. https://doi.org/10.1161/JAHA.122.025784

Baptie, G., Andrade, J., Bacon, A.M., and Norman, A. (2020). Birth trauma: The mediating effects of perceived support. *British Journal of Midwifery, 28*(10), 724–730. https://doi.org/10.12968/bjom.2020.28.10.724

Benton, M., Wittkowski, A., Edge, D., Reid, H.E., Quigley, T., Sheikh, Z., et al. (2024). Best practice recommendations for the integration of trauma-informed approaches in maternal mental health care within the context of perinatal trauma and loss: A systematic review of current guidance. *Midwifery, 131*, 103949. https://doi.org/10.1016/j.midw.2024.103949

Berry, S.N. (2022). The trauma of perinatal loss: A scoping review. *Trauma Care, 2*, 392–407. https://doi.org/10.3390/traumacare2030032

Berry, S.N., Winsor, T., and Huene, L. (2023). A proposed framework for perinatal loss trauma informed care. *Journal of Neonatal Nursing, 29*(6), 916–921. https://doi.org/10.1016/j.jnn.2023.08.004

Boyle, M. (ed.) (2024). *Emergencies Around Childbirth: A handbook for midwives*. London: Routledge.

British Association of Perinatal Medicine (BAPM) (2026). *Perinatal management of extreme preterm birth before 27 weeks of gestation*. https://www.bapm.org/resources/perinatal-management-of-extreme-preterm-birth-before-27-weeks-of-gestation (accessed 20 August 2025).

Bryant, A., Mhyre, J.M., Leffert, L.R., Hoban, R.A., Yakoob, M.Y., and Bateman, B.T. (2012). The association of maternal race and ethnicity and the risk of postpartum hemorrhage. *Anesthesia and Analgesia, 115*(5), 1127–1136. https://doi.org/10.1213/ANE.0b013e3182691e62

Carfoot, S., Williamson, P., and Dickson, R. (2005). A randomised controlled trial in the north of England examining the effects of skin-to-skin care on breast feeding. *Midwifery, 21*(1), 71–79. https://doi.org/10.1016/j.midw.2004.09.002

Chainarong, N., Deevongkij, K., and Petpichetchian, C. (2022). Secondary postpartum hemorrhage: Incidence, etiologies, and clinical courses in the setting of a high cesarean delivery rate. *PLoS One, 17*(3), e0264583. https://doi.org/10.1371/journal.pone.0264583

Chakkarapani, A.A., Roehr, C.C., Hooper, S.B., te Pas, A.B., and Gupta, S. (2024). Transitional circulation and hemodynamic monitoring in newborn infants. *Pediatric Research, 96*(3), 595–603. https://doi.org/10.1038/s41390-022-02427-8

Di Martino, D.D., Sabattini, E., Parasiliti, M., Viscioni, L., Zaccone, E., Cerri, S., et al. (2025). Exploring new predictors for hypertensive disorders of pregnancy. *Best Practice and Research Clinical Obstetrics and Gynaecology, 100*, 102598. https://doi.org/10.1016/j.bpobgyn.2025.102598

Donnellan, D., Moore, Z., Patton, D., O'Connor, T., and Nugent, L. (2020). The effect of thermoregulation quality improvement initiatives on the admission temperature of premature/very low birth-weight infants in neonatal intensive care units: A systematic review. *Journal for Specialists in Pediatric Nursing, 25*(2), e12286. https://doi.org/10.1111/jspn.12286

Dumas, L., Lepage, M., Bystrova, K., Matthiesen, A-S., Welles-Nyström, B., and Widström, A-M. (2013). Influence of skin-to-skin contact and rooming-in on early mother–infant interaction: A randomized controlled trial. *Clinical Nursing Research, 22* (3), 310–336. https://doi.org/10.1177/1054773812468316

Elser, H., Mumford, S.L., Grantz, K.L., Pollack, A.Z., Mendola, P., Mills, J.L., et al.. (2025). Postpartum haemorrhage and long-term mortality. *Paediatric and Perinatal Epidemiology, 39*(3), 244–253. https://doi.org/10.1111/ppe.13166

Escobar, M.F., Nassar, A.H., Theron, G., Barnea, E.R., Nicholson, W., Ramasauskaite, D., et al. (2022). FIGO recommendations on the management of postpartum hemorrhage 2022. *International Journal of Gynecology and Obstetrics, 157*(suppl. 1), 3–50. https://doi.org/10.1002/ijgo.14116

Felker, A., Patel, R., Kotnis, R., Kanyon, S., and Knight, M. (eds.) (2024). *Saving Lives, Improving Mothers' Care: Lessons learned to inform maternity care from the UK and Ireland Confidential Enquiries into Maternal Deaths and Morbidity 2020–22.* Oxford: National Perinatal Epidemiology Unit, University of Oxford. https://www.npeu.ox.ac.uk/mbrrace-uk/reports/maternal-reports/maternal-report-2020-2022 (accessed 20 August 2025).

Findlay, H.J., Anderson, J.K., Francis, K.L., Clegg, L.M., and Maria, S.J. (2024). The significance of paramedic communication during women's birth experiences: A scoping review, *Australasian Emergency Care, 27*(3), 218–226. https://doi.org/10.1016/j.auec.2024.04.002

Flanagan, B., Lord, B., Reed, R., and Crimmins, G. (2019). Women's experience of unplanned out-of-hospital birth in paramedic care. *BioMed Central Emergency Medicine, 19*(1), 54. https://doi.org/10.1186/s12873-019-0267-9

Ford, J.. and Pett, G. (2008). 'BBA' birth: Analysis of one year's 'born before arrival' births (n = 29) and trends in BBA birth 2000–07 in a large English maternity unit. *MIDIRS Midwifery Digest, 18*(2), 217–223.

Gerry, S., Bedford, J., Redfern, O.C., Rutter, H., Chester-Jones, M., Knight, M., et al. (2024). Development of a national maternity early warning score: Centile based score development and Delphi informed escalation pathways. *BMJ Medicine, 3*, e000748. https://doi.org/10.1136/bmjmed-2023-000748

Ghosh, J., Papadopoulou, A., Devall, A.J., Jeffery, H.C., Beeson, L.E., Do, V., et al. (2021). Methods for managing miscarriage: A network meta-analysis. *Cochrane Database of Systematic Reviews, 6*, CD012602. https://doi.org/10.1002/14651858.CD012602.pub2

Goodwin, L., Hunter, B., and Jones, A. (2018). The midwife–woman relationship in a South Wales community: Experiences of midwives and migrant Pakistani women in early pregnancy. *Health Expectations, 21*(1), 347–357. https://doi.org/10.1111/hex.12629

Goodwin, L., Voss, S., McClelland, G., Beach, E., Bedson, A., Black, S., et al. (2022). Temperature measurement of babies born in the pre-hospital setting: Analysis of ambulance service data and qualitative interviews with paramedics. *Emergency Medicine Journal, 39*(11), 826–832. https://doi.org/10.1136/emermed-2021-211970

Graves, B.W., and Haley, M.M. (2013). Newborn transition. *Journal of Midwifery and Women's Health, 58*(6), 662–670. https://doi.org/10.1111/jmwh.12097

Heath, M., Hvass, A.M.F., and Wejse, C.M. (2023). Interpreter services and effect on healthcare: A systematic review of the impact of different types of interpreters on patient outcome. *Journal of Migration and Health, 7*, 100162. https://doi.org/10.1016/j.jmh.2023.100162

Hendriks, E., Rosenberg, R., and Prine, L. (2020). Ectopic pregnancy: Diagnosis and management. *American Family Physician, 101*(10), 599–606. PMID: 32412215.

Henriksen, L., Grimsrud, E., Schei, B., and Lukasse, M. (2017). Factors related to a negative birth experience: A mixed methods study. *Midwifery, 51*, 33–39. https://doi.org/10.1016/j.midw.2017.05.004

Hill, M., Miles, A., Flanagan, B., Hansen, S., Mills, B., and Hopper, L. (2025). Out-of-hospital births and the experiences of emergency ambulance clinicians and birthing parents: A scoping review of the literature. *BMJ Open, 15*, e086967. https://doi.org/10.1136/bmjopen-2024-086967

Human, M., Groenewald, C., Odendaal, H.J., Green, S., Goldstein, R.D., and Kinney, H.C. (2014). Psychosocial implications of stillbirth for the mother and her family: A crisis-support approach. *Social Work/Maatskaplike Werk, 50*(4). https://doi.org/10.15270/50-4-392

Jardine, J., Walker, K., Gurol-Urganci, I., Webster, K., Muller, P., Hawdon, J., et al., (2021). Adverse pregnancy outcomes attributable to socioeconomic and ethnic inequalities in England: A national cohort study. *The Lancet, 398*(10314), 1905–1912. https://doi.org/10.1016/S0140-6736(21)01595-6

Joint Royal Colleges Ambulance Liaison Committee (JRCALC) (2024). *JRCALC clinical guidelines update*, January. https://jrcalc.org.uk/publication-date-january-2024/ (accessed 11 December 2025).

Joint Royal Colleges Ambulance Liaison Committee (JRCALC) (2025). *JRCALC clinical guidelines update*, July. https://jrcalc.org.uk/publication-date-july-2025/ (accessed 11 December 2025).

Kiyak, S. (2024). The relationship of depression, anxiety, and stress with pregnancy symptoms and coping styles in pregnant women: A multi-group structural equation modeling analysis. *Midwifery, 136*, 104103. https://doi.org/10.1016/j.midw.2024.104103

Kramer, M.S., Dahhou, M., Vallerand, D., Liston, R., and Joseph, K.S. (2011). Risk factors for postpartum hemorrhage: Can we explain the recent temporal increase? *Journal of Obstetrics and Gynaecology Canada, 33*(8), 810–819. https://doi.org/10.1016/S1701-2163(16)34984-2

Li, X.L., Guo, P.L., Xue, Y., Gou, W.L., Tong, M., and Chen, Q. (2016). An analysis of the differences between early and late preeclampsia with severe hypertension. *Pregnancy Hypertension: An International Journal of Women's Cardiovascular Health, 6*(1), 47–52. https://doi.org/10.1016/j.preghy.2015.12.003

Linton, S. (2025). Why are black women still more likely to die in childbirth? *British Medical Journal, 388*, r226. https://doi.org/10.1136/bmj.r226

Loughney, A., Collis, R., and Dastgir, S. (2006). Birth before arrival at delivery suite: Associations and consequences. *British Journal of Midwifery, 14*(4), 204–208. https://doi.org/10.12968/bjom.2006.14.4.20786

Marin Gabriel, M.A., Llana Martin, I., Lopez Escobar, A., Fernandez Villalba, E., Romero Blanco, I., and Touza Pol, P. (2010). Randomized controlled trial of early skin-to-skin contact: Effects on the mother and the newborn. *Acta Paediatrica, 99*(11), 1630–1634. https://doi.org/10.1111/j.1651-2227.2009.01597.x

Marshall, J.E., and Raynor, M.D. (eds.) (2020). *Myles Textbook for Midwives* (17th edition). Amsterdam: Elsevier.

Marx, W., Penninx, B.W.J.H., Solmi, M., Furukawa, T.A., Firth, J., Carvalho, A.F., et al. (2023). Major depressive disorder. *Nature Reviews Disease Primers, 9*, 44. https://doi.org/10.1038/s41572-023-00454-1

Mavrides, E., Allard, S., Chandraharan, E., Collins, P., Green, L., Hunt, B.J., et al., on behalf of the Royal College of Obstetricians and Gynaecologists (2016). Prevention and management of postpartum haemorrhage. *BJOG: An International Journal of Obstetrics and Gynaecology, 124*, e106–e149. https://doi.org/10.1111/1471-0528.14178

MBRRACE (2024). *The Ectopic Pregnancy Trust's statement on the MBRRACE-UK 2024 report.* https://ectopic.org.uk/blog/the-epts-statement-on-the-mbrrace-uk-report-2024 (accessed 25 November 2025).

McClelland, G., Burrow, E., and McAdam, H. (2019). Babies born in the pre-hospital setting attended by ambulance clinicians in the north east of England. *British Paramedic Journal, 4*(3), 43–48. https://doi.org/10.29045/14784726.2019.12.4.3.43

McLelland, G., McKenna, L., Morgans, A., and Smith, K. (2018). Epidemiology of unplanned out-of-hospital births attended by paramedics. *BMC Pregnancy and Childbirth, 18*, 15. https://doi.org/10.1186/s12884-017-1638-4

McLelland, G.E., Morgans, A.E., and McKenna, L.G. (2014). Involvement of emergency medical services at unplanned births before arrival to hospital: A structured review. *Emergency Medicine Journal, 31*, 345–350. https://emj.bmj.com/content/31/4/345

Nakimuli, A., Jasper, B.A., Nakubulwa, S., Adroma, M., Akello, J., Namagembe, I., et al. (2025). Risk factors associated with progression from pre-eclampsia to eclampsia: A prospective cohort study and population-wide data analysis. *Acta Obstetricia et Gynecologica Scandinavica, 104*(8), 1487–1495. https://doi.org/10.1111/aogs.15154

National Institute for Health and Care Excellence (NICE) (2023a). *Ectopic pregnancy and miscarriage: Diagnosis and initial management* (NG126). London: NICE. https://www.nice.org.uk/guidance/ng126 (accessed 11 December 2025).

National Institute for Health and Care Excellence (NICE) (2023b). *Hypertension in pregnancy: Diagnosis and management* (NG133). London: NICE. https://www.nice.org.uk/guidance/ng133 (accessed 25 November 2025).

O'Donnell, C.P.F., Kamlin, C.O., Davis, P.G., Carlin, J.B., and Morley, C.J. (2007). Clinical assessment of infant colour at delivery. *Archives of Disease in Childhood: Fetal and Neonatal Edition, 92*, F465–F467. https://doi.org/10.1136/adc.2007.120634

Resuscitation Council UK (RCUK) (2025). *Newborn resuscitation and support of transition of infants at birth guidelines.* https://www.resus.org.uk/professional-library/2025-resuscitation-guidelines/newborn-resuscitation-and-support-transition-infants-birth (accessed 25 November 2025).

Royal College of Obstetricians and Gynaecologists (RCOG) (2011). *Antepartum haemorrhage.* https://www.rcog.org.uk/guidance/browse-all-guidance/green-top-guidelines/antepartum-haemorrhage-green-top-guideline-no-63/ (accessed 25 November 2025).

Royal College of Obstetricians and Gynaecologists (RCOG) (2015). *Reducing the risk of thrombosis and embolism during pregnancy and the puerperium.* https://www.rcog.org.uk/guidance/browse-all-guidance/green-top-guidelines/reducing-the-risk-of-thrombosis-and-embolism-during-pregnancy-and-the-puerperium-green-top-guideline-no-37a/ (accessed 25 November 2025).

Royal College of Obstetricians and Gynaecologists (RCOG) (2016). *Prevention and management of postpartum haemorrhage.* https://www.rcog.org.uk/guidance/browse-all-guidance/green-top-guidelines/prevention-and-management-of-postpartum-haemorrhage-green-top-guideline-no-52/ (accessed 25 November 2025).

Ruiz, M.T., Azevedo, N.F., Raponi, M.B.G., Fonseca, L.M.M., Wernet, M., Silva, M.P.C., et al. (2023). Skin-to-skin contact in the third stage of labor and postpartum hemorrhage prevention: A scoping review. *Maternal and Child Health Journal, 27*, 582–596. https://doi.org/10.1007/s10995-022-03582-4

SANDS (2021). *Sands Bereavement Support Book.* https://www.sands.org.uk/support bereavement-support/sands-bereavement-support-book (accessed 25 November 2025).

Smith, L., Ortega, M., and Whitley, A.G. (2025). Ambulance clinicians' preparedness for unplanned pre-hospital childbirth: A rapid evidence review. *British Paramedic Journal, 10*(1), 47–55. https://doi.org/10.29045/14784726.2025.6.10.1.47

Sotiropoulos, J., Kapadia, V., Ramachandran, S., and Oei, J.L. (2022). Ten minutes to save a baby: A narrative review of newborn assessment during first minutes of life and relationship to outcomes. *Pediatric Medicine, 5.* https://doi.org/10.21037/pm-21-84

Thornton, C.E., and Dahlen, H.G. (2018). Born before arrival in NSW, Australia (2000–2011): A linked population data study of incidence, location, associated factors and maternal and neonatal outcomes. *BMJ Open, 8*, e019328. https://doi.org/10.1136/bmjopen-2017-019328

Ubom, A.E., Muslim, Z., Beyeza-Kashesya, J., Schlembach, D., Malel, Z.J., Begum, F., et al. (2025). Postpartum hemorrhage: Findings of a global survey by the World Association of Trainees in Obstetrics and Gynecology (WATOG). *International Journal of Gynaecology and Obstetrics, 171*(2), 593–600. https://doi.org/10.1002/ijgo.70512

Widström, A., Brimdyr, K., Svensson, K., Cadwell, K., and Nissen, E. (2019). Skin-to-skin contact the first hour after birth, underlying implications and clinical practice. *Acta Paediatrica, 108*(7), 1192–1204. https://doi.org/10.1111/apa.14754

World Health Organization (WHO) (2012). *WHO recommendations for the prevention and treatment of postpartum haemorrhage.* https://www.who.int/publications/i/item/9789241548502 (accessed 11 December 2025).

6 Women's health and wellbeing: Gendered care needs

Jane-Louise Reid and Yuet Wah Patrick

Introduction

Women's health within the pre-hospital and paramedic context encompasses a broad spectrum of acute, urgent, and complex presentations shaped by interactions between biological sex, gendered social structures, and persistent inequities in healthcare research and delivery. Epidemiological evidence demonstrates that women experience diagnostic delays and poorer outcomes across numerous conditions due to the historic prioritisation of male physiological baselines in clinical research and guideline development (Criado Perez, 2019; Mauvais-Jarvis et al., 2020). Cardiovascular data illustrate this clearly, as women are more likely to present with atypical symptoms during myocardial infarction, increasing the risk of non-recognition by both patients and healthcare professionals (Hsu et al., 2021). The consequences of non-recognition in the pre-hospital setting include prolonged delays, reduced adherence to protocol-driven treatment, and higher mortality rates (MINAP, 2025). These disparities persist in part because female-specific manifestations of acute coronary syndromes remain under-represented in the evidence guiding practice (Pompei et al., 2024).

Similar inequities extend to other health domains, including oncology and musculoskeletal disease, where rising breast cancer incidence and the high burden of osteoporosis and arthritis significantly shape women's long-term health trajectories (Cancer Research UK, 2023). Paramedics, as the first point of clinical contact, play a critical role in mitigating these inequities through early recognition, gender-informed clinical reasoning, and trauma-informed communication (McLelland et al., 2016; Withanarachchie et al., 2025). The gender health gap in the UK reflects long-standing inequalities in healthcare access and outcomes, with women reporting higher morbidity but experiencing delayed diagnosis and unmet healthcare needs (NHS Digital, 2022; Jeffrey, 2025). As women age, particularly beyond 40, multi-morbidity becomes increasingly prevalent and is associated with reduced functional capacity, poorer quality of life, and higher rates of depression and anxiety (Skou et al., 2022).

These inequities are amplified for women from lower socioeconomic and marginalised backgrounds and may contribute to hesitancy in seeking emergency care, particularly when women report feeling unheard or dismissed during healthcare encounters (NIHR, 2022; Pompei et al., 2024).

This chapter aims to provide a comprehensive, evidence-informed exploration of women's health within pre-hospital care. It synthesises current literature and UK guidance to highlight epidemiological patterns, physiological considerations, trauma-informed assessment strategies, and implications for clinical practice. Through discussion of common presentations, integrated assessment frameworks, and a detailed case study, the chapter seeks to support paramedics, educators, and students in delivering safe, equitable, and person-centred care for women experiencing acute health crises. By focusing on gender-specific evidence and drawing attention to areas where knowledge remains incomplete, the chapter supports the ongoing development of pre-hospital care that more effectively meets the needs of women throughout their lives.

Common women's health conditions encountered in pre-hospital care

Women access ambulance services for a wide range of emergency presentations that intersect physiological, reproductive, psychological, and social domains. Paramedics must therefore draw upon an integrated understanding of women's health that encompasses both gender-specific pathology and gendered influences on symptom reporting and access to care. Many of the conditions described in this section are under-represented within paramedic education and training or are complicated by atypical presentation patterns, making awareness essential for accurate and timely management.

Gynaecological emergencies

Gynaecological emergencies commonly present with acute pelvic pain, abdominal pain, bleeding, dizziness, collapse, or signs of sepsis. Although often perceived as complex or anxiety-provoking due to concerns around intimate examination and unfamiliarity, these presentations require methodical assessment and trauma-informed communication.

Ovarian torsion

Ovarian torsion occurs when the ovary rotates on its ligamentous axis, compromising blood flow and causing acute, severe unilateral pelvic pain with nausea and vomiting (Baron and Mathai, 2023). The condition is frequently misinterpreted as renal colic or appendicitis, leading to potential delays in surgical intervention. Since ovarian viability diminishes rapidly once arterial flow is compromised, prompt recognition and expedited transport are key. Paramedics are encouraged to avoid downplaying pain severity, deliver timely and appropriate analgesia, and keep a broad diagnostic perspective when symptoms overlap (Bedekar et al., 2025).

Ovarian cyst rupture may present with variable pain intensity, signs of peritoneal irritation, and in some cases, haemodynamic changes if intra-abdominal bleeding occurs (Lim et al., 2022). Paramedics should exercise caution when interpreting apparently stable observations, as significant pathology can be present despite normal vitals. Management focuses on analgesia, supportive care, and close monitoring for deterioration. Peritoneal involvement is suggested by features such as rebound tenderness, involuntary guarding, abdominal rigidity, and pain exacerbated by movement, percussion, or coughing. Systemic indicators, including tachycardia, hypotension, fever, or altered consciousness, may reflect evolving sepsis or haemorrhage.

Pelvic inflammatory disease

Pelvic inflammatory disease (PID) involves ascending infection of the uterus, fallopian tubes, and ovaries, resulting in pelvic pain, fever, abnormal discharge, and deep dyspareunia. Shame or fear of judgement may impede disclosure of sexual history, thus a trauma-informed, non-judgemental approach supports more accurate assessment. Paramedics should screen for sepsis, provide appropriate analgesia and antiemetics, and facilitate urgent referral for antibiotic therapy whenever PID is suspected, particularly in the presence of red-flag features such as severe clinical illness, pregnancy, vomiting, or suspicion of tubo-ovarian abscess (NICE, 2018).

Endometriosis

Endometriosis is a chronic systemic inflammatory condition characterised by ectopic endometrial tissue growth, severe dysmenorrhoea, pain crises, nausea, vomiting, and sometimes syncope. Women with endometriosis frequently report years of disbelief or inadequate pain management within healthcare encounters, making validation critical to building trust. Acute exacerbations may mimic appendicitis, torsion, or ectopic pregnancy, requiring careful assessment and the avoidance of anchoring bias.

Dysmenorrhoea

Primary dysmenorrhoea involves painful menstruation in the absence of pathology, while secondary dysmenorrhoea results from underlying conditions such as fibroids, adenomyosis, or endometriosis. Severe cases can lead to hyperventilation, vasovagal episodes, or vomiting. Best practice requires the paramedic to distinguish between benign menstrual pain and pain indicating acute pathology. Supportive communication and analgesia are central to care.

Menopause and perimenopause

Perimenopause may begin several years before menopause and is associated with hormonal fluctuations affecting the cardiovascular system, thermoregulation, mood, the pattern of sleep, and cognition. Symptoms include palpitations, chest discomfort, dizziness, anxiety, panic, hot flushes, and 'brain fog'. These presentations often mimic acute coronary syndromes (ACS), arrhythmias, respiratory disease, dehydration, or anxiety disorders (NICE, 2024).

Paramedics should refrain from prematurely attributing symptoms solely to menopause but recognise that perimenopause increases cardiovascular risk that may amplify the severity or perception of other health issues. Sensitive communication and reassurance, combined with appropriate clinical caution, support accuracy and reduce distress.

Mental health and psychosocial crises

Women are disproportionately affected by anxiety and depressive disorders, particularly between the ages 45 of 54. Emergency presentations may reflect acute psychological distress, chronic stress, trauma, perimenopausal symptoms, or the cumulative burden of caregiving responsibilities. Symptoms often include hyperventilation, chest tightness, dizziness, non-cardiac chest pain, or dissociative sensations, which can complicate differentiation from cardiopulmonary disease.

Women experiencing domestic abuse or coercive control may present with vague or somatic symptoms, reluctance to speak freely, or inconsistent histories. The paramedic is encouraged to create opportunities for private conversation, use non-leading questions, and document disclosures carefully. Trauma-informed principles of safety, choice, collaboration, trust, and empowerment are essential in these encounters.

Cardiovascular disease

Cardiovascular disease (CVD) is the leading cause of mortality in women. Women often present with non-classic ACS symptoms such as fatigue, nausea, dyspnoea, or discomfort in the jaw, back, or epigastric region (Pompei et al., 2024). Risk factors, such as diabetes, obesity, and menopause-related endothelial changes, further complicate presentation (NICE, 2024). Failure to recognise atypical ACS contributes to delayed treatment and increased morbidity. Effective care depends on the paramedic's ability to maintain a low threshold for ECG acquisition and escalation.

Cancer-related complications

Women with cancer may present with sepsis, neutropenia, pathological fractures, spinal cord compression, airway compromise, pain crises, or complications from chemotherapy or endocrine therapy. Rapid recognition and pre-alerting are essential, particularly for neutropenic sepsis, a time-critical emergency (Cancer Research UK, 2023).

Breast cancer is the most common form of cancer in women and its diagnosis and treatment can have a profound psychological impact on the woman's wellbeing. Survivors of breast cancer are more likely to experience severe symptoms of anxiety and depression for at least 10 years after diagnosis (Maass et al., 2019).

Musculoskeletal and bone health

Osteoporosis is highly prevalent among post-menopausal women and substantially increases the risk of fragility fractures. Women experience a markedly higher incidence of neck of femur fractures than men, with international epidemiological data demonstrating that hip fractures occur approximately two to three times more frequently in women due to lower bone mineral density and accelerated post-menopausal bone loss (International Osteoporosis Foundation, 2023). Falls may result in hip fractures, vertebral collapse, or impaired mobility. Best practice requires the paramedic to employ gentle handling techniques, provide adequate analgesia, and consider safeguarding concerns in frail or isolated women.

Prognosis after hip fractures is poor with a global mortality rate of 22% (Downey et al., 2019). After a hip fracture, individuals commonly experience diminished functional status, reduced social autonomy, and impaired mobility, accompanied by an increase in depressive symptoms, most notably during the first year after the injury (Swayambunathan et al., 2021).

Clinical presentation and pre-hospital assessment

Assessment of women's health presentations in the pre-hospital environment demands a synthesis of physiological knowledge, trauma-informed communication, clinical reasoning, and an awareness of gender-specific symptom patterns. Women's presentations are often subtle, atypical, or complicated by psychological or social dimensions. Paramedics must therefore adopt a blended approach that integrates structured assessment with sensitivity to context and lived experience, recognising that conventional clinical heuristics may not align with women's symptoms and disease patterns. This section outlines key principles and adaptations relevant to assessing women in emergency settings, emphasising both the technical and relational components of care.

The importance of trauma-informed assessment

A trauma-informed assessment recognises that many women have experienced previous medical, psychological, physical, or sexual trauma that may influence their reactions to emergency encounters (Molloy et al., 2020). Flashbacks, fear, shame, or dissociation may be triggered by intimate questioning, physical touch, exposure of the body, or perceived loss of control. Trauma-informed practice does not alter clinical priorities but enhances them by maximising patient cooperation, improving the accuracy of information, and enhancing safety.

Trauma-informed communication begins with establishing psychological safety. This includes explaining each step of the assessment, seeking permission before touching or exposing any part of the body, and offering choices where possible, such as whether a support person is present or whether assessment occurs sitting or lying. Women who have previously felt dismissed or disbelieved may also require additional reassurance that their symptoms are legitimate and deserving of care (Molloy et al., 2020). These practices support rapport building, reduce distress, and create a collaborative atmosphere that enhances clinical reasoning. Paramedics support patient wellbeing when they are aware that women experiencing acute physiological symptoms may also simultaneously experience emotional triggers unrelated to the immediate pathology, and sensitivity to this interaction is central to trauma-informed assessment (NICE, 2019).

Recognising key signs and symptoms in women's emergency presentations

Women frequently exhibit different symptom clusters than men for several high-risk emergency conditions. For example, in acute coronary syndromes (ACS), women may present with dyspnoea, nausea, fatigue, indigestion-like discomfort, jaw pain, or back pain rather than classic chest pain. These atypical patterns contribute to misdiagnosis and delayed intervention, reinforcing the need for heightened vigilance among paramedics. Diabetes, obesity, and menopausal status may further obscure ACS presentation by blunting pain perception or modifying autonomic responses. A thorough history and repeated physiological observations are critical to identifying deterioration.

Gynaecological red flags, such as sudden severe pelvic pain, abnormal bleeding, fever with adnexal tenderness, or pain disproportionate to findings, require paramedics to consider torsion, ectopic pregnancy, cyst rupture, or pelvic inflammatory disease. Many of these symptoms overlap with non-gynaecological conditions, including renal colic or appendicitis, requiring broad differential reasoning.

Menopause-related presentations commonly include palpitations, dizziness, hot flushes, anxiety, shifts in mood, and difficulties with clear thinking (NICE, 2024). These symptoms can mimic arrhythmias, panic attacks, hypoglycaemia, or respiratory distress and require careful differentiation. Paramedics ought to minimise anchoring prematurely on 'anxiety' without ruling out physical causes.

Mental health presentations also require a focused assessment. Panic attacks, hyperventilation, dissociative symptoms, and acute distress may be precipitated by psychosocial stressors, hormonal fluctuations, or trauma triggers. Clinical guidance recommends that the paramedic will assess risk of self-harm, suicidal ideation, and safeguarding concerns, particularly in women experiencing coercive control or domestic abuse.

An adapted ABCDE framework for women's health

While the ABCDE model remains the cornerstone of paramedic assessment, gender-specific adaptations enhance its utility in women's health emergencies.

A – Airway: Women generally have smaller airway diameters than men of similar body size, increasing the risk of airway resistance and difficulty during ventilation or intubation (Mann et al., 2021). They also experience a higher prevalence of conditions that reduce cervical mobility, such as rheumatoid arthritis, autoimmune disease, and metastatic involvement, as well as greater susceptibility to radiation-related airway changes. Obesity, which affects women more than men in many populations, further narrows the upper airway and reduces respiratory reserve. Paramedics should therefore anticipate increased airway difficulty in women presenting with sepsis, anaphylaxis, cancer-related disease, or trauma, while communicating in a manner sensitive to discomfort, fear, or prior trauma (American Heart Association, 2020).

B – Breathing: Women experience breathlessness from a wide differential, and anxiety may co-exist with or obscure serious pathology. Anaemia arising from heavy menstrual bleeding or fibroids can lead to tachypnoea and fatigue, while pulmonary embolism risk is elevated in women using hormonal contraception, undergoing fertility treatment, or experiencing perimenopausal prothrombotic changes. Paramedics should balance reassurance with clinical vigilance, avoiding premature attribution of breathlessness to psychological causes.

C – Circulation: Women have higher rates of atypical ACS presentations and are at greater risk of underdiagnosis, with additional risk modifiers linked to hormonal transitions across the life span. Early ECG acquisition is recommended, even without chest pain, alongside comparison with previous traces where available (Byrne et al., 2023). Concealed haemorrhage from gynaecological causes, postpartum complications, or ruptured ovarian cysts warrants careful circulatory assessment; sepsis related to PID, cancer therapy, or urinary infections may present subtly (NICE, 2020).

D – Disability: Neurological assessment should integrate awareness of sex-linked conditions such as migraine (which is more prevalent in women), autoimmune diseases including lupus and multiple sclerosis, and hormonal influences that may exacerbate neurological symptoms. Emotional distress or cognitive fog may complicate evaluation but should not be assumed psychological until organic causes have been excluded.

E – Exposure: Exposure requires balancing clinical necessity with dignity, cultural sensitivity, and explicit consent. Paramedics should recognise key clinical findings such as bruising patterns, surgical scars, drainage devices, ports, lymphoedema, or indicators of metastatic disease. Consent is fundamental when exposing intimate areas, and alternative strategies should be offered where appropriate.

Focused history-taking in women's emergencies

History-taking is a core clinical skill that requires expanded domains when assessing women, with attention to menstrual, hormonal, and reproductive factors that may shape presentation. Sensitive health history-taking should be patient-centred, culturally aware, and trauma-informed to ensure accurate disclosure and safe care. Paramedics should prioritise privacy, confidentiality, and rapport, explaining the purpose and voluntary nature of sensitive questions whilst respecting patient autonomy throughout the encounter. Creating an environment built on respect and trust is essential for facilitating open discussion, particularly about personal or intimate subjects such as sexual health, experiences of trauma, and intimate partner violence, which are common yet often under-addressed aspects of women's health history (WHO, 2014). Effective practice includes using neutral, open-ended questions to avoid judgement or assumptions, and being mindful of language that may cause discomfort or inhibit disclosure. For example, guidance on sexual history-taking emphasises starting with permission statements and avoiding assumptions about sexual behaviour, orientation, or relationship status to gain trust and reduce stigma.

Culturally sensitive history-taking is a critical component of high-quality health care that ensures paramedics actively recognise and respond to the diverse cultural backgrounds, values, and communication preferences of patients, particularly women from minority cultural groups. It involves paramedics becoming aware of their own cultural beliefs and biases and adapting their communication styles and questioning to respect patients' cultural worldviews and health beliefs, rather than assuming a one-size-fits-all approach to care (Brooks et al., 2019). Culturally sensitive communication incorporates not only linguistic competence such as the use of interpreters or culturally appropriate language but also adaptive questioning that recognises cultural differences in beliefs in health and illness and expectations of care. This approach helps to avoid misinterpretations, build rapport, and gain more accurate and meaningful patient histories. Strategies include asking patients about their personal explanations for illnesses, their preferred treatments, and any traditional or community health practices that might influence care, promoting shared understanding and trust.

In women's health, culturally sensitive history-taking also requires sensitivity to gender-specific cultural norms around modesty, roles within the family, and community expectations. Evidence indicates that ethnic minority women may experience barriers to accessing care when cultural nuances are not understood, and that culturally adapted approaches can improve engagement, satisfaction, and health outcomes (Gardner et al., 2024).

Overall, culturally sensitive history-taking is not merely about acquiring factual information; it is a relational process that honours patients' cultural identities, reduces bias, and enhances the accuracy and relevance of clinical histories, leading to improved health equity and personalised care (Kurtz et al., 2017). Throughout, documentation must remain factual, objective, and free from inference, supporting clinical reasoning while respecting dignity and autonomy.

Integrating UK guidelines into assessment

In addition to 'Working Together to Safeguard Children' (HM Government, 2018) and the Domestic Abuse Act 2021, several safeguarding frameworks guide risk identification and referral pathways for women. The Care Act 2014 establishes statutory duties for adult safeguarding, particularly for women at risk of abuse, neglect, coercion, or exploitation. Multi-Agency Risk Assessment Conferences (MARAC) and Multi-Agency Public Protection Arrangements (MAPPA) provide coordinated responses for individuals experiencing high-risk domestic abuse or those threatened by high-risk offenders. Legislative protections, such as the Female Genital Mutilation Mandatory Reporting Duty (Serious Crime Act 2015), the Modern Slavery Act 2015, with its National Referral Mechanism, and the Forced Marriage (Civil Protection) Act 2007, extend safeguarding to women affected by culturally specific or criminally driven harm. National strategies such as the 'Violence Against Women and Girls' (VAWG) Strategy (HM Government, 2021), alongside NICE guidance on safeguarding, domestic abuse, and trauma-informed practice, further strengthen multi-agency responsibilities and ensure that clinicians, including paramedics, can recognise vulnerability, respond safely, and facilitate timely referral (Health and Care Act 2022; NICE, 2016, 2018).

High-quality pre-hospital care involves the paramedic recognising that women remain underrepresented in validation studies for many diagnostic tools and guidelines, requiring caution in interpretation (Pompei et al., 2024).

Summary of assessment principles

Effective assessment in women's health emergencies requires:

- Integration of physiological and psychosocial reasoning.
- Avoidance of diagnostic bias and minimisation of symptoms.
- Trauma-informed communication at all stages.
- Consistent use of guidelines with awareness of their limitations.
- Careful documentation and patient involvement in decision-making.

These principles support equitable, person-centred, and clinically robust pre-hospital care.

Case study: A women's health emergency

Case study: Narrative

A 47-year-old woman, Sarah, calls 999 late in the evening reporting sudden palpitations, chest tightness, breathlessness, and a profound sense of impending doom. Her voice is shaky, her breathing rapid, and she states that she 'feels like something terrible is happening'. The call handler dispatches a Category 2 ambulance due to concerns about potential ACS or respiratory compromise. Sarah lives alone and has no documented cardiac history. She notes increased stress over recent months and describes deteriorating sleep, irregular menstrual cycles, intermittent hot flushes, and escalating anxiety.

Initial paramedic assessment

Upon arrival, the paramedic crew finds Sarah seated on the floor, leaning against the sofa, trembling and visibly distressed. She is hyperventilating, tearful, and repeatedly apologising for calling the ambulance. This apologetic behaviour is common among women who fear their symptoms will be dismissed or perceived as non-urgent. Establishing psychological safety is the first priority.

ABCDE assessment

Airway: Sarah's airway is patent. No signs of obstruction or stridor are present.

Breathing: Her respiratory rate is elevated at 28 breaths per minute. Breathing is shallow and rapid, but she is able to complete short sentences. No other abnormalities are noted. Hyperventilation is likely but cannot be assumed. Differential diagnoses include ACS, pulmonary embolism, anxiety-related hyperventilation, anaemia, arrhythmia, or metabolic acidosis.

Circulation: Heart rate is 120bpm and regular. Blood pressure is 154/92mmHg. Her skin is warm and slightly diaphoretic. A 12-lead ECG demonstrates sinus tachycardia with no acute ischaemic changes.

Disability: Sarah is alert with a Glasgow Coma Scale score of 15. She describes tingling around her mouth and in her hands, a sensation frequently associated with low CO_2 levels during hyperventilation. She reports 'foggy thoughts' but no focal neurological deficits.

Exposure: She feels warm and flushed, consistent with vasomotor symptoms of perimenopause. No rashes, injuries, or visible signs of domestic violence are present. Her temperature is within normal limits.

Throughout this assessment, paramedics use trauma-informed communication: asking permission before touching, explaining each step, and providing clear reassurance that her concerns are being taken seriously. This approach improves cooperation, reduces distress, and strengthens diagnostic accuracy by enabling a more complete history (NICE, 2022; HM Government, 2023).

Focused history

The paramedic engages Sarah with calm, slow-paced questioning.

- *Symptom history*: She reports sudden onset palpitations, chest tightness, nausea, shaking, and a sensation of 'losing control'. Symptoms began while preparing for bed. She denies sharp chest pain, exertional triggers, or radiation, though such absences do not rule out ACS in women.
- *Psychosocial stressors*: She has been caring for an ageing parent, managing increased workload demands, and experiencing relational strain. She denies alcohol misuse and takes no recreational drugs.
- *Menstrual and reproductive history*: Periods have become irregular over the past year. She experiences hot flushes, night sweats, sleep disturbance, and fluctuating mood. She has not previously associated these symptoms with perimenopause.
- *Mental health background*: No diagnosed anxiety or depression, but she reports escalating worry and emotional instability over the last six months.

Clinical reasoning and differential diagnosis

Several time-critical conditions must be considered.

- *Thromboembolism* leading to *acute coronary syndrome* (ACS) or *pulmonary embolism*: Tachycardia, dyspnoea, and nausea are common symptoms of anxiety, but they are also symptomatic of ACS and of a pulmonary embolism, making pre-hospital diagnosis challenging, particularly due to the absence of testing facilities to detect changes in biomarkers in the pre-hospital setting.
- *Cardiac arrhythmia*: Sinus tachycardia currently present. Palpitations and fear may reflect adrenergic surge rather than cardiac pathology.
- *Anaemia*: Heavy menstrual bleeding sometimes associated with perimenopause could cause anaemia in severe circumstances. Symptoms of anaemia include tachycardia, palpitations, and dyspnoea, which is a similar presentation to anxiety.

Synthesis of objective clinical data, such as vital signs and ECG findings, with subjective indicators, including the person's emotional state, recent psychosocial stressors, and menstrual history, is necessary to formulate a comprehensive clinical assessment. This assessment should adopt a holistic approach that accounts for the complex interplay of physiological, psychological, and social factors contributing to the presentation. Anxiety, in particular, exhibits a complex relationship with physical health conditions, often obscuring symptom aetiology and complicating the differentiation between primary psychological distress and underlying medical pathology.

Management and intervention

Communication and de-escalation: The paramedic employs grounding interventions by delivering clear and structured instructions to guide and coach breathing with the aim of reducing physiological arousal and re-orienting Sarah to the present moment. Efforts are made to alleviate emotional distress through calm and supportive communication. Validating statements such as, '*Many people having strong physical sensations during hormonal changes can feel this way. You're not alone, and we are here to keep you safe*', reassures Sarah that what she is feeling is normal, creating a sense of safety, which in turn tells her that her symptoms and concerns are being taken seriously. This approach supports anxiety reduction while reinforcing person-centred care.

Clinical management:

- Repeat ECG to confirm no evolving ischaemic changes.
- Monitor vital signs for trend-based assessment.
- Encourage slow diaphragmatic breathing.
- Offer assistance to reduce hyperventilation-induced discomfort.
- Evaluate safeguarding concerns sensitively and privately.

As her chest symptoms are new, midlife-onset, and potentially cardiac in origin, conveyance is discussed.

Shared decision-making: Women often feel that they are not taken seriously and that their needs are misunderstood or are dismissed. Giving them a voice by listening to their concerns and making decisions based on their needs will restore their faith in health care and empower them to take control over their own health. In Sarah's case, it is not possible to rule out underlying medical causes for her symptoms, so conveyance to hospital for further investigation will validate her concerns and enforce patient trust.

Emergency department outcome

At hospital, Sarah undergoes blood tests, cardiac biomarkers, repeat ECGs, and chest imaging. All results are within normal limits. The emergency physician attributes her presentation to:

- perimenopausal hormonal fluctuations
- vasomotor instability
- stress-related autonomic arousal
- panic and hyperventilation episode

She receives a referral to her GP for menopause support, including potential hormone replacement therapy. She is given discharge advice on panic management and safety-netting regarding future cardiac symptoms. This underscores the profound impact of pre-hospital clinician behaviour on women's emotional wellbeing and trust in healthcare systems (NHS Digital, 2022; DHSC, 2022; NICE 2024).

Case study: Lessons

High-quality pre-hospital care for women relies on effective communication, empathy, cultural humility, and the ability to interpret symptoms within broader psychosocial contexts. Women's emergency presentations often include complex intersections between biology, trauma, chronic disease, and gendered expectations. Best practice frameworks, therefore, support paramedics in moving beyond narrow biomedical interpretations and looking to encompass the woman's experiences of events that led up to her medical emergency (Criado Perez, 2019; Mauvais-Jarvis et al., 2020; Skou et al., 2022; Jeffrey, 2025).

Communication is an essential component of clinical assessment, particularly in women's health where symptoms may be ambiguous, emotionally charged, or shaped by previous negative healthcare experiences. Women frequently report that their pain or distress has been dismissed or reframed as psychological, which can impair help-seeking behaviour and compromise engagement with healthcare professionals (Criado Perez, 2019; NHS Digital, 2022). Paramedics therefore play a pivotal role in disrupting these patterns by validating women's symptoms, actively listening, and avoiding language that minimises severity. Effective communication includes explaining procedures, seeking explicit consent before examination, using gender-sensitive terminology, and providing reassurance without prematurely attributing symptoms to anxiety. These practices create psychological safety, support more complete histories, and enhance diagnostic accuracy (Kurtz et al., 2017; Molloy et al., 2020).

Women continue to experience disparities in emergency diagnosis, pain management, and access to care. For example, women often wait longer for analgesia, are misdiagnosed more frequently during ACS episodes, and experience gaps in mental health support related to midlife transitions. These inequalities arise from implicit bias, male-centric clinical research, and inequitable access to healthcare resources. Best practice requires paramedics to adopt an equity-focused lens, widening differential diagnoses, considering atypical symptom patterns, and resisting assumptions about the emotional nature of women's presentations. Recognising that women may delay care because of caregiving responsibilities, fear of judgement, or cultural stigma supports more effective communication and safety-netting. In addition, limited awareness and understanding of women-specific conditions, including gynaecological disorders and perimenopause, contribute to a significant knowledge gap among both healthcare professionals and women themselves (NICE, 2024). This deficit can result in delayed recognition, misinterpretation of symptoms, and suboptimal management of these conditions (Pompei et al., 2024; Hsu et al., 2021; DHSC, 2022).

Women's health emergencies frequently intersect with vulnerability, including domestic abuse, coercive control, financial hardship, mental health crises, substance use disorders, chronic illness, and social isolation. Domestic abuse presentations may appear subtle: hesitation to speak, inconsistent histories, injuries inconsistent with mechanisms, or a partner who dominates conversation. Paramedics must create opportunities for private discussion, use non-leading questions, and be prepared for disclosures at unexpected moments. Compassionate, non-judgemental responses are critical, alongside appropriate safeguarding referrals and accurate documentation. For older women, frailty, cognitive impairment, or neglect may also underlie repeated emergency calls, requiring holistic assessment and consideration of social support needs (WHO, 2014; HM Government, 2021; Care Act 2014; Domestic Abuse Act 2021).

Women's emergency presentations often involve intimate histories, examinations, or safeguarding disclosures, making ethical clarity essential. Consent must be explicit, continuous, and informed. Women should understand why an examination is needed, what it entails, and their right to decline. Cultural and religious considerations may influence preferences regarding clinician gender or bodily exposure. Confidentiality is fundamental but not absolute; safeguarding concerns may require information-sharing in the patient's best interests. Paramedics should maintain professional boundaries to avoid overstepping into counselling or reassurance-seeking roles beyond their clinical remit. Clear, factual documentation is essential for continuity of care and legal protection (Kurtz et al., 2017; Brooks et al., 2019).

Future directions and challenges

The landscape of women's health within pre-hospital care is evolving rapidly. Persistent inequities, gaps in evidence, and a growing recognition of sex-specific needs underscore the importance of expanding paramedic education, refining clinical guidelines, and strengthening system-level integration. The future of women's health in emergency care will depend on the profession's ability to address long-standing deficits and embrace new opportunities for research, collaboration, and innovation.

Advancing paramedic education and workforce development

Current discussions in paramedic education highlight limited historical attention to sex-specific physiology, atypical ACS presentations, menopause, chronic pelvic pain, and trauma-informed approaches. Analytical reviews indicate that emerging curricula are beginning to incorporate evidence on cardiovascular risk variation, endocrine transitions, and chronic disease patterns relevant to women. Simulation-based learning is also being used to represent presentations such as perimenopausal anxiety resembling ACS, endometriosis pain crises, and cancer-related emergencies. Continuing professional development initiatives provide a mechanism for updating practitioners trained prior to gender-inclusive educational frameworks (Mauvais-Jarvis et al., 2020; DHSC, 2022; Pompei et al., 2024).

System-level integration and policy development

System analysis shows that women's emergency care often spans multiple services, including primary care, acute hospitals, mental health, oncology, gynaecology, and community organisations. Fragmentation across these sectors has been associated with delays and communication challenges. Telemedicine models such as real-time consultation with gynaecology or menopause specialists are being considered as potential mechanisms to support decision-making in pre-hospital settings. Policy documents, including the 'Women's Health Strategy for England' (DHSC, 2022), identify professional training, safeguarding, and recognition of women's symptoms as priority areas. Paramedic services are positioned within these frameworks as stakeholders able to contribute operational insight into service gaps and patterns of inequity (DHSC, 2022; HM Government, 2021).

Addressing research gaps

Analyses of the evidence base indicate continued underrepresentation of women in clinical trials informing ACS, sepsis, respiratory care, and analgesia guidance. Pre-hospital literature offers limited examination of perimenopause, despite its influence on symptom interpretation and healthcare utilisation. Further investigation is also required to understand how chronic conditions such as osteoporosis, diabetes, cancer, and autoimmune disease shape emergency presentations. Research focused on underserved groups including minoritised ethnic communities, migrants, and socioeconomically disadvantaged women remains limited. Although trauma-informed practice is frequently referenced, empirical evaluation in pre-hospital contexts is sparse. Paramedic-led studies using mixed-methods designs present opportunities to address these gaps (Criado Perez, 2019; Pompei et al., 2024; Skou et al., 2022).

The evolving role of paramedics

As paramedic practice continues to develop clinically and academically, discussions have emerged regarding potential roles linked to women's health. These include specialist women's health paramedics, community follow-up teams, and contributions to menopause-related urgent care pathways. Telehealth may also enable real-time links with gynaecology, sexual health, or mental health specialists. Paramedics' interface position between community and acute care provides opportunities for involvement in system-level developments relating to women's health (DHSC, 2022; Jeffrey, 2025).

Conclusion

Women's health in the pre-hospital environment is shaped by the complex interaction of biological sex, psychosocial factors, structural inequities, and multimorbidity. This chapter has demonstrated that women's emergency presentations frequently reflect a convergence of acute symptoms and chronic health burdens, influenced by endocrine transitions, cardiovascular risk, musculoskeletal vulnerability, cancer-related complications, and mental health conditions. These intersecting factors demand that paramedics integrate cross-disciplinary clinical knowledge with sensitivity to the lived realities of women's health. As frontline clinicians, paramedics are uniquely positioned to recognise atypical presentations, reduce diagnostic delay, and facilitate equitable, evidence-informed care at the earliest point of contact.

A central theme has been the persistence of diagnostic inequities affecting women. Symptoms associated with conditions such as acute coronary syndromes, chronic pelvic pain, and menopause are often subtle, variable, or misattributed to emotional causes, contributing to delays in recognition and treatment. Addressing this requires a gender-aware approach to clinical reasoning that challenges male-normed assumptions, incorporates sex-specific physiology, and prioritises careful exploration of non-classical symptom patterns. Such practice enhances diagnostic safety while upholding ethical principles of equity and inclusivity.

Trauma-informed care in emergency practice incorporates experiences of interpersonal violence, reproductive health events, medical trauma, and systemic marginalisation, which can significantly shape women's responses to acute illness and clinical encounters. Trauma-informed approaches, characterised by psychological safety, validation, and patient choice, support effective history-taking, reduce re-traumatisation, and build trust, ultimately improving clinical outcomes.

Future progress in women's pre-hospital health requires sustained investment in research, education, and system integration. Enhancing paramedic education, addressing women's underrepresentation in research, and strengthening links between urgent care and specialist services align with the 'Women's Health Strategy for England' (DHSC, 2022) and are essential to advancing equitable care. As the profession continues to evolve, paramedics hold significant potential to influence how women's health is recognised and respected across emergency care settings (Criado Perez, 2019; Mauvais-Jarvis et al., 2020; DHSC, 2022).

Further learning materials

Multiple-choice questions

MCQ1: *Gender health gap*: Which factor most strongly contributes to diagnostic delay and poorer outcomes for women in emergency care?

A. Women experience fewer acute illnesses than men

B. Female physiology is always represented in clinical trials

C. Male baselines have historically shaped research and guidelines

D. Women present with identical symptoms to men

Correct answer: C

Rationale: Male-centric evidence and assumptions contribute to missed or delayed recognition in women.

MCQ2: *Atypical ACS presentation*: Which symptom cluster should raise concern for ACS in women even without 'classic' chest pain?

A. Fatigue, nausea, and dyspnoea

B. Localised rib pain on palpation

C. Itchy rash and wheeze

D. Isolated headache relieved by rest

Correct answer: A

Rationale: Women may present with non-classical symptoms such as fatigue, nausea, and breathlessness.

MCQ3: *Gynaecological time-critical emergency*: Sudden severe unilateral pelvic pain with vomiting is most consistent with:

A. Constipation

B. Ovarian torsion

C. Menopause

D. Panic attack

Correct answer: B

Rationale: Ovarian torsion is time-critical; early recognition and urgent transport are essential.

MCQ4: *Menopause/perimenopause and risk*: Which is the safest paramedic approach to perimenopausal presentations such as palpitations and chest discomfort?

A. Assume anxiety if the patient is tearful
B. Attribute symptoms to menopause once hot flushes are reported
C. Rule out physical causes first, while acknowledging hormonal transitions may contribute
D. Provide reassurance only and no further assessment

Correct answer: C

Rationale: Perimenopause can mimic acute illness, but can also coincide with increased cardiovascular risk.

MCQ5: *Trauma-informed assessment*: Which practice most supports trauma-informed care during intimate history-taking or assessment?

A. Proceeding quickly to minimise embarrassment
B. Asking permission, explaining each step, and offering choices
C. Avoiding all sensitive questions
D. Using humour to reduce tension

Correct answer: B

Rationale: Safety, consent, and choice reduce distress and improve disclosure.

MCQ6: *Domestic abuse indicators*: Which feature should increase suspicion of coercive control or domestic abuse?

A. Patient asks for analgesia
B. Partner insists on answering all questions and will not leave
C. Patient is upset and crying
D. Patient has a chronic condition

Correct answer: B

Rationale: Limited privacy, controlling behaviour, and restricted communication are all red flags.

Guided clinical reasoning questions

Q1: *Assessment and differentials*: In Sarah's case, what features support a broad differential (ACS/pulmonary embolism/arrhythmia/anaemia/hyperventilation), and what cannot be excluded pre-hospital?

Q2: *Assessment and differentials*: Which immediate assessments should be prioritised for women with breathlessness and chest symptoms (ECG, trend vitals, risk factors, red flags)?

Q3: *Avoiding bias*: What are the risks of premature diagnostic closure on 'panic/anxiety' in midlife women?

Q4: *Avoiding bias*: How does gender bias influence pain assessment and escalation decisions in the pre-hospital setting?

Q5: *Trauma-informed practice*: What language helps validate symptoms without implying 'it's all psychological'?

Q6: *Trauma-informed practice*: How would you ask about menstrual/hormonal factors and sexual health in a trauma-informed, culturally sensitive way?

Q7: *Safeguarding*: What practical steps enable safe enquiry about domestic abuse (privacy, non-leading questions, documentation)?

Q8: *Safeguarding*: When and how should safeguarding frameworks be activated (Care Act, MARAC/MAPPA, Modern Slavery/NRM, FGM duty)?

Q9: *Decision-making and safety-netting*: What makes conveyance appropriate for Sarah even if ECG is non-ischaemic?

Q10: *Decision-making and safety-netting*: What safety-net advice would you give if symptoms recur or evolve?

Reflective questions for learners

Q1: When have you minimised (or might you minimise) women's symptoms, and what would help you notice this in the moment?

Q2: How do you balance reassurance with clinical caution when symptoms overlap with anxiety or menopause?

Q3: What helps you maintain dignity, consent, and cultural sensitivity during intimate assessment?

Q4: How can paramedics use their first-contact role to reduce the gender health gap in outcomes?

Teaching commentary

This chapter addresses women's health emergencies through an equity lens, highlighting how male-normed evidence and gendered assumptions contribute to diagnostic delay, undertreatment, and poor outcomes. The content supports paramedics to recognise atypical symptom patterns (especially ACS), maintain broad differentials for pelvic pain and midlife presentations, and avoid premature attribution of symptoms to anxiety or menopause. Teaching can focus on trauma-informed assessment (consent, choice, privacy), culturally sensitive history-taking, and safeguarding competence in contexts such as domestic abuse, exploitation, and culturally specific harm. The case study reinforces trend-based assessment, shared decision-making, and safety-netting as practical tools for person-centred, diagnostically safe pre-hospital care.

References

American Heart Association (2020). *American Heart Association guidelines for cardio-pulmonary resuscitation and emergency cardiovascular care.* Dallas, TX: American Heart Association.

Baron, S.L., and Mathai, J. (2023). *Ovarian torsion.* Treasure Island, FL: StatPearls Publishing. https://www.ncbi.nlm.nih.gov/books/NBK560675/ (accessed 14 December 2025).

Bedekar, K., McInnes, A., and Burgess, W. (2025). Ovarian torsion: Presenting features and delays in recognition. *New Zealand Medical Journal, 138*(1613), 79–86. https://nzmj.org.nz/media/pages/journal/vol-138-no-1613/ovarian-torsion-determining-the-presenting-features-and-where-the-delays-occur/ba2754b33b-1744167860/6809.pdf.

Brooks, L.A., Manias, E., and Bloomer, M.J. (2019). Culturally sensitive communication in healthcare: A concept analysis. *Collegian, 26*(3), 383–391. https://doi.org/10.1016/j.colegn.2018.09.007

Byrne, R.A., Rossello, X., Coughlan, J.J., Barbato, E., Berry, C., Chieffo, A., et al. (2023). ESC guidelines for the management of acute coronary syndromes. *European Heart Journal, 44*(38), 3720–3826. https://doi.org/10.1093/eurheartj/ehad191

Cancer Research UK (2023). *Breast cancer statistics.* https://www.cancerresearchuk.org (accessed 1 December 2025).

Care Act 2014, c. 23. https://www.legislation.gov.uk/ukpga/2014/23 (accessed 1 December 2025).

Criado Perez, C. (2019). *Invisible Women: Data bias in a world designed for men.* London: Chatto & Windus.

Department of Health and Social Care (DHSC) (2022). *Women's health strategy for England.* London: DHSC. https://www.gov.uk/government/publications/womens-health-strategy-for-england

Domestic Abuse Act 2021, c. 17. https://www.legislation.gov.uk/ukpga/2021/17/contents (accessed 1 December 2025).

Downey, C., Kelly, M., and Quinlan, J.F. (2019). Changing trends in the mortality rate at 1-year post hip fracture. *World Journal of Orthopedics, 10*(3), 166–175. https://doi.org/10.5312/wjo.v10.i3.166

Forced Marriage (Civil Protection) Act 2007, c. 20. https://www.legislation.gov.uk/ukpga/2007/20 (accessed 1 December 2025).

Gardner, A., Oduola, S., and Teague, B. (2024). Culturally sensitive perinatal mental health care. *Health Expectations, 27*(4), e14160. https://doi.org/10.1111/hex.14160

Health and Care Act 2022, c. 15. https://www.legislation.gov.uk/ukpga/2022/15/contents (accessed 16 December 2025).

HM Government (2018). *Working together to safeguard children.* London: Department for Education.

HM Government (2021). *Tackling violence against women and girls strategy 2021–2024.* London: Home Office.

HM Government (2023). *Trauma-informed approaches in health and social care.* London: UK Government.

Hsu, B., Carcel, C., Wang, X., Peters, S., Randall, D., Havard, A., et al. (2021). Sex differences in emergency medical services management of patients with myocardial infarction. *American Heart Journal, 241*, 87–91. https:doi.org/10.1016/j.ahj.2021.07.009

International Osteoporosis Foundation (2023). *Facts and statistics.* https://www.osteoporosis.foundation (accessed 10 December 2025).

Jeffrey, G. (2025). Barriers to women accessing healthcare in the UK. *LSE Public Policy Review, 3*(4), 1–12. https://doi.org/10.31389/lseppr.122

Kurtz, S., Silverman, J., and Draper, J. (2017). *Teaching and Learning Communication Skills in Medicine* (3rd edition). Boca Raton, FL: CRC Press.

Lim, W.H., Woods, N., and Lamaro, V. (2022). Trends and outcomes of ruptured ovarian cysts. *Postgraduate Medical Journal, 98*(1161), e9. https://doi.org/10.1136/postgradmedj-2020-138833

Maass, S.W.M.C., Boerman, L.M., Verhaak, P.F.M., Du, J., de Bock, G.H., and Berendsen, A.J. (2019). Long-term psychological distress in breast cancer survivors. *Maturitas, 130*, 6–12. https://doi.org/10.1016/j.maturitas.2019.09.003

Mann, L.M., Angus, S.A., Doherty, C.J., and Dominelli, P.B. (2021). Evaluation of sex-based differences in airway size and physiological implications. *European Journal of Applied Physiology, 121*(11), 2957–2966. https://doi.org/10.1007/s00421-021-04778-2

Mauvais-Jarvis, F., Merz, N.B., Barnes, P.J., Brinton, R.D., Carrero, J-J., DeMeo, D.L., et al. (2020). Sex and gender: Modifiers of health, disease, and medicine. *The Lancet, 396*(10250), 565–582. https://doi.org/10.1016/S0140-6736(20)31561-0

McLelland, G., McKenna, L., Morgans, A., and Smith, K. (2016). Antenatal emergency care provided by paramedics. *Prehospital Emergency Care, 20*(4), 531–538. https://doi.org/10.3109/10903127.2015.1128030

MINAP (2025). *Myocardial Ischaemia National Audit Project annual report*. London: NHS Digital.

Modern Slavery Act 2015, c. 30. https://www.legislation.gov.uk/ukpga/2015/30/contents (accessed 1 December 2025).

Molloy, L., Fields, L., Trostian, B., and Kinghorn, G. (2020). Trauma-informed care for people presenting to the emergency department with mental health issues. *Emergency Nurse, 28*(2), 30–35. https://doi.org/10.7748/en.2020.e1990

National Institute for Health and Care Excellence (NICE) (2016). *Domestic violence and abuse* (QS116). London: NICE. https://www.nice.org.uk/guidance/qs116 (accessed 16 December 2025).

National Institute for Health and Care Excellence (NICE) (2018). *Heavy menstrual bleeding: Assessment and management* (NG88). London: NICE. https://www.nice.org.uk/guidance/ng88 (accessed 16 December 2025).

National Institute for Health and Care Excellence (NICE) (2019). *Endometriosis: Diagnosis and management* (NG73). London: NICE. https://www.nice.org.uk/guidance/ng73 (Accessed: 16 December 2025).

National Institute for Health and Care Excellence (NICE) (2022). *Self-harm: Assessment, management and preventing recurrence* (NG225). London: NICE. https://www.nice.org.uk/guidance/ng225 (accessed 16 December 2025).

National Institute for Health and Care Excellence (NICE) (2024). *Menopause: Diagnosis and management* (NG23). London: NICE. https://www.nice.org.uk/guidance/ng23 (accessed 16 December 2025).

National Institute for Health and Care Research (NIHR) (2022). *Improving women's health: Addressing inequalities in access and outcomes*. London: NIHR.

NHS Digital (2022). *Health survey for England: Cardiovascular health*. Leeds: NHS Digital.

Pompei, G., van de Hoef, T.P., den Ruijter, H.M., and Kunadian, V. (2024). Gaps in evidence for women in acute coronary syndrome guidelines. *European Journal of Clinical Investigation, 54*(2), e14148. https://doi.org/10.1111/eci.14148

Serious Crime Act 2015, c. 9. https://www.legislation.gov.uk/ukpga/2015/9 (accessed 1 December 2025).

Skou, S.T., Mair, F.S., Fortin, M., Guthrie, B., Nunes, B.P., Miranada, J.J., et al. (2022). Multimorbidity. *Nature Reviews Disease Primers, 8*(1), 48. https://doi.org/10.1038/s41572-022-00376-4

Swayambunathan, J., Dasgupta, A., and Bhattacharyya, T. (2021). The impact of hip fractures on psychosocial wellbeing. *Journal of the American Academy of Orthopaedic Surgeons, 29*(1), e22–e30. https://doi.org/10.5435/JAAOS-D-19-00530

Withanarachchie, V., Todd, V., Dicker, B., and Maessen, S.E. (2025). Navigating emotions, communication and pain during prehospital labour. *BMC Emergency Medicine, 25*(1), 83. https://doi.org/10.1186/s12873-025-01236-6

World Health Organization (WHO) (2014). *Health Care for Women Subjected to Intimate Partner Violence or Sexual Violence: A clinical handbook*. Geneva: WHO.

7 Severe and enduring mental illness: Psychosis, schizophrenia, and eating disorders

Jo Augustus and Kaitee Robinson

Introduction

Severe and enduring mental illness (SMI) encompasses a group of complex psychiatric conditions (e.g. schizophrenia, bipolar disorder, personality disorders, and eating disorders) that significantly affect cognition, mood, behaviour, and functioning across the life course (Schinnar et al., 1991; Ruggeri et al., 2000; Zumstein and Riese, 2020; Gonzales et al., 2022; NHS England, 2025). For paramedics, these presentations are among the most challenging encountered in pre-hospital practice, requiring a nuanced blend of clinical reasoning, trauma-informed communication, legal literacy, and the ability to navigate acute risk under pressure (Phillips et al., 2023; Zumstein and Riese, 2020). SMI crises seldom occur in isolation; they emerge in the context of social adversity, a history of trauma, poverty, discrimination, system fragmentation, and unmet relational needs (Nelson, 2002; Padgett, 2020). As NHS England continues to reshape crisis care pathways, paramedics increasingly form part of the essential mental health response workforce, often serving as the first and sometimes the only clinicians to encounter individuals at their most vulnerable (Abdulmalik et al., 2019; Ebrahimi et al., 2018; NHS England, 2023). Whilst the traditional role of the paramedic has been tailored towards emergency care (Evashkevich and Fitzgerald, 2014), the profession has now started to address gaps in the healthcare system (Emond et al., 2019) with the role now being solely degree-based (Royal College of Paramedics, 2019), culminating in a variety of health conditions being managed successfully (Shaban, 2005) due to the paramedic being able to assess and manage numerous complaints.

O'Meara et al. (2017) found that paramedics are capable of contributing to the effective assessment and management of patients with an array of mental illnesses; however, negative attitudes, stigma, and biases have prevented a significant change in how paramedics deliver quality care. Whilst in the pre-hospital context paramedics are called upon to manage an increasing number of mental health presentations (Lowthian et al., 2010), it was found that inadequate training and education contributed to the poor care of this patient group (Rees et al., 2015; Hou et al., 2013), alongside organisational processes and protocols preventing an organic clinical decision-making process in mental health (Parsons and O'Brien, 2011).

Understanding severe and enduring mental illness

Severe and enduring mental illness is a term used to describe psychiatric conditions characterised by chronicity, relapse, functional impairment, and significant personal, social, and clinical impact (Lagomasino et al., 1999; Patel et al., 2016). Unlike milder or episodic mental health problems, SMI typically involves long-term patterns of disruption to cognition, affect, interpersonal functioning, and physical health. Many individuals experience repeated crises, fluctuating capacity, a complex trauma history, and vulnerability to exploitation or neglect (Nelson, 2002). Paramedics frequently enter individuals' lives at precisely the moment when symptoms have escalated beyond what community care can contain, often in environments marked by confusion, distress, fear, or conflict.

Several themes cut across SMI conditions. First, individuals often experience complex health inequalities. The rates of homelessness, unemployment, social isolation, poverty, and discrimination are significantly higher among those living with SMI (Padgett, 2020). These structural pressures increase the likelihood of deterioration and reliance on emergency services. Second, SMI is strongly associated with risk of suicide. People with schizophrenia, bipolar disorder, or a personality disorder experience a substantially elevated lifetime risk of suicide compared with the general population (Hor and Taylor, 2010). Third, SMI conditions frequently interact with physical health deterioration. Antipsychotic medications increase the risk of metabolic syndrome, cardiovascular disease, and diabetes (De Hert et al., 2011). Mood stabilisers such as lithium require regular renal and thyroid monitoring, and toxicity can present as a medical emergency (Geddes and Miklowitz, 2013). Eating disorders present life-threatening risks of electrolyte disturbance, arrhythmia, dehydration, and multi-organ impairment (Mehler and Andersen, 2022).

In the context of these complexities, pre-hospital care is rarely straightforward. Individuals may appear calm yet be physiologically compromised; articulate yet lacking capacity; agitated yet terrified; withdrawn yet at high risk. Paramedics must therefore integrate medical and mental health assessment, adopting a formulation-driven approach that acknowledges both symptoms and the wider psychosocial context. The following sections apply this orientation to each core SMI diagnosis, beginning with schizophrenia and psychotic disorders.

The impact of receiving a diagnosis of severe and enduring mental illness

A diagnosis of severe and enduring mental illness can have profound psychological, social, and practical consequences for an individual, influencing how they see themselves and how they are treated by others. While diagnostic labels can offer clarity, access to treatment, and validation of lived experience, they can also carry stigma, evoke fear, and shape expectations of what a person is capable of. Becker's labelling theory highlights how being assigned a psychiatric label may alter not only public perceptions, but also an individual's self-identity, contributing to what he describes as a 'self-fulfilling prophecy' in which people internalise the negative assumptions associated with their diagnosis (Becker, 1963). This can lead to withdrawal, shame, or a reluctance to seek help, especially in a system where mental health stigma remains a significant barrier to care.

For paramedics, recognising the impact of labelling is essential. Many people with SMI have experienced judgement, coercion, or discrimination in healthcare settings, which can heighten mistrust during crisis encounters. A diagnostic label may also overshadow physical health needs, increasing the risk of diagnostic overshadowing, where physical symptoms are incorrectly attributed to mental illness (Jones et al., 2008). Paramedics therefore play a critical role in counteracting the negative effects of labelling by adopting a trauma-informed, person-centred approach that focuses on the individual rather than the diagnosis. Validating distress, using non-stigmatising language, and remaining curious about the person's experience can improve engagement, reduce escalation, and support more equitable care.

Exemplar: Schizophrenia and psychotic disorders

Schizophrenia is a severe mental disorder involving significant disturbances in cognition, perception, emotion, and behaviour. Common symptoms include hallucinations, delusions, disorganised thinking, disorganised behaviour, and negative symptoms such as social withdrawal and flattened emotions. In the pre-hospital environment, psychosis may present as fear, confusion, agitation, mutism, or intense distress. Individuals may misinterpret paramedics' intentions, perceive threat where none exists, or withdraw from communication entirely. These behaviours are not signs of wilfulness but the result of profound perceptual and cognitive disruption (Williams and Shepherd, 2000).

Clinical presentation: Paramedics often encounter individuals in acute psychosis during periods of relapse, medication non-adherence, or heightened stress. Hallucinations – particularly auditory hallucinations – may cause the person to respond to voices or commands encouraging self-harm or harm to others. Delusions may take paranoid, persecutory, or referential forms, leading individuals to misinterpret everyday events as threatening. Disorganised thinking can manifest as tangential speech or difficulty following simple instructions, while negative symptoms may mimic depression or intoxication. Cognitive impairment affecting attention, memory, and executive function is common, and contributes to difficulties with capacity, engagement, and adherence.

Assessment and risk formulation: Assessment should begin with non-intrusive observation: environmental cues, behaviour, posture, pacing, withdrawal, or fearfulness. Paramedics must balance clinical curiosity with safety, avoiding sudden movements or unnecessary proximity. Communication should be slow, calm, and concrete. Validating distress without reinforcing delusions (e.g. 'I can hear this feels very real for you') helps create psychological safety.

Risk formulation is central. Individuals with psychosis are vulnerable to self-harm, accidental injury, self-neglect, exploitation, and sudden medical deterioration. Paramedics must assess for command hallucinations, persecutory beliefs, suicidal ideation, agitation, confusion, and signs of medical compromise such as dehydration, infection, or toxicity. In addition, paramedics must establish current prescribed medication and when it was last taken (Table 7.1). Physical health assessment is essential to rule out delirium, intoxication, or metabolic disturbance.

Pre-hospital management: Management requires a combination of de-escalation, environmental control, and clinical assessment. Collaborative decision-making is ideal, but individuals may lack capacity, necessitating MCA- or MHA-supported conveyance. Under Right Care, Right Person (RCRP), police involvement should be limited to situations involving imminent violence or weapons (NHS England, 2023). Clear documentation of risk, capacity, and rationale is crucial. Paramedics' emotional labour in psychosis-related incidents should not be underestimated; supervision, debriefing, and reflective practice are essential to prevent burnout (McCann et al., 2018).

Table 7.1: Schizophrenia and psychotic disorders: Examples of commonly prescribed medications

First generation – 'typical'	Second generation – 'atypical'
Chlorpromazine hydrochloride 25mg TDS	Amisulpride 400–800mg QID
Levomepromazine 25–50mg	Asenapine 5mg BID
Prochlorperazine 12.5mg BID	Clozapine 12.5mg QID/BID
Flupentixol 3–9mg BID	Olanzapine 10mg QID
Haloperidol 2–10mg QID	Quetiapine 25mg BID
Sulpiride 200–400mg BID	Risperidone 2mg QID

Abbreviations: BID, twice daily; TDS, three times a day; QID, four times a day.

Summary

Severe and enduring mental illness is shaped not only by psychiatric symptomatology but by structural inequalities, trauma history, and the cumulative impact of social and environmental stressors. For paramedics, recognising these intersecting influences is essential for safe, person-centred care. The discussion of schizophrenia and psychosis introduces one of the most acute and high-risk areas of mental health crisis work, illustrating how perceptual disturbances, disorganised thinking, and impaired insight challenge pre-hospital assessment and communication. This reinforces the need for slow, compassionate engagement, dynamic risk formulation, and an approach that integrates physical, psychological, and contextual understanding. These foundations set the stage for the more detailed exploration of diagnostic categories and clinical complexities that follow.

Other key conditions

Bipolar disorder

Bipolar disorder is a complex and cyclical mood disorder characterised by significant fluctuations between depressive, manic, hypomanic, and mixed affective states. For paramedics, bipolar presentations can pose considerable challenges, particularly when individuals are experiencing elevated arousal, reduced inhibition, impaired judgement, or profound depression. Mood episodes often arise in response to stress, trauma, interpersonal conflict, or disruptions to medication, sleep, or routine. As with schizophrenia, individuals with bipolar disorder are at significantly increased risk of suicide, self-harm, and physical health complications (McIntyre et al., 2022). Paramedics frequently encounter patients during periods of acute behavioural dysregulation, intense distress, or exhaustion, and must be prepared to assess mood states with sensitivity, clarity, and respect.

Clinical presentation: Manic episodes typically present with elevated, irritable, or expansive mood, increased energy, and reduced need for sleep. Individuals may exhibit pressured speech, racing thoughts, distractibility, agitation, or grandiosity, and may misinterpret events or interactions due to heightened emotional intensity. Behaviour often becomes risky or impulsive, including excessive spending, unsafe sexual practices, reckless driving, or sudden long-distance travel. Psychotic symptoms may also emerge, commonly involving grandiose, religious, or persecutory delusions. Paramedics may be called when behaviour becomes visibly unsafe, alarming to others, or disruptive to the environment.

Hypomania, while less severe, can still lead to impaired judgement and heightened risk. Because individuals often enjoy the elevated mood and increased productivity of hypomania, they may resist intervention or deny deterioration. By contrast, bipolar depression can be overwhelming, involving profound hopelessness, guilt, anhedonia, psychomotor retardation, and suicidal ideation. Mixed episodes where manic and depressive symptoms co-exist are particularly dangerous, combining high energy with despair and impulsivity. Such presentations are unpredictable and carry the highest risk of suicide.

Assessment and risk formulation: Paramedics should adopt a structured and empathetic approach, beginning with calm engagement and clear introductions. Observational assessment is essential: pacing, rapid movements, irritability, slowed speech, tearfulness, exhaustion, or signs of self-neglect provide important clinical cues. Individuals in mania may appear confident and articulate but could still lack the capacity to make safe decisions. Depression, conversely, may be masked by social withdrawal or minimised when shame is present.

Risk formulation should consider contextual triggers such as bereavement, relational conflict, financial stress, or medication non-adherence. Important questions include recent sleep patterns, changes in behaviour, whether the individual has acted on impulsive ideas, and the presence of suicidal thoughts. Wider information from family members or carers can be invaluable in assessing baseline functioning and the degree of deviation from the person's usual presentation. This should include current prescribed medication, and when it was last taken:

Examples of commonly prescribed medications: quetiapine 50mg QID, lamotrigine 25mg QID, lithium 0.52–1.56g QID, asenapine 5mg BID, carbamezapine 400mg QID, sodium valproate 750mg QID.

Pre-hospital management: Management focuses on providing structure, clarity, and emotional containment. Paramedics should speak slowly, avoid confrontation, and provide simple explanations of next steps. Offering choices wherever possible helps preserve autonomy and reduces escalation. Conveyance is often necessary when risk is high, capacity is impaired, or psychosis is present. For individuals experiencing depression, particularly with suicidal ideation, conveyance to a place of safety with mental health assessment is essential. Non-conveyance should only be considered when risk is low, capacity is intact, and immediate follow-up by crisis or community teams is guaranteed. Paramedic wellbeing is also a concern during intense bipolar presentations, especially when individuals display volatile or unpredictable behaviour. Regular clinical supervision and reflective practice should be encouraged.

Personality disorders

Personality disorders involve enduring and pervasive patterns of emotional, interpersonal, and behavioural difficulties that begin in early adulthood and persist across contexts. The ICD-11 conceptualises personality disorder in terms of severity – mild, moderate, or severe – with optional trait qualifiers such as borderline, dissocial, avoidant, or anankastic (WHO, 2022). For paramedics, personality disorder presentations are among the most emotionally complex, often involving acute crises precipitated by relational conflict, trauma triggers, or overwhelming feelings of abandonment. These crises may involve self-harm, suicidal statements, dissociation, or intense emotional dysregulation.

Clinical presentation: Characteristic features include rapid shifts in mood, difficulty regulating emotions, impulsive behaviour, fear of abandonment, unstable relationships, and chronic feelings of emptiness. Individuals may present with self-inflicted injuries, overdoses, extreme agitation, or withdrawal. Crises often arise following arguments, perceived rejection, or interpersonal stress, and may fluctuate rapidly in intensity. Dissociation ranging from mild detachment to severe disconnection may occur under stress, affecting memory, perception, and engagement. Individuals may struggle to articulate their distress and may feel deeply misunderstood or judged by clinicians.

Assessment and risk formulation: In their assessment, paramedics should be curious, empathic, and non-judgemental. Emotional dysregulation should not be interpreted as manipulation or attention-seeking; rather, these behaviours reflect profound distress and attempts to cope with overwhelming emotions (Linehan, 2015). Risk assessment must consider both immediate danger and contextual vulnerabilities, including recent conflict, trauma history, patterns of self-harm, and social instability. Because intent can fluctuate rapidly, risk formulation must remain dynamic, incorporating both the individual's verbal statements and their observed behaviour.

Capacity assessment can be challenging during intense emotional states. While strong emotions alone do not remove capacity, dissociation, impulsivity, or cognitive overload may impair the ability to understand, weigh, or communicate decisions. A decision-specific, time-specific MCA assessment is therefore essential.

Pre-hospital management: Best practice involves maintaining calm, consistent boundaries while validating the person's emotions: 'I can see this feels overwhelming'. Avoiding power struggles, ultimatums, or invalidating language reduces escalation. Paramedics should offer clear, predictable information and avoid promising outcomes that cannot be guaranteed. Where self-harm has occurred, physical assessment should proceed sensitively and without judgement. Conveyance may be required due to significant self-harm, suicide risk, or capacity concerns. For lower-risk presentations, collaborative safety planning and referral to crisis teams may suffice, but only where follow-up is reliable.

Personality disorder crises can be emotionally demanding for paramedics. Feelings of helplessness, frustration, or concern for personal safety are not uncommon. Support, reflective practice and psychologically safe team cultures are therefore vital components of workforce sustainability (Parsons and O'Brien, 2011; McCann et al., 2018).

Eating disorders

Eating disorders represent some of the most medically serious and psychologically complex conditions within SMI. They include anorexia nervosa, bulimia nervosa, binge eating disorder, and avoidant/restrictive food intake disorder. Unlike many mental illnesses, eating disorders can present with severe physiological instability even when individuals appear outwardly calm or deny the severity of their condition. The Medical Emergencies in Eating Disorders (MEED) guidance (Royal College of Psychiatrists, 2022) emphasises that medical risk is not determined by body mass index alone; individuals of any weight may be critically unwell.

Clinical presentation: Anorexia nervosa involves severe restriction of food intake, intense fear of weight gain, and distorted body image. Individuals may present with profound weight loss, bradycardia, hypotension, hypothermia, dehydration, or electrolyte imbalance. However, denial of risk is common, often due to cognitive rigidity or fear of losing control. Bulimia nervosa involves recurrent bingeing followed by compensatory behaviours such as vomiting or laxative misuse. Medical complications include hypokalaemia, metabolic alkalosis, dental erosion, and oesophageal damage. Binge eating disorder involves recurrent binge episodes accompanied by shame and distress, and increases long-term risks of obesity, diabetes, and cardiovascular disease. Avoidant/restrictive food intake disorder involves restricted eating not motivated by weight concerns but by sensory sensitivities, fear of choking, or lack of interest in food. Individuals may present with fainting, nutritional deficiencies, or acute deterioration.

Assessment and risk formulation: Assessment must combine sensitivity with clinical vigilance. Individuals often minimise symptoms, fear hospital admission, or experience shame around eating behaviours. Paramedics should inquire gently about recent intake, purging behaviours, dizziness, chest pain, or palpitations. Objective measurements of heart rate, blood pressure, capillary glucose, and temperature are central to identifying MEED red flags. Collateral information from carers may illuminate patterns of deterioration, avoidance, or rapid weight loss.

Capacity assessment is nuanced. Cognitive distortion surrounding food, shape, and weight may impair decision-making even when the person is articulate. Individuals may understand information but be unable to weigh it appropriately due to overwhelming fear or entrenched beliefs (Mehler and Andersen, 2022). When medical instability is present, the least restrictive but safest option is urgent hospital conveyance.

Pre-hospital management: Management focuses on minimising physiological risk, maintaining emotional safety, and facilitating urgent medical assessment when indicated. Paramedics should communicate with empathy, avoid comments about weight or appearance, and explain the rationale for hospital assessment in plain language: ‘Your heart rate is very low, and we need to make sure you're safe'. Where transfer to hospital is refused and capacity is questioned, MCA provisions may be necessary. In all cases, documentation must clearly evidence risk factors, capacity considerations, and the reasoning behind decisions. Eating disorder crises can also be emotionally taxing for clinicians; reflective practice and support are essential.

Summary

This section has explored bipolar disorder, personality disorder, and eating disorders, which are often linked to trauma, relational instability, and significant physical health risk. Each presents distinct challenges in pre-hospital care, requiring strong assessment skills, emotional awareness, and legal understanding. Paramedics must manage fluctuating capacity, rapid shifts in mood or risk, communication difficulties, and, particularly in eating disorders, potential medical deterioration. The section also emphasised validating distress, maintaining clear and respectful communication, and avoiding stigma that may escalate crises. Together, these discussions reinforce that effective paramedic involvement in severe mental illness requires both clinical competence and relational sensitivity, setting the foundation for the risk and best-practice principles that follow.

Associated risks and medical complications in SMI

Severe and enduring mental illnesses involve an extensive range of risks that are clinically significant for paramedics working in pre-hospital environments. These risks span physical deterioration, psychological distress, social vulnerability, self-harm, and safeguarding concerns. Importantly, risk is rarely unidimensional; instead, it tends to emerge through the interplay of symptoms, social circumstances, trauma history, and the absence of timely support (Nelson, 2002; Padgett, 2020). For paramedics, understanding these intersecting layers is crucial, as crisis presentations often mask underlying medical instability or emergent risk.

One of the most notable risks across SMI is suicide. Individuals with schizophrenia, bipolar disorder, or a personality disorder experience substantially elevated lifetime suicide rates compared with the general population (Hor and Taylor, 2010). Suicide risk is particularly heightened during periods of acute psychosis, mixed affective states, recent discharge from psychiatric care, or significant psychosocial stress. Paramedics must therefore conduct dynamic risk formulations that consider both expressed intent and behavioural indicators such as withdrawal, agitation, impulsivity, or sudden calmness following intense distress.

Physical health risks are equally prominent. Individuals taking antipsychotic medication may experience metabolic syndrome, obesity, cardiovascular complications, or diabetes due to pharmacological side effects (NHS England, 2025; De Hert et al., 2011). Lithium, although not routinely so, is used to manage bipolar disorder. Lithium carries risks of toxicity that can present subtly through confusion, tremors, vomiting, or ataxia (Geddes and Miklowitz, 2013, NICE, 2025). These risks underscore the importance of holistic assessment: vital signs, hydration status, and neurological observations help differentiate psychiatric presentations from medical emergencies.

Eating disorders, particularly anorexia nervosa, present some of the most dangerous medical complications encountered in SMI. The Medical Emergencies in Eating Disorders (MEED) guidance (2022) emphasises that individuals can be critically unwell irrespective of body mass index. Bradycardia, hypotension, hypothermia, electrolyte imbalance, and arrhythmia require urgent intervention (Mehler and Andersen, 2022; Pennick et al., 2023). Paramedics must therefore adopt a low threshold for conveyance when vital signs are abnormal or when individuals refuse care despite clear evidence of medical risk.

Social vulnerabilities also compound clinical risk. Homelessness, poverty, exploitation, and social isolation increase exposure to harm, reduce access to routine health care, and exacerbate crisis presentations (Padgett, 2020). Individuals with SMI may also be at risk of domestic abuse, financial control, sexual exploitation, or coercion. Paramedics are often the first professionals to identify these safeguarding concerns, making sensitive questioning and thorough documentation vital.

Legal and ethical considerations further shape risk management. The Mental Capacity Act 2005 requires clinicians to assess whether individuals can understand, retain, weigh, and communicate information relevant to decisions about their care. Conditions such as delirium, psychosis, severe mood disturbance, or starvation can impair these cognitive processes. When capacity is lacking and risk is high, paramedics may need to use statutory frameworks such as the MCA or Mental Health Act 1983 (as amended 2007), always prioritising the least restrictive option.

Recognising that SMI crises also affect paramedic wellbeing is essential. Exposure to emotionally intense scenarios such as suicide attempts, violent incidents, or high-risk self-neglect can contribute to burnout, moral distress, and compassion fatigue (McCann et al., 2018; Parsons and O'Brien, 2011). Organisational support, reflective practice, and clinical supervision are therefore important components of safe and sustainable practice.

Treatments, interventions, and the role of the multidisciplinary team

Although paramedics do not provide long-term psychiatric treatment, an understanding of core interventions is essential for safe, effective pre-hospital care. Treatments for SMI typically combine pharmacological, psychological, and social interventions delivered across multiple settings and involving a wide range of professionals.

Antipsychotic medication is central to the treatment of schizophrenia and other psychotic disorders. While first- and second-generation antipsychotics reduce hallucinations and delusions, they also carry risks of extrapyramidal symptoms, sedation, metabolic syndrome, and, in rare cases, neuroleptic malignant syndrome (De Hert et al., 2011). Paramedics who understand these side effects can more effectively assess whether physical symptoms reflect medication toxicity, acute psychosis, or emerging medical deterioration.

Mood stabilisers, including lithium, valproate, and lamotrigine, underpin treatment for bipolar disorder. Lithium requires stringent monitoring due to its narrow therapeutic index and vulnerability to dehydration, infection, and drug interactions (Geddes and Miklowitz, 2013). When paramedics identify lithium toxicity symptoms, urgent conveyance becomes essential, even when individuals minimise their symptoms or appear stable.

Personality disorders are most effectively treated through structured psychological therapies such as dialectical behaviour therapy, mentalisation-based therapy, and schema therapy. These approaches focus on emotion regulation, interpersonal effectiveness, and trauma processing (Linehan, 2015). Awareness of these therapeutic principles helps paramedics adopt communication strategies that are validating, predictable, and non-judgemental, reducing escalation during crisis.

Eating disorder treatment is multidisciplinary, combining nutritional rehabilitation, medical monitoring, and psychotherapy. The MEED guidance (2022) highlights the risk of rapid physiological collapse, making early recognition vital for paramedics. Collaborative care involving specialist eating disorder teams, mental health services, GPs and dietitians ensures continuity of treatment once the immediate crisis has passed.

The multidisciplinary team (MDT) includes psychiatrists, psychologists, community psychiatric nurses, approved mental health professionals (AMHPs), social workers, liaison psychiatrists, crisis teams, and voluntary sector partners. Paramedics often act as the bridge between crisis presentations in the community and secondary mental health services. High-quality handovers including the individual's history, observed risks, physical findings, communication style, stressors, and social context support accurate, timely decision-making within the MDT (Evashkevich and Fitzgerald, 2014; McCann et al., 2018).

Best practice for paramedics responding to SMI

Best practice in SMI care involves a synthesis of trauma-informed communication, clinical reasoning, legal literacy, and relational safety. Trauma-informed care is foundational: many individuals with SMI have an extensive history of childhood adversity, interpersonal trauma, or systemic marginalisation (Nelson, 2002). Recognising trauma's impact on behaviour helps paramedics avoid misattributing fear or dissociation as hostility or non-compliance. Clear explanations, predictable actions, and consent-based interactions reduce re-traumatisation.

Cultural humility is equally important. People from racialised, marginalised, or neurodivergent communities often experience disparities in access to care and may be disproportionately subjected to coercive interventions (NHS England, 2023). Paramedics should adopt a stance of curiosity, avoid assumptions, and consider inequality as part of risk formulation.

Communication should be slow, clear, and collaborative. For individuals experiencing psychosis, grounding statements and non-confrontational clarification reduce fear. For those with eating disorders, avoiding weight-based comments and focusing on physiological safety help reduce shame. For emotionally dysregulated individuals, validation (e.g. 'I can see this is overwhelming') can de-escalate crises.

Legal frameworks guide safe decision-making. The Mental Capacity Act requires decision-specific assessments and encourages the least restrictive options. Where risks are imminent or capacity is impaired, the Mental Health Act may provide authority for conveyance. Right Care, Right Person requires police involvement only when risks clearly exceed the threshold for health-led intervention.

Finally, paramedic wellbeing is central to best practice. Access to debriefing, supervision, and psychologically safe team cultures supports resilience and reduces the risk of burnout (McCann et al., 2018).

Case study: Delusion, neglect, and distress

Case study: Narrative

Amira, a 23-year-old woman, is reported by her neighbour to be 'behaving oddly' and 'wandering around outside in slippers despite the cold'. It is early evening in late autumn; temperatures have begun to fall, and the caller reports that Amira appears confused, unsteady, and talking to herself. The neighbour sounds anxious, stating, 'She's usually quiet but very polite. Tonight, she looks frightened and keeps checking behind her.'

When the paramedic crew arrive, they find Amira sitting on the doorstep of her shared accommodation. She is wearing thin clothing and appears visibly underweight. Her posture is hunched and protective, and she is shivering. She looks up only briefly when approached, then lowers her gaze to the ground. Her skin is pale, and she appears fatigued. A half-empty mug of cold tea sits beside her. The surrounding area is cluttered with takeaway containers that others in the household may have left, but it gives the impression of neglect or chaotic living.

Initial engagement

The lead paramedic introduces herself gently. Amira responds quietly, with minimal eye contact: 'I'm okay. I don't need hospital. I can't go there', she whispers. Her speech is slow and soft. The crew notice subtle delays in her responses, as if she is hearing or processing something else at the same time. Her foot taps rhythmically, and she keeps glancing to her left, as though responding to an unseen stimulus.

When asked what brought her outside, Amira replies, 'They know. They're inside. I had to leave before they hurt me.' She does not specify who 'they' are, but she appears fearful and mistrustful. Her body tenses when the second crew member steps closer.

Collateral information

A housemate emerges and speaks quietly to the crew while keeping a respectful distance: 'She's been getting worse for months. Barely eats. She hasn't been sleeping. She thinks the news presenters are sending her messages. Some days she won't leave her room. She hasn't been to the mental health team in ages.' Her housemate also adds: 'She fainted last week. She refused to let anyone call for help.'

Clinical assessment

The crew gently encourage Amira into the ambulance for privacy and warmth. She agrees reluctantly but only after the door is kept open, explaining, 'I need to see who's coming.'

Her vital signs show:

- Heart rate: 42 beats per minute
- Blood pressure: 86/54 mmHg
- Temperature: 34.8°C
- Capillary glucose: 3.2 mmol/L
- Respiratory rate: 16 breaths per minute
- Oxygen saturation: 98% on air

Her hands are cold to the touch. She insists she has 'eaten earlier', though the housemate is seen to shake their head subtly behind her.

During conversation, Amira intermittently pauses mid-sentence, turning her head towards her left, sometimes whispering responses under her breath. She appears to be experiencing auditory hallucinations. Her thought processes are tangential; when asked simple questions about her wellbeing, she diverts to unrelated topics such as the news, 'hidden messages', and a belief that the neighbours are 'controlling my thoughts'.

When the paramedic gently asks about eating, she becomes defensive and tearful: 'I do eat. I don't need as much as other people. My body doesn't work like yours. If I eat more, I'll get sick. I can feel it changing me.'

Her BMI, estimated visually, appears very low. Her clothing hangs loosely on her frame. Her hair is brittle, and her skin shows signs of dehydration.

Risk indicators include:

- bradycardia
- hypotension
- hypothermia
- possible prolonged starvation
- delusional beliefs
- auditory hallucinations
- possible fainting episodes

- self-neglect
- difficulty engaging with reality-based questions
- fear that hospital will 'hurt her'
- diminished insight into physical risk

Amira refuses conveyance, stating firmly, 'I can't go to the hospital. They'll see me. They'll take control.' And she becomes increasingly distressed at the mention of admission. Her hands begin to shake, and she starts pacing within the vehicle. Her fear is palpable, and the paramedics recognise that her distress stems from terror, not defiance.

Capacity considerations

When the crew assess her ability to understand the seriousness of her physical symptoms, she shifts between evasive responses and fixed, delusional explanations. She cannot accurately reflect the consequences of refusing treatment. Statements such as 'My heart is strong; it's just beating quietly so they can't track me' indicate severe cognitive distortion.

Her ability to weigh information is impaired by psychosis and entrenched eating disorder beliefs. She repeatedly states, 'If I go there, I won't survive', revealing that fear not reason is driving her decision.

Clinical decision-making

Given ample evidence of MEED red flags, psychosis, significant self-neglect, and impaired insight, the crew conclude:

- She lacks capacity to refuse care.
- She is at risk of rapid medical deterioration.
- The least restrictive safe option is urgent hospital conveyance under the Mental Capacity Act 2005.

They communicate this clearly, compassionately, and slowly. Her distress escalates briefly but settles with grounding, reassurance, and the presence of her housemate, who accompanies her to hospital.

Case study: Lessons

The case reinforces that refusal does not equal capacity, particularly when delusions and starvation impact cognition. It also demonstrates how trauma histories may shape behaviour: avoidance, mistrust, hypervigilance, and emotional shutdown should be understood as protective strategies rather than 'challenging behaviour'. Finally, it underscores the importance of interprofessional collaboration, with paramedics acting as the bridge between community presentation and specialist mental health and medical services.

The future of mental health and paramedic practice

From an educational perspective, this chapter has highlighted the need for enhanced mental health training throughout the paramedic curriculum. Pre-registration programmes must move beyond traditional biomedical models to include deeper exploration of psychosis, affective disorders, personality disorder, eating disorders, trauma-informed care, cultural humility, and mental capacity assessment. Students require opportunities to practise complex communication, de-escalation strategies, and multidisciplinary collaboration through simulation. Exposure to lived-experience narratives, reflective writing, case-based learning, and supervised practice can further support the development of clinical judgement and empathy. Professional standards, such as the HCPC Standards of Proficiency (2023), underline that mental health competence and clinician wellbeing are no longer 'optional' but integral to safe practice.

Future clinical practice will increasingly demand system-level changes. As NHS England expands community crisis pathways and embeds RCRP, paramedics will play a pivotal role in health-led crisis responses, strengthening collaboration with crisis teams, liaison psychiatry, AMHPs, and specialist services. The profession will need ambition and leadership to shape new models of care, including integrated mental health response vehicles, telepsychiatry-supported decision-making, and more consistent access to specialist eating disorder advice (NHS England 2025). There is a pressing need for research to understand disparities in crisis responses, including racial, socioeconomic, and gender inequalities; to examine non-conveyance pathways; to evaluate paramedic-led interventions; and to explore the long-term outcomes of pre-hospital decision-making (McCann et al., 2018). Equally, research must address paramedic wellbeing, moral injury, and psychological load, acknowledging evidence that repeated exposure to high-risk mental health presentations can impact clinician mental health (Parsons and O'Brien, 2011).

Conclusion

Severe and enduring mental illness represents one of the most challenging areas of paramedic practice, requiring clinical vigilance, compassionate communication, legal literacy, and trauma-informed care. This chapter has highlighted the intersection of biological vulnerability, psychological distress, social adversity, and structural inequality that shapes the lived experience of individuals with conditions such as psychosis, bipolar disorder, personality disorder, and eating disorders (Lagomasino et al., 1999; Nelson, 2002; Padgett, 2020). Effective paramedic responses therefore demand more than technical competence; they require an understanding of the person behind the diagnosis and an awareness of the emotional labour inherent in crisis care.

A central theme is the significant medical risk associated with severe mental illness. Physical deterioration due to medication effects, toxicity, malnutrition, or self-neglect frequently co-exists with psychological distress and may be overlooked through diagnostic overshadowing. Frameworks such as MEED (Royal College of Psychiatrists, 2022) emphasise the importance of integrating physical and mental health assessment, particularly where subtle physiological changes may signal life-threatening deterioration. Alongside this, trauma-informed and relational approaches help paramedics interpret distress-driven behaviours with empathy, reduce escalation and preserve dignity, while legal frameworks such as the Mental Capacity Act 2005 and Right Care, Right Person (NHS England, 2023) support proportionate, person-centred decision-making.

In summary, this chapter positions severe and enduring mental illness as both a complex clinical challenge and a critical opportunity for compassionate, equitable paramedic care. Strengthening mental health expertise, interdisciplinary working, cultural humility, and clinician wellbeing will be central to future practice, ensuring paramedics remain equipped to provide safe, lawful, and dignified care at moments of profound vulnerability.

Further learning materials

Multiple-choice questions

MCQ1: *Psychosis recognition*: During the assessment, Amira frequently pauses mid-sentence, responds to unseen stimuli, and whispers replies under her breath. These features are most consistent with?

A. Thought insertion

B. Auditory hallucinations

C. Tactile hallucinations

D. Grandiose delusions

Correct answer: B

Rationale: Pausing, responding to unseen stimuli, whispering replies, and glancing sideways toward an imagined source strongly indicate auditory hallucinations. Thought insertion involves beliefs that thoughts are being placed into one's mind (not observed here). There is no evidence of tactile hallucinations or grandiose delusions.

MCQ2: *MEED red flags*: Which of the following findings represents the strongest immediate MEED red flag requiring urgent medical assessment?

A. Mild anxiety about eating

B. Heart rate of 42 bpm

C. BMI estimated at 17

D. Refusing to talk about weight

Correct answer: B

Rationale: Bradycardia <50 bpm is an immediate red flag in MEED (2022). BMI alone does not determine risk. Refusal to discuss weight and mild anxiety are concerning but not acute red flags. Amira's HR of 42 bpm is life-threatening.

MCQ3: *Capacity assessment*: Which element of the Mental Capacity Act 2005 is most impaired in Amira's decision-making?

A. Understanding the information

B. Retaining the information

C. Weighing the information

D. Communicating a decision

Correct answer: C

Rationale: Amira can communicate and understand basic information, but cannot weigh risks due to delusions ('my heart is beating quietly so they can't track me') and eating disorder cognitions ('if I eat, I will get sick'). This is the hallmark of impaired capacity in SMI.

MCQ4: *Legal decision-making*: Which framework is most appropriate for facilitating hospital conveyance in this scenario?

A. Mental Health Act Section 136

B. Mental Health Act Section 2

C. Common law

D. Mental Capacity Act 2005

Correct answer: D

Rationale: Amira is experiencing impaired capacity regarding her medical needs and refusing life-saving care. The MCA supports acting in her best interests to prevent harm. Section 136 applies only in public places (and via police). Section 2 is for assessment of mental illness but would require AMHP/doctor involvement. Common law no longer applies where MCA covers the situation.

MCQ5: *Trauma-informed practice*: Which response is most consistent with trauma-informed communication?

A. 'You must go to hospital or things will get worse.'

B. 'We are trying to help, but we need you to cooperate.'

C. 'I can see this feels frightening. I will explain each step before I do anything.'

D. 'Your fears are not real – we need to focus on your physical health.'

Correct answer: C

Rationale: Trauma-informed practice emphasises predictability, validation, and choice. Option C acknowledges distress while maintaining clarity. Options A and B risk escalation; option D invalidates her subjective experience.

MCQ6: *Safeguarding*: Which factor in Amira's presentation raises specific safeguarding concerns?

A. Her refusal to answer weight-related questions

B. Her fixation on news presenters

C. Her housemate reporting she 'barely eats and fainted last week'

D. Her quiet, withdrawn demeanour

Correct answer: C

Rationale: Repeated fainting + severe restriction = self-neglect, which is a safeguarding issue. Other features are clinically relevant but not explicit safeguarding triggers.

MCQ7: *RCRP application*: Under Right Care, Right Person, when would police involvement be appropriate?

A. When the patient refuses conveyance

B. When the patient is experiencing psychosis

C. When there is an imminent risk of violence or a weapon present

D. When the patient is malnourished

Correct answer: C

Rationale: RCRP states police should only be involved when there is immediate threat, violence, or criminal concerns. Refusal, psychosis, or malnutrition alone *do not* justify a police presence.

MCQ8: *Medical-psychiatric interaction*: Which interaction is contributing most significantly to Amira's impaired mental state?

A. Her neighbour's distress

B. Malnutrition worsening cognitive function and emotional regulation

C. The cold weather

D. Her housemate's frustration

Correct answer: B

Rationale: Starvation severely affects cognition, attention, judgement, and increases vulnerability to psychosis. This is a well-known risk in anorexia (Mehler and Andersen, 2022). The other factors do not cause acute cognitive impairment.

MCQ9: *Risk formulation*: Which combination best describes the primary risks in Amira's situation?

A. Emotional distress + low mood

B. Delusions + poor sleep

C. Medical instability + psychosis + impaired capacity

D. Limited social support + anxiety

Correct answer: C

Rationale: These three risks interact dangerously: medical instability (bradycardia, hypoglycaemia, hypothermia); psychosis (hallucinations, delusions); impaired capacity (cannot weigh information). This combination mandates urgent intervention.

MCQ10: *Paramedic professionalism*: Which paramedic action best supports professional wellbeing after this call?

A. Immediately attending the next call without discussion

B. Reassuring oneself that distress is 'part of the job'

C. Participating in a structured reflective debrief with a colleague

D. Reviewing the legal paperwork alone later

Correct answer: C

Rationale: Reflective, supportive debriefing reduces moral distress and burnout (McCann et al., 2018). Options A and B increase emotional pressure; D lacks relational support.

Guided clinical reasoning questions

Q1: *Assessment*: What features of Amira's presentation indicate acute psychosis?

Q2: *Assessment*: Which physical observations suggest a high-risk eating disorder emergency according to MEED (2022)?

Q3: *Assessment*: How did the environment and collateral information help shape your risk formulation?

Q4: *Assessment*: Which symptoms could indicate imminent medical collapse?

Q5: *Risk formulation*: Identify the interacting physical, psychological, and social risks in this scenario.

Q6: *Risk formulation*: How does self-neglect present differently from self-harm, and how does it influence your risk assessment?

Q7: *Risk formulation*: What safeguarding considerations are present?

Q8: *Capacity*: Using the MCA stages (understand/retain/weigh/communicate), identify which areas of capacity are impaired.

Q9: *Capacity*: Does Amira demonstrate insight into her physical health? Why or why not?

Q10: *Capacity*: Would her fear of hospital constitute a 'reasonable rationale' for refusal?

Q11: *Legal/ethical*: Why is the MCA more appropriate than the MHA in this scenario?

Q12: *Legal/ethical*: Under Right Care, Right Person, would police involvement be appropriate at any stage?

Q13: *Legal/ethical*: How would you document your decision-making?

Q14: *Communication*: What trauma-informed strategies helped reduce distress during engagement?

Q15: *Communication*: How can paramedics avoid inadvertently reinforcing delusional content?

Q16: *Paramedic wellbeing*: What emotional responses might clinicians experience during this encounter?

Q17: *Paramedic wellbeing*: What follow-up or reflective practices would support clinician wellbeing?

Reflective questions for learners

Q1: How did your own assumptions influence your interpretation of Amira's behaviour?

Q2: Did you feel more urgency around the psychosis or the eating disorder? Why?

Q3: How might cultural, gender, or social factors shape Amira's experience?

Q4: What biases might clinicians hold about who 'should' have an eating disorder or psychosis?

Q5: How would you ensure dignity and respect while enforcing MCA-based conveyance?

Teaching commentary

This case study illustrates the complexity of SMI presentations, particularly where psychosis and eating disorders co-exist. Psychosis masks insight and distorts reasoning, while anorexia-related cognitive rigidity intensifies fear around nutrition and medical intervention.

The paramedic role requires:

- balancing clinical urgency with empathic communication
- conducting rapid but accurate capacity assessments
- navigating legal frameworks
- identifying MEED red flags
- working within RCRP principles
- managing distress without escalation
- protecting patient dignity
- safeguarding physical and psychological safety
- ensuring clinician psychological safety

References

Abdulmalik, J., Olayiwola, S., Docrat, S., Lund, C., Chisholm, D., and Gureje, O. (2019). Sustainable financing mechanisms for strengthening mental health systems in Nigeria. *International Journal of Mental Health Systems, 13*, 38. https://doi.org/10.1186/s13033-019-0293-8

Becker, H.S. (1963). *Outsiders: Studies in the sociology of deviance.* New York: Free Press of Glencoe.

De Hert, M., Detraux, J., van Winkel, R., Yu, W., and Correll, C.U. (2011). Metabolic and cardiovascular adverse effects associated with antipsychotic drugs. *Nature Reviews Endocrinology, 8*(2), 114–126. https://doi.org/10.1038/nrendo.2011.156

Ebrahimi, H., Seyedfatemi, N., Namdar Areshtanab, H., Ranjbar, F., Thornicroft, G., Whitehead, B., et al. (2018). Barriers to family caregivers' coping with patients with severe mental illness in Iran. *Qualitative Health Research, 28*(6), 987–1001. https://doi.org/10.1177/1049732318758644

Emond, K., O'Meara, P., and Bish, M. (2019). Paramedic management of mental health related presentations: A scoping review. *Journal of Mental Health, 28*(1), 89–96. https://doi.org/10.1080/09638237.2018.1487534

Evashkevich, M., and Fitzgerald, M. (2014). *A framework for implementing community paramedic programs in British Columbia.* Richmond, BC: Ambulance Paramedics of British Columbia. https://doi.org/10.13140/RG.2.1.1611.5445

Geddes, J.R., and Miklowitz, D.J. (2013). Treatment of bipolar disorder. *The Lancet, 381*(9878), 1672–1682. https://doi.org/10.1016/S0140-6736(13)60857-0

Gonzales, L., Kois, L.E., Chen, C., López-Aybar, L., McCullough, B., and McLaughlin, K.J. (2022). Reliability of the term 'serious mental illness': A systematic review. *Psychiatric Services, 73*(11), 1255–1262. https://doi.org/10.1176/appi.ps.202100661

Health and Care Professions Council (HCPC) (2023) *Standards of Proficiency: Paramedics.* London: HCPC. https://www.hcpc-uk.org/standards/standards-of-proficiency/paramedics/ (accessed 27 November 2025).

Hor, K., and Taylor, M. (2010). Suicide and schizophrenia: A systematic review of rates and risk factors. *Journal of Psychopharmacology, 24*(4 suppl.), 81–90. https://doi.org/10.1177/1359786810385490

Hou, X-Y., Rego, J., and Service, M. (2013). Review article: Paramedic education opportunities and challenges in Australia. *Emergency Medicine Australasia, 25*(2), 114–119. https://doi.org/10.1111/1742-6723.12034

Jones, S., Howard, L., and Thornicroft, G. (2008). 'Diagnostic overshadowing': Worse physical health care for people with mental illness. *Acta Psychiatrica Scandinavica, 118*(3), 169–171. https://doi.org/10.1111/j.1600-0447.2008.01211.x

Lagomasino, I., Daly, R., and Stoudemire, A. (1999). Medical assessment of patients presenting with psychiatric symptoms in the emergency setting. *Psychiatric Clinics of North America, 22*(4), 819–850.

Linehan, M.M. (2015). *DBT® Skills Training Manual* (2nd edition). New York: Guilford Press.

Lowthian, J.A., Curtis, A.J., Cameron, P.A., Stoelwinder, J.U., Cooke, M.W., and McNeil, J.J. (2010). Systematic review of trends in emergency department attendances: An Australian perspective. *Emergency Medicine Journal, 28*(5), 373–377. https://doi.org/10.1136/emj.2010.099226

McCann, T.V., Savic, M., Ferguson, N., Bosley, E., Smith, K., Roberts, L., et al. (2018). Paramedics' perceptions of their scope of practice in caring for patients with non-medical emergency-related mental health and/or alcohol and other drug problems: A qualitative study. *PLoS One, 13*(12), e0208391. https://doi.org/10.1371/journal.pone.0208391

McIntyre, R.S., Ismail, Z., Watling, C.P., Weiss, C., Meehan, S.R., Musingarimi, P., et al. (2022). Patient-reported outcome measures for life engagement in mental health: A systematic review. *Journal of Patient-Reported Outcomes, 6*, 62. https://doi.org/10.1186/s41687-022-00468-5

Mehler, P.S., and Andersen, A.E. (2022). *Eating Disorders: A comprehensive guide to medical care and complications* (4th edition). Baltimore, MD: Johns Hopkins University Press.

Mental Capacity Act 2005, c. 9. https://www.legislation.gov.uk/ukpga/2005/9/contents (accessed 27 November 2025).

Mental Health Act 1983, c. 20 (as amended by the Mental Health Act 2007). https://www.legislation.gov.uk/ukpga/1983/20 (accessed 27 November 2025).

National Institute for Health and Care Excellence (NICE) (2025). *Bipolar disorder: Lithium.* https://cks.nice.org.uk/topics/bipolar-disorder/prescribing-information/lithium/ (accessed 12 December 2025).

Nelson, A. (2002). *Unequal Treatment: Confronting racial and ethnic disparities in health care.* Washington, DC: National Academies Press.

NHS England (2023). *National Partnership Agreement: Right Care, Right Person (RCRP).* https://www.gov.uk/government/publications/national-partnership-agreement-right-care-right-person (accessed 27 November 2025).

NHS England (2025). *Improving the physical health of people living with severe mental illness: Guidance for integrated care systems.* https://www.england.nhs.uk/long-read/improving-the-physical-health-of-people-living-with-severe-mental-illness/ (accessed 12 December 2025).

O'Meara, P.F., Furness, S., and Gleeson, R. (2017). Educating paramedics for the future: A holistic approach. *Journal of Health and Human Services Administration, 40*(2), 219–251. https://doi.org/10.1177/107937391704000204

Padgett, D.K. (2020). Homelessness, housing instability and mental health: Making the connections. *BJPsych Bulletin, 44*(5), 197–201. https://doi.org/10.1192/bjb.2020.49

Parsons, V., and O'Brien, L. (2011). Paramedic clinical decision-making in mental health care: A new theoretical approach. *International Paramedic Practice, 3*(10), 72–79. https://doi.org/10.12968/jpar.2011.3.10.572

Patel, K., Tchanturia, K., and Harrison, A. (2016). An exploration of social functioning in young people with eating disorders: A qualitative study. *PLoS One, 11*(7), e0159910. https://doi.org/10.1371/journal.pone.0159910

Pennick, H., Cousins, L., and Marikar, D. (2023). Medical emergencies in eating disorders. *Archives of Disease in Childhood: Education and Practice, 108*(6), 410–415. https://doi.org/10.1136/archdischild-2022-324484

Phillips, R., Durkin, M., Engward, H., Cable, G., and Iancu, M. (2023). The impact of caring for family members with mental illnesses on the caregiver: A scoping review. *Health Promotion International, 38*(3), daac049. https://doi.org/10.1093/heapro/daac049

Rees, N., Rapport, F., and Snooks, H. (2015). Perceptions of paramedics and emergency care staff about the care they provide to people who self-harm: A qualitative systematic review. *Journal of Psychosomatic Research, 78*(6), 529–535. https://doi.org/10.1016/j.jpsychores.2015.03.007

Royal College of Paramedics (2019). *Become a Paramedic.* https://collegeofparamedics.co.uk/COP/COP/BecomeAParamedic/Become_a_Paramedic.aspx?hkey=f10838de-b67f-44a0-83b7-8140d8cdba83 (accessed 27 November 2025).

Royal College of Psychiatrists (2022). *Medical Emergencies in Eating Disorders (MEED): Guidance on recognition and management* (CR233). London: Royal College of Psychiatrists. https://www.rcpsych.ac.uk/improving-care/campaigning-for-better-mental-health-policy/college-reports/2022-college-reports/cr233

Ruggeri, M., Leese, M., Thornicroft, G., Bisoffi, G., and Tansella, M. (2000). Definition and prevalence of severe and persistent mental illness. *British Journal of Psychiatry, 177*(2), 149–155. https://doi.org/10.1192/bjp.177.2.149

Schinnar, A.P., Rothbard, A.B., and Kanter, R. (1991). Adding state counts of the severely and persistently mentally ill. *Administration and Policy in Mental Health and Mental Health Services Research, 19*(1), 3–12. https://doi.org/10.1007/BF00710514

Shaban, R.Z. (2005). Paramedic clinical judgment of mental illness: Representations of official accounts. *Journal of Emergency Primary Health Care, 3*(4). https://doi.org/10.33151/ajp.3.4.340

Williams, E.R., and Shepherd, S.M. (2000). Medical clearance of psychiatric patients. *Emergency Medicine Clinics of North America, 18*(2), 185–198. https://doi.org/10.1016/s0733-8627(05)70117-6

World Health Organization (WHO) (2022). *International Statistical Classification of Diseases and Related Problems* (11th edition), ICD-11. https://icd.who.int/en/

Zumstein, N., and Riese, F. (2020). Defining severe and persistent mental illness – a pragmatic utility concept analysis. *Frontiers in Psychiatry, 11*, 648. https://doi.org/10.3389/fpsyt.2020.00648

8 Self-harm and suicidality: Paramedic responses to risk and distress

Seb Brown, Corina Downing, Paula Gardner, and Jo Augustus

Introduction

Self-harm, or non-suicidal self-injury, encompasses deliberate actions intended to inflict harm on oneself without the explicit aim of suicide. Intentional self-harm is defined as any deliberate act of self-poisoning or self-injury irrespective of the apparent purpose of the act. This includes behaviours undertaken with and without suicidal intent. These behaviours often emerge as coping strategies in response to circumstances such as intense emotional distress, psychological trauma, or overwhelming situations. Individuals who engage in self-harm may do so for a wide range of reasons, which can vary greatly from person to person and even from one episode to another. The motivations are often complex and multifaceted. Reasons why people self-harm include:

- *Express inexpressible emotions*: translating complex or unspoken feelings into tangible actions.
- *Externalise internal pain*: manifesting emotional suffering through physical means.
- *Alleviate emotional numbness*: counteracting feelings of detachment or dissociation.
- *Regain a sense of control*: asserting autonomy in situations perceived as uncontrollable.
- *Punish oneself*: enacting self-punishment for perceived faults or experiences.
- *Create a reason for care*: establishing a basis for receiving physical attention or care.
- *Communicate distress*: signalling emotional turmoil to others when verbal communication is challenging.

These behaviours may provide temporary relief; however, they often lead to a cycle of repetition. The transient nature of the relief can reinforce the behaviour, making cessation increasingly difficult. Moreover, subsequent feelings of guilt, shame, or self-criticism may exacerbate the underlying emotional distress, perpetuating the cycle of self-harm.

For paramedic science, understanding intentional self-harm is particularly relevant because paramedics are often the first point of contact for people in crisis, frequently dealing with acute presentations that require rapid assessment, medical intervention, and decisions around mental health risk and safeguarding. Their role is not just to manage physical injuries but also to engage with complex psychosocial dimensions under time pressure and in uncontrolled settings.

In the UK, self-harm is a substantial public health issue. According to NICE (2025), among 11–16-year-olds in England, around 7.3% of girls and 3.6% of boys report having self-harmed or attempted suicide at some point. Among 17–19-year-olds, these figures rise to 21.5% for girls and 9.7% for boys.

Most people who self-harm do not present to hospital services. However, self-harm remains one of the main reasons for hospital attendance for poisoning or injury and repeat visits are common, with approximately 20% re-presenting within one year. The incidence is particularly high among young people: data from Wales shows that among those aged 10–24, there are high rates of presentation in primary care, emergency departments, and other hospital settings. Females are more likely than males to be admitted following self-harm, especially in younger age groups (Marchant et al., 2020).

Risk factors are multifactorial, spanning clinical, demographic, psychosocial, and situational dimensions. Some of the more notable risk factors include:

- *Previous self-harm history*: people who have self-harmed before are at high risk of doing so again.
- *Mental health disorders*: depression, anxiety, personality disorders, and other psychiatric comorbidity are strongly associated with self-harm.
- *Substance misuse*: including alcohol, appears in many episodes of self-harm that present to emergency departments.
- *Family history of suicide or self-harm*: early life adversity (abuse, neglect), social isolation, and socioeconomic disadvantage are prominent risk factors.
- *Physical illness or multi-morbidity*: associated with increased odds of self-harm, even after controlling for depression and other mental health variables.
- *Protective factors*: less studied but include strong social support, good problem-solving skills, stable relationships, and hopefulness or a positive outlook.

Impact on patients, families, and healthcare providers

For patients, intentional self-harm carries immediate risks, including physical injury, poisoning/toxicity, infection, and potentially life-threatening complications. Beyond the physical, there are psychological consequences: shame, guilt, stigma, isolation, repeated episodes, and elevated risk of suicide especially following hospital presentation.

Families and carers can be deeply affected. Qualitative research by O'Keeffe et al. (2021) conducted with the parents of young people who self-harm, shows that they often experience profound emotional responses such as shock, anger, guilt, anxiety, depression, and social isolation. Their daily lives may become disrupted balancing work, caring responsibilities, and other children, and sometimes facing financial burdens. They also found that siblings can also be significantly impacted. There is also often a sense of uncertainty and lack of understanding about what self-harm means, how to help, and fears about the future.

Healthcare providers, including paramedics, face specific challenges. Research shows that caring for people who self-harm can be emotionally draining and morally distressing, particularly when encountering repeat cases, when patients decline further care, or where there is limited mental health support available. In one qualitative UK study, paramedics described gaps in training, uncertainty in roles, and emotional burden when dealing with self-harm cases (Rees et al., 2018).

The demands are not only clinical but also ethical, as paramedics must weigh up respect for autonomy, patient safety, capacity issues, safeguarding, and consent, in settings often with limited privacy or time.

Paramedics operate in high-pressure environments, often the very first healthcare contact for individuals engaging in self-harm. Their assessment, response, and behaviour can shape immediate outcomes such as physical health, prevention of further harm, and longer-term trajectories, for example, whether people engage with follow-up mental health support, risk of repetition or suicide.

Understanding epidemiology and risk factors helps paramedics anticipate which patients may be at higher risk, which informs triage, referral, and risk management decisions. Furthermore, an awareness of the psychosocial dimensions – for instance, how stigma, shame, and family/carer context matter – can improve communication, empathy, and patient experience.

Finally, failing to understand or address self-harm adequately may contribute to negative outcomes. For patients, this may include repeated self-harm or escalation and for families distress and breakdown. Providers may also experience burnout, compassion fatigue, and potential legal/ethical risks. Given the rising rates of self-harm among certain demographic groups, and the cost to the NHS of repeat emergency presentations, it is essential that paramedic science integrates robust evidence on self-harm into education, practice protocols, and system-level policies.

Different perspectives: Pathophysiological and psychological

Self-harm is a complex phenomenon that encompasses biological, psychological, and social dimensions. For paramedics, understanding the underlying mechanisms is essential not only for immediate clinical management, but also for sensitive engagement with patients whose behaviour may be misinterpreted as irrational or attention-seeking. This section explores the physiological and psychological mechanisms, the common methods encountered in the pre-hospital setting, and the broader context of mental health, substance use, and trauma that frequently underpins self-injurious acts.

Although self-harm is often approached as a psychological or behavioural issue, there are important physiological mechanisms at play. Some research suggests that individuals who self-harm often exhibit altered pain thresholds. One study found that adolescents aged 12–17 who had self-harmed five or more times showed significantly higher pain thresholds (thermal and pressure thresholds) compared with peers who had never self-harmed (Cummins et al., 2021). Endorphin release during injury can blunt pain perception, producing temporary relief or even a sense of calm. Dysregulation of the hypothalamic-pituitary-adrenal (HPA) axis has been observed, linking self-harm with stress reactivity and cortisol imbalance. A recent meta-analysis titled 'Physiological stress reactivity and self-harm' (Goreis et al., 2023), which included 29 studies with nearly 1,000 individuals with a history of self-harm and controls, found that those who self-harmed showed significantly lower cortisol responses to stress (e.g. a blunted HPA-axis reaction), as well as lower parasympathetic activity overall.

Case study: Refusing help

Case study: Narrative

It is 2:00am and a paramedic crew consisting of a registered paramedic and a recently employed level 3 emergency care assistant (ECA) are dispatched to a 47-year-old woman, Maria, who lives alone. Maria reports that at approximately 1:00am, around an hour prior to their arrival, she ingested 200 over-the-counter paracetamol tablets with water.

Maria states that she has not consumed alcohol or any other substances and has remained at home throughout the day. She reports having felt increasingly hopeless and low in mood over the previous two weeks but has not discussed this with anyone, although she describes having a positive relationship with her GP. Over recent months, she has experienced increased anxiety, particularly about driving and becoming unwell, and describes a general sense of not 'being herself'. She wonders whether these changes may be related to the menopause.

Maria has no significant past medical history and has not undergone surgery in the last 25 years. She is not prescribed regular medication and has no known drug or food allergies. She exercises regularly and identifies physical activity as one of her main interests, alongside reading and attending the cinema.

She reports no previous history of psychiatric illness, self-harm, or suicidal ideation. She does not smoke, drinks alcohol occasionally, and does not use recreational drugs. On assessment, her affect is consistent with low mood; however, she engages appropriately with the clinicians and demonstrates insight into her situation. She is alert, orientated, and communicates clearly.

Her vital signs are within normal limits, with a respiratory rate of 20 breaths per minute and a capillary blood glucose level of 4.8 mmol/L.

Maria has no surviving parents, both having died from smoking-related illnesses. She separated from her partner two years previously. Her sister lives in the United States; although their relationship has been strained, they have recently resumed contact. Maria believes her sister may have contacted out-of-hours services or NHS 111, which may have led to the ambulance being dispatched. She is currently undertaking a doctorate and has spent her career in research science, specialising in immunology.

Maria states that she took the overdose with the explicit intention of ending her life. She demonstrates detailed knowledge of paracetamol metabolism, explaining that approximately 90% is metabolised by hepatic microsomes and that a proportion generates the toxic metabolite *N*-acetyl-*p*-benzoquinoneimine (NAPQI), which, if untreated, can lead to oxidative hepatocyte injury, liver failure, and death (Schaffer et al., 2025).

Maria willingly discusses her medical and social history and consents to physiological observations being recorded. However, she firmly declines conveyance to hospital or any treatment to reverse the overdose. She states clearly and consistently that her intention is to remain at home and die. She declines assistance and politely asks the clinicians to leave the property. Maria's presentation raises a central pre-hospital dilemma: how to respond when a patient describes clear suicidal intent after a potentially fatal overdose, yet refuses conveyance and treatment. The sections that follow use this case to structure clinical reasoning around safety planning, capacity, proportionality, and lawful escalation.

Safety planning 'in the ambulance or at the doorstep'

In Maria's case, a brief safety plan may support engagement while capacity and immediate medical risk are being clarified. Safety planning is a collaborative, short-term intervention that can reduce immediate risk and support engagement with ongoing care. In pre-hospital settings, safety plans should be simple, practical, and achievable within the next 24 hours.

Practical safety planning prompts for paramedics

P1: Triggers and warning signs
What usually makes things worse?
What signs tell you that you're starting to struggle?

P2: Internal coping strategies
What has helped even a little before (e.g. breathing, grounding, distraction, movement)?

P3: People or places for distraction
Who could you be with, or where could you go, to feel less alone?

P4: Trusted contacts
Who can you call or message if things escalate (friend, family member, neighbour)?
P5: Professional support routes
Crisis line numbers
Local crisis team or mental health services
GP or out-of-hours services
P6: Reducing access to means
Can medications, sharps, or ligatures be moved, locked away, or supervised?
Is someone able to help with this?
P7: Clear escalation plan
What should you do if the urge to self-harm or die becomes stronger tonight?
P8: Agreement and review
Confirm understanding and agreement
Document the plan and provide written information where possible

Safety plans should never replace appropriate conveyance when medical or psychiatric risk is high, but when used appropriately, they can foster hope, preserve autonomy, and reduce immediate harm.

On-scene clinical reference for paramedic management of self-harm and suicidality

Table 8.1 provides a structured, JRCALC-aligned framework to support paramedic clinical reasoning, communication, legal decision-making, and documentation when managing self-harm and suicidality in pre-hospital settings (JRCALC, 2022).

Table 8.1: JRCALC-aligned framework

Stage of care	Key considerations	Practice focus for paramedics
1. Scene safety and immediate risk	JRCALC emphasises clinician and patient safety as the first priority in mental health emergencies	Assess scene safety (sharps, ligatures, medications, aggression, intoxication, environmental risks) Remove or reduce access to means where possible using non-confrontational approaches Consider police support if there is immediate risk to life or safety

(continued)

Table 8.1: *(continued)*

Stage of care	Key considerations	Practice focus for paramedics
2. Primary survey and time-critical physiology	Mental health presentations do not preclude life-threatening physical pathology (JRCALC, 2022)	Conduct ABCDE assessment and treat immediate physiological threats Identify time-critical risks (e.g. overdose, haemorrhage, head injury, airway compromise) Seek early clinical advice (e.g. clinical hub, toxicology services) if indicated
3. Clarifying the self-harm episode	JRCALC recommends understanding the context and intent of self-harm to inform risk management	Establish method(s), timing, dose (if overdose), and whether ingestion was single or staggered Explore the patient's stated intention (to die, to cope, or ambivalent) Identify what the self-harm was intended to achieve (e.g. relief, control, communication)
4. Suicide risk: Dynamic formulation	JRCALC discourages reliance on predictive tools alone and promotes holistic assessment	Assess current suicidal intent (active, passive, or none) Identify plans, access to means, and immediacy of risk Consider dynamic risk factors (hopelessness, entrapment, intoxication) Identify protective factors present at the time of assessment
5. Mental capacity and consent (Mental Capacity Act 2025)	JRCALC highlights the importance of MHA assessments in refusal of care	Assess capacity for the specific decision at that time (understand, retain, weigh, communicate) Consider factors impairing capacity (acute distress, psychosis, intoxication, cognitive impairment) If capacity is lacking or unclear, act in the patient's best interests using the least restrictive option

(continued)

Table 8.1: *(continued)*

Stage of care	Key considerations	Practice focus for paramedics
6. Communication and de-escalation	Effective communication and emotional containment are core JRCALC competencies	Use calm, non-judgemental, trauma-informed language Validate distress without endorsing self-harm or suicide Avoid coercive or dismissive language Offer choices where possible to preserve autonomy and reduce escalation
7. Disposition and care planning	JRCALC supports conveyance, referral, or on-scene management based on risk and capacity	Determine the safest next step: ED conveyance, mental health pathway, primary care referral, or crisis support If not conveyed, develop a collaborative short-term safety plan Ensure the patient knows when and how to seek urgent help if risk escalates
8. Safeguarding considerations	Safeguarding responsibilities apply regardless of patient age or presentation	Identify risks to children, vulnerable adults, or others in the household Consider domestic abuse, coercive control, neglect, or exploitation Escalate safeguarding concerns according to local and national policy
9. Documentation and handover	JRCALC stresses accurate, contemporaneous documentation to support continuity of care	Record the patient's own words regarding intent and refusal Document capacity assessment and rationale clearly Note options offered, decisions made, and safety advice given Use structured handover (e.g. SBAR) including psychosocial risk factors

(continued)

Table 8.1: *(continued)*

Stage of care	Key considerations	Practice focus for paramedics
10. Post-incident reflection and support	JRCALC recognises the emotional impact of mental health emergencies on clinicians	Seek debrief or senior support after high-risk or distressing incidents Reflect on moral distress and uncertainty Access occupational and peer support where needed

'Refusal to Go' toolkit: Capacity, persuasion, proportionality, and action

Refusal of conveyance or treatment following self-harm represents one of the most ethically and clinically challenging scenarios in paramedic practice. These encounters often involve high emotional intensity, uncertainty regarding suicide risk, fluctuating mental capacity, and limited access to specialist mental health support. Paramedics must balance respect for patient autonomy with their duty of care to preserve life, while acting lawfully and proportionately in time-pressured, non-clinical environments (JRCALC, 2022).

A structured conversation approach to refusal

A structured, compassionate conversation can reduce escalation and support safer decision-making. The following sequence is recommended:

Validate – Explore – Offer choices – Clarify consequences – Revisit

- *Validate distress*: Acknowledge the patient's emotional experience without endorsing self-harm or suicidal intent (e.g. 'I can hear how overwhelming this feels for you').
- *Explore the refusal*: Seek to understand the patient's reasons for declining care (e.g. fear of hospital, loss of control, stigma, previous negative experiences).
- *Offer choices*: Where possible, present alternatives that preserve autonomy (e.g. ED conveyance vs. mental health assessment, staying while advice is sought, contacting a trusted person).
- *Clarify consequences*: Provide clear, factual information about risks of refusal in plain language, avoiding coercion or moral pressure.
- *Revisit the decision*: Allow time for reflection; decisions may change once distress reduces or understanding improves.

Applied to Maria, this structure helps explore her reasons for refusing hospital, communicate medical risk in plain language, and create space for reconsideration as distress settles. This approach aligns with trauma-informed care principles and supports proportionality by prioritising engagement over coercion.

Capacity assessment in the context of self-harm

When a patient refuses care, paramedics must assess capacity in relation to this specific decision at this specific time, in line with the Mental Capacity Act 2005. Capacity should not be assumed or dismissed solely on the basis of mental illness or suicidal ideation.

Capacity assessment template (self-harm specific)
The patient must be able to:

1. **Understand:**
   – the nature of their self-harm or overdose
   – the proposed treatment or conveyance
   – the likely consequences of refusing care (including risk of death or serious harm)
2. **Retain:**
   – the relevant information long enough to make a decision
3. **Use or weigh:**
   – the information as part of a reasoning process
   – this includes appreciating personal risk, not merely repeating facts
4. **Communicate:**
   – the decision clearly by speech, writing, or other means

Capacity is decision-specific and time-specific. A patient may have capacity for some decisions but not others.

Fluctuating or unclear capacity

Capacity may be impaired or fluctuate due to:

- acute emotional distress or panic
- intoxication (alcohol or drugs)
- psychosis or severe depression
- trauma responses or dissociation
- hypoglycaemia, head injury, or metabolic disturbance

Where capacity is unclear or fluctuating, paramedics should:

- treat reversible physiological causes where possible
- allow time for de-escalation and reassessment
- seek senior clinical advice (clinical hub, on-call manager)
- act in the patient's best interests if urgent risk to life is present

In such circumstances, preserving life may justify temporary restriction of autonomy, provided actions are lawful and proportionate.

Escalation and multi-agency support

Paramedics should consider escalation when:

- there is ongoing suicidal intent with refusal of care
- capacity is absent or disputed
- there is immediate risk to life
- safeguarding concerns are present

Escalation options include:

- on-call clinical advice or senior paramedic support
- mental health crisis teams (where accessible)
- police support where necessary to prevent immediate harm or facilitate Mental Health Act assessment

Police involvement should be framed as a safety intervention, not a punitive measure, and used only when proportionate and necessary.

Least restrictive and proportionate action

Any intervention that restricts liberty must meet the principles of:

- *Necessity*: Is action required to prevent serious harm?
- *Proportionality*: Is the level of restriction justified by the risk?
- *Least restrictive option*: Is there a safer alternative that preserves autonomy?

Where possible, persuasion, collaboration, and safety planning should precede coercive measures. Clear documentation of reasoning is essential. The next section builds on this, outlining assessment and referral principles that support defensible decisions in cases like Maria's.

Paramedic management and treatment approaches

Pre-hospital assessment techniques and risk evaluation tools

The National Institute of Health and Clinical Excellence states that any person presenting in primary care following an episode of self-harm should have a psychosocial assessment conducted as soon as possible (NICE, 2025). This includes evaluation of any injury and requirement for treatment; this aspect may at least be relatively uncomplicated, as the focus of paramedic education is often noted as being on physical conditions rather than mental health issues (Rees et al., 2018). Once any wounds have been managed, the clinician's next steps should be to evaluate the patient's mental status and any degree of distress: any pressing safety concerns or need for specialist psychiatric referral should be considered at this stage (NICE, 2025). For Maria, the immediate priority is that the psychosocial conversation occurs alongside urgent management of overdose risk, including escalation for clinical advice and clear documentation of refusal and capacity. The Joint Royal Colleges Ambulance Liaison Committee recommends that this involves assessing the patient's behaviour, speech, and non-verbal cues, like appearance, mood, or affect (JRCALC, 2025). Herein lies a frequent challenge to practitioners, as many paramedics lack targeted mental health education, with relatively few feeling confident caring for self-harm patients (McCabe, 2023).

However, the use of fundamental skills like appropriate communication strategies is crucial to successfully working with someone who presents in crisis with a mental health problem (JRCALC, 2025); the Committee suggests that basic emotional intelligence should aid in potentially explaining behaviours, and allow the implementation of suitable management approaches, like reducing anxiety. It is worth noting the importance of the paramedic role in these cases: paramedics are likely to be the first professionals encountered after self-harm, and effective management can be critical in mitigating risk of future episodes (Mughal and Clarke, 2023). Nonetheless, a range of factors beyond the professional's control may adversely impact outcomes of the initial assessment: a person's feelings of shame, especially in the presence of relatives, can prevent paramedics gathering necessary findings to inform care decisions (Rees et al., 2018). Similarly, health inequalities can play a role: regional irregularities in the implementation of self-harm pathways correlate with areas of economic and social deprivation, meaning that patients who self-harm and live in areas of high poverty are likely to report adverse experiences of clinical services (Lever et al., 2025).

Notwithstanding this, appropriate referral remains at the centre of recommended approaches. An elemental evaluation is required, as noted above: beyond this, a specialist assessment, exploring broad psychosocial aspects such as individual strengths and personal needs, is indicated by NICE (2025).

Furthermore, a range of risk assessment strategies may be implemented for the self-harm patient. The close correlation between suicide and self-harm is well-known (Parker et al., 2022). This suggests this approach should form a central element of the approach, and many paramedics will be familiar with simple tools like IPAP - Intent, Plans, Actions, Protection (JRCALC, 2025). Whilst these may potentially form part of a more comprehensive psychosocial evaluation, equally they may serve to promote patient stigmatisation among clinicians and increase ensuing microaggressions from staff; also, there is scepticism as regards the use of 'tick-box' questioning style (Lever et al., 2025). Patients often feel risk assessments are used to protect clinicians and employers rather than being used in their own interests and safety – it is common for practitioners to spend far longer documenting assessments than actually doing them (O'Keeffe et al., 2021). NICE (2025) specifically excludes their use to grade potential risk of self-harm or suicide, similarly stating that they should not be used to inform treatment or discharge decisions. Whilst their use is controversial, the potential association between self-harm and subsequent adverse psychiatric outcomes is acknowledged (Bettis et al., 2020). Indeed, the setting itself may pose its own challenge: the presentation of suicidal ideation in the context of emergency care is associated with higher lethality (Hammarbäck et al., 2023).

In any case, when considering paramedic approaches to self-harm and suicide, analysis often returns to challenges faced in this context for a variety of reasons. Both ability and confidence in delivery of mental health support amongst paramedics could be improved by better access to education and senior clinical advice (Romeu et al., 2023). Ongoing focus on medical care leaves pre-hospital emergency services poorly equipped to manage psychiatric crisis cases (McCann et al., 2018). Moreover, such services that exist are subject to inconsistencies in the levels of care available in different parts of the UK (Phillips, 2024).

Outline of best practices for managing patients manifesting self-harm behaviours

Self-harm behaviours are a result of emotion, and emotional response – the paramedic must manage this to allow rapport to be established (JRCALC, 2022). Paramedics need to be aware of their own perceptions of self-harm, whilst also seeking to understand the patient's emotions and how these may influence behaviour (Kool et al., 2014). JRCALC (2025) suggest empathy is key to this, using active listening and a respectful, compassionate approach. However, appropriate assessment and referral continue to challenge paramedics used to more biomedical methods and they may lack both confidence and competence in this field (Rees et al., 2018).

Service users emphasise the importance of an unbiased attitude from professionals; those who perceive their presentation to be considered an invalid reason for emergency care unsurprisingly report poor experiences (O'Keeffe et al., 2021). Moreover, for practitioners, the challenges of potential misunderstanding coupled with low confidence in their ability to provide satisfactory outcomes can lead to frustration: this obstructs the development of the therapeutic relationship (Kool et al., 2014).

Exploring the nature of this relationship (or 'alliance') may help paramedics develop their approach to patients who self-harm. Key elements include a respectful, open, and collaborative approach, which seeks to promote trust and empathy: these are vital in promoting communication and mutual understanding between service user and professional (Iversen et al., 2025). Indeed, the measured use of these 'soft' skills, particularly empathy, may have greater impact than the use of more specific assessment tools (Opland and Torrico, 2024). It is, however, important to note that being able to engage fully with the conversation is critical: communication barriers or fatigue can limit the professional's ability to achieve this connection (Hammarbäck et al., 2023).

An effective therapeutic relationship allows practitioners to assess risk more accurately and gain better insights into patients' needs (O'Keeffe et al., 2021). Establishing rapport is important to allow the subject of self-harm to be broached, but building *trust* is key to supporting the patient through their care journey, from assessment to referral (Leather et al., 2023). The patient's positive perception of the alliance is widely considered conducive to better outcomes; conversely, where therapeutic relationships are not developed, disengagement and feelings of coercion are more likely (Iversen et al., 2025). On occasion, professional and patient may be 'mismatched' – this can limit potential development of the alliance, leading to disengagement (Opland and Torrico, 2024). Repeated suboptimal experiences where practitioners are seen as authority figures cause service users to feel vulnerable (Iversen et al., 2025). Nonetheless, non-physician professionals like paramedics can be seen as more approachable and open to discuss challenging topics including self-harm (Leather et al., 2023). The paramedic should ultimately protect and acknowledge the patient, but this may be further complicated by being emotionally affected, and caring 'too much' (Parker et al., 2022).

Key aspects of developing a therapeutic relationship are known to support this approach. Using active listening skills, showing empathy and respect, allow professionals to show that they value and understand their patients and their feelings, which in turn builds trust and supports engagement with shared treatment plans (Opland and Torrico, 2024). It is crucial for the provider to appreciate the importance of the life story being shared with them: professionals need to validate the patient's concerns and feelings, as this can facilitate difficult conversations around suicide whilst simultaneously reducing distress (Hammarbäck et al., 2023).

Clearly, being open and transparent is important here. Some debate has developed around the issue of self-disclosure by professionals. Zamir et al. (2022) note that many studies show that this can act as a model of recovery and source of hope for service users. Sharing vulnerability is neither weak nor a sign of weakness; rather, it shows compassion and a willingness to confront challenge and pain with the patient (Hammarbäck et al., 2023). Though there is potential that the practitioner may be perceived as impaired, further patient benefits of self-disclosure include reducing perceived isolation and feelings of shame (Howe, 2011); such advantages may outweigh any drawbacks but on balance this approach would need to be managed carefully and tailored to each individual case.

Though the therapeutic alliance is clearly crucial to fostering meaningful interventions with this patient group, more traditional frameworks are equally valid. The maxim that the clinical history provides the foundation of diagnostic decisions may apply even more in psychiatric presentations as it does in physical health (Moldawsky, 2020). This should include findings from both the patient's personal recollection and story, and more structured frameworks; both should be synthesised through the lens of professional judgement (Bohman, 2023). The use of structured tools like the Patient Health Questionnaire (PHQ-9; see below) should be encouraged and integrated: these can be reliably applied by paramedics in the practice setting (Pretorius and Padmanabhanunni, 2024).

It is important to note that assessment of the self-harm patient's presentation should be mindful of potential negative stereotyping, unconscious biases, or dismissal of the patient's lived experience. Avoiding being judgemental cannot be emphasised enough, as patients who perceive that their presentation is validated have better experiences than those made to feel that their self-harm does not warrant emergency treatment (O'Keeffe et al., 2021). Again, developing a mutual connection is important, and care should focus on understanding the individual context of the patient's actions, feelings, and behaviours (Kool et al., 2014). Indeed, the patient's expectations may well be realistic, that all their issues cannot be 'fixed', and that it is enough that they are listened to and communicated with meaningfully (O'Keeffe et al., 2021). Practitioner education should focus on adopting an altruistic, unbiased, and inclusive approach as a priority in such cases (Parker et al., 2022).

Suicide and self-harm

Of the people who complete suicide, the Royal College of Psychiatrists (2020) state that around half (with a higher proportion among younger people) have engaged in self-harm before. Increased frequency and variety in methods of self-harm are associated with higher incidence, and medical severity, of suicide attempts (Chesin et al., 2017). Although it is important to recognise this close link, some studies suggest paramedics may overestimate (and assume) the suicidal intent amongst self-harm patients, regardless of the severity of injury involved (Rees et al., 2018).

Suicidal ideation

Though it may appear obvious, it is worth clarifying the degree to which suicidal ideation – the desire to cause oneself harm and end life – is indeed a mental 'disorder', to use the language of the Mental Health Act 1983. Harmer et al. (2024) consider suicidal ideation a major mental health concern with potential for catastrophic consequences if not managed appropriately. It has largely been categorised as a symptom of depressive illness rather than been considered an independent subtype (Reeves et al., 2022). Suicidal ideation may also arise when a person feels they simply cannot carry on with their life, rather than them specifically having a mental illness (Hammarbäck et al., 2023)

Predictive aspects of self-harm and suicide

Whilst previously downplayed or under-recognised, today a proactive approach to helping self-harm patients is regarded as crucial in preventing escalation to suicidal behaviour (Royal College of Psychiatrists, 2020). More young people die by suicide than any other cause (Duncan et al., 2019); this should serve only to validate this view.

The likelihood of people who self-harm completing suicide is one hundred times higher compared with the general population (Rees et al., 2018). Self-harm may predict suicidal behaviours in both adolescents and young adults (Chesin et al., 2017). The risk is exacerbated in the presence of a psychiatric co-morbidity, particularly if characterised by psychosis (Beckman, 2018).

Risk assessment

NICE (2022) is unequivocal in its prohibition of the use of prescribed risk assessment scales and frameworks to inform prognosis for future suicide attempts or self-harm. Confusingly, for paramedics at least, the JRCALC (2022) guidelines used to advocate the use of the IPAP Suicide Risk Assessment, which has since been replaced by the 'IPPA' tool in managing these patients. Reluctance to recommend such tools stems from the 'low-risk paradox' as noted by NHS England (2025) that the majority of patients who complete suicide who have been screened by such tools were categorised as low risk. Uncertainty in this area may be further exacerbated by specific paramedic concerns, such as perceived personal accountability (as well as their compassion) should a patient attempt suicide after discharge from their care (Rees et al., 2018). The potential of screening tools to generate false positives is noted by O'Rourke et al. (2023); this could further impact upon any tendency for defensive decision-making.

Nonetheless, while risk assessment frameworks are not perfect, there is support for a consistent approach to conducting a psychiatric assessment, considering both risk and mitigating factors, as this helps establish key patient information (Oquendo and Bernanke, 2017). Adopting a holistic, person-centred approach will integrate aspects of the therapeutic alliance. Such risk assessment should only be conducted in conjunction with sufficient understanding of the patient and their psychiatric history (O'Rourke et al., 2023). NHS England (2025) validate this further, suggesting practitioners should focus on seeking to understand the context of the patient's life and safeguarding their mental health. Safety plans, developed in collaboration with the patient, play a crucial role in this, seeking to mitigate risk factors, rather than predict or manage these (Royal College of Psychiatrists, 2020).

Awareness of factors associated with the likelihood of completed suicide attempts is beneficial. The presence of a psychiatric condition – particularly one involving psychosis – elevates this, as does violent self-harm and elevated aggressive or impulsive behaviour (Beckman, 2018). Furthermore, patients who use a variety of methods to self-harm, and those who present with repeated episodes, should be considered as a 'red flag' in decision-making approaches (Royal College of Psychiatrists, 2020).

Example assessment tools

The Columbia-Suicide Severity Rating Scale (C-SSRS) seeks to distinguish suicidal thoughts from actions, by assessing (separately) the intensity and severity of the ideation itself, as well as related behaviours and their capacity to cause harm; this expands previous linear approaches, which suggested an 'ideation to attempt' progression (Salvi, 2019). It is considered useful in separating active suicidal ideation from more passive thoughts in patients with psychiatric diagnoses (Xiao et al., 2025). Furthermore, it has predictive benefit in terms of classifying suicidality, especially the immediate threat thereof (Bjureberg et al., 2021). However, the importance of the person-centred approach cannot be overstated, and it is worth noting that suicide risk assessment may offer little beyond what a more basic depression score may elicit (Mann et al., 2021).

Similarly, the Patient Health Questionnaire (PHQ-9) was devised to combine practical efficacy with a degree of reliability to assess the frequency of depressive symptoms experienced over the preceding two weeks (Ford et al., 2020). The tool is considered to have both high internal consistency and convergent validity (Rahman et al., 2022). Any assessment tool is of course subject to discrepancies due to inter-operator variability; it has further been observed that variations in how responses are offered by the assessor can cause over-triage of depression (Ford et al., 2020). As noted above, any findings should be considered in the context of the patient's lived experiences and their current presentation, often obtained from the development of a strong therapeutic alliance.

Onward psychiatric care

Clearly, the professional relationship between paramedic and person forms the cornerstone of the approach to the self-harm patient in the field of pre-hospital care. An approach that values empathy, transparency, and integrity should enable the patient to feel that their experience is validated, thus fostering mutual trust and a foundation upon which to develop onward treatment and recovery. It is crucial to maintain an awareness of the close association between self-harming behaviours and suicidal ideation. Central to the concept of supporting these patients is the idea of 'safety management', care that is co-created by patient and professional and focuses on a biopsychosocial approach that addresses both immediate and longer-term safety concerns (NHS England, 2025). Suicidal episodes are frequently characterised by hopelessness and lack of escape from the crisis: having access to a toolkit of coping mechanisms and resources has been found to make a significant difference in breaking harmful cycles (Michail, 2021). The Royal College of Psychiatrists (2020) suggests the 'safety plan' be personalised and include activities to promote feelings of hope, appropriate distraction techniques, and signposting to sources of support. Quantitative research suggests such an approach improves suicidal thoughts, reduces hopelessness, and improves engagement with treatment initiatives (Ferguson et al., 2022). Though this approach will underpin ongoing care strategies, it is important for the paramedic to have an appreciation of the positive impact of safety plans in the immediate management of crisis, as they can offer hope and a foundation upon which to build recovery.

Review of initial paramedic interventions and care in other settings

Despite widespread awareness of NICE guidance in primary care settings, suboptimal practice in the care of self-harm patients continues (Lever et al., 2025). The significance of the paramedic role should not be overlooked, as paramedics are likely to be the first point of contact for a person in crisis, who may well be highly distraught; dealing with this stress is crucial to achieving positive outcomes (JRCALC, 2022). The role of paramedics is further validated by their encounters with patients at different points in their suicide journey (Hammarbäck et al., 2023). As noted above, the significance of empathy in the approach to the self-harm patient, whilst treating them both compassionately and respectfully, cannot be overstated (Mughal and Clarke, 2023).

Furthermore, Phillips (2024) stresses the importance of de-escalation techniques and suicide risk assessment as part of the collaborative approach. Facilitators of high-quality treatment interventions include previous exposure to psychiatric patients, senior practitioner support, and specialist mental health education (Romeu et al., 2023). Such training should encompass both patient assessment and referral decision-making, as well as explore the underlying causes of self-harm behaviours (Zayed et al., 2020). Though the desire for further development is widely expressed, this may have unwelcome consequences. There are concerns that this may manifest itself as overtreatment in psychiatric care by paramedics (Phillips, 2024).

Handover strategies

Effective patient handover remains an area of potential improvement in paramedic practice. Risk is inherent in the process itself: stress, environmental factors, and distractions leave the paramedic handover susceptible to error and poor shared communication (Najafi Kalyani et al., 2017). Furthermore, a lack of standardised models and lack of clarity around responsibility may be detrimental to patient safety (Dúason et al., 2021; Asurlekar, 2025).

Factors such as burnout and exposure to frequent callers can harden practitioner feelings towards self-harm patients (O'Keeffe et al., 2021). These attitudes may be manifested during the handover, and should be avoided: negativity towards patients, particularly around labelling them and being judgemental, inevitably compromises ongoing care and may have severe consequences (Hunt et al., 2011). These include disjointed care, treatment delays, and a lack of understanding of the patient's needs; nonetheless, this risk could be mitigated by improving the structure of handovers (Asurlekar, 2025). The application of a simple and familiar framework like 'SBAR' (Situation, Background, Assessment, Recommendation) may well be effective here (Park, 2020). Evidence from psychiatric inpatient settings suggests a closer involvement of patients in handovers may offer potential benefits, although research in this area is limited. While some nurses struggle with appropriate language and data-sharing, patient experience has been shown to improve when they take a more active role in the handover process, as active collaboration in decision-making and co-creation of care is fostered (Van de Velde et al., 2024). Although the adoption of this approach in a paramedic context may be some way off, it offers potential to develop further person-centred approaches.

Referral pathways and interprofessional collaboration with mental health services

If safe to do so, the self-harm patient should be referred to primary care within a 48-hour period (NICE, 2022). Indeed, it is this destination where most of this patient group receive treatment, whether pharmacological or social prescribing is used: this emphasises how important it is for paramedics to develop close working relationships with both GPs and community psychiatric professionals (Phillips, 2024). However, there remains an issue since the long-established primacy of physical over psychiatric care in paramedicine means practitioners may not be well-equipped to adequately respond to self-harm patients (McCann et al., 2018). A lack of certainty around referral processes and destinations remains a challenge to patient management (Leather et al., 2023). The frequent inability to liaise with crisis teams compounds this; essentially, the desire to do better is there, yet often the means to achieve this are not (Rees et al., 2018). Clearly there is a need for high-quality pathways into primary care so paramedics can facilitate onward care journeys for this vulnerable patient group (Phillips, 2024).

Beyond primary care, national guidance suggests that UK Trusts providing ambulance, psychiatric, and casualty services should collaborate to improve pathways for self-harm-patients (Zayed et al., 2020). A potential issue here is the transition of care ensuring a consistent approach is maintained. Paramedic patient encounters are relatively brief whilst other providers have a longer-term focus: differing priorities may mean working together to achieve these goals is a significant challenge (Phillips, 2024).

The Department of Health and Social Care (DHSC, 2023) notes significant investment in psychiatric acute services, including innovative solutions like mental health ambulances and crisis cafes and hubs. Whilst this is a welcome intervention, it is a long-term strategy, and it may be some years before any benefits are widely felt.

Currently, there remains wide variation in the provision of appropriate services for self-harm patients. Whilst ambulance Trusts have been proactive in developing creative pathway solutions, the success of these depends largely upon whether mental health teams are available (Zayed et al., 2020). For people requiring specialist interventions, services may differ dependent on location and specific patient need (Phillips, 2024). There are fewer admissions to inpatient care for self-harm patients from deprived areas than in more affluent areas, with consequential adverse experiences reported (Lever et al., 2025). Concern around such potential variations, and their preparedness to navigate these, remains an issue for paramedics (McCann et al., 2018). Overall, it is widely agreed that pathways for patients who self-harm need alternatives to emergency departments, more resourcing and staffing, and education for paramedics, particularly for patients who decline hospital attendance (Romeu et al., 2023).

Ethical and legal considerations

Caring for self-harm patients remains a challenge, not least due to the established association with suicidal behaviours. One area of concern is the suicidal patient who refuses help or onward referral, particularly if they appear to have capacity. The doctrine of self-determination is a central tenet of English law, and patients have the right to decline aid, however irrational or dangerous the intention (Muzaffar, 2011). Hammarbäck et al. (2023) note that paramedics struggle to form a concept of their duty of care in these cases; the ethical conflict between an expectation of beneficence potentially at odds with respect for autonomous self-direction, remains at the heart of this. Maria's scenario illustrates this conflict clearly: she communicates a consistent wish to die following a potentially lethal act, yet also appears calm, articulate, and informed, making lawful, proportionate decision-making essential.

One study found that of the patients presenting at the emergency department with self-harming behaviours who had capacity, just under a third expressed a desire to refuse life-saving care (Nowland et al., 2019). This suggests a significant number of patients who may present paramedics with this clear dilemma. The straightforward onus to preserve life is provided further rationale by JRCALC (2022), who note that some survivors of highly lethal suicide attempts later stated they were acting impulsively, often as a reaction to adverse life events.

The lack of a leading case in this area does little to clarify the legal standing of paramedics in these circumstances. The case of Karen Woolterton is perhaps the best example. Having attempted suicide on multiple occasions previously, she presented at the emergency department having ingested antifreeze, though on her last attendance she had an advance directive to refuse life-saving interventions; her treating doctors assessed her as having capacity to refuse care (Beale et al., 2024). The case was subject to a coroner's inquest, who found no issue with this decision (Owen et al., 2019). Nonetheless, it was noted that the question remained as to whether the patient should have been admitted for assessment under s. 63 of the Mental Health Act 1983, for treatment of a mental disorder without consent (Craigie and Bortolotti, 2014). The case was not further discussed in court: the Court of Protection may well have judged it differently to the coroner, but this will never be known (Beale et al., 2024).

Though a complex area, Rees et al. (2018) note that many paramedics feel they have a reasonable working knowledge of the legal parameters around self-harm, though they are equally acutely aware of the potential ethical challenges and may not be confident in addressing these. The suicidal patient with capacity, clear means and intent brings two key articles of the Human Rights

Act 1998 into direct conflict: Article 2 (right to life) and Article 5 (right to liberty). Beale et al. (2024) note that both the Mental Health Act 2007 and Mental Capacity Act 2005 (MCA) were drafted to observe these principles: central to both is the idea of *proportionality*. This means that any decision made that interferes with such rights must have adequate justification.

Proportionality requires that decision-makers considering an interference with a Convention right must balance the severity of the interference with the intensity of the social need for action. In essence, they must decide whether interference with a person's rights is justified. The emergency nature of much paramedic work, particularly in mental health care, should be considered here. The MCA Code of Practice (Department for Constitutional Affairs, 2007) notes that definitions of 'reasonable' are different in emergency settings from those in different clinical settings (at 6.35), and that suicidal ideation at time of writing an Advance Decision may suggest a lack of capacity (at 9.9). Indeed, a competent person freely deciding to end their life represents the most compelling example of autonomy (Fontalis et al., 2018). In person-centred care, after all, self-determination should overarch even beneficence in decision-making (Cave, 2017).

The key question to consider is whether acute suicidal ideation alone represents an adequate insult to cognitive function to invoke a best interest decision under the MCA 2005. In *King's College NHS Foundation Trust v. C and V*, the Court of Protection clearly ruled that the presence of psychiatric illness should not allow practitioners to assume inability to make a decision. In practice, whilst not all patients with depression lack capacity, up to a third may well be impaired: in patients who attempted suicide, up to 60% were found to have impaired decision-making insight (Olié et al., 2023). In a range of settings, a person's wish to end their life may be a rational decision (Fontalis et al., 2018). Conversely, in suicide, the preserve of autonomy should not be the clinician's focus: whilst similar arguments may be proposed, the setting of a paramedic exercising their duty of care to a patient presenting with acute suicidal ideation is very different to the wider 'right to die' debate. In suicide risk patients, clinicians should act positively to protect life rather than consider mental capacity as the principal factor (Beale et al., 2024). The European Court of Human Rights (ECHR) explicitly states this in *Fernandes De Oliveira v. Portugal* (2019), noting that it would be unconscionable for the state to leave the vulnerable to end their lives in respect of their personal autonomy.

Conclusion

Self-harm and suicidality are common and complex presentations in pre-hospital care, often shaped by psychological distress, trauma, social adversity, and fluctuating risk. Returning to Maria, the chapter's principles translate into three priorities: manage time-critical overdose risk, assess capacity for refusal in the moment, and, where non-conveyance is not lawful or safe, escalate and act proportionately in the patient's best interests. For paramedics, the challenge lies in working simultaneously across two domains: urgent physical risk management (e.g. poisoning, injury, physiological deterioration) and person-centred mental health crisis care, including distress containment, risk formulation, safeguarding, and collaborative safety planning. These calls frequently occur in time-pressured, unpredictable environments where privacy is limited and access to specialist mental health services varies.

This chapter has sought to emphasise that effective paramedic responses depend less on 'perfect prediction' and more on good clinical reasoning and proportionate decision-making. This includes establishing immediate safety, clarifying the function and context of self-harm, assessing current suicidal intent and access to means, considering dynamic protective factors, and making defensible decisions about conveyance or referral. In high-stakes cases, particularly where life-saving treatment is refused, paramedics must balance ethical principles of autonomy and beneficence within the legal frameworks of the Mental Capacity Act and Mental Health Act, ensuring that any interference with liberty is necessary, proportionate, and least restrictive.

A consistent, compassionate approach is also clinically important. Many patients report that the manner of the first professional contact after self-harm can influence whether they engage with ongoing support. Paramedics therefore have a pivotal role not only in preventing immediate harm, but also in shaping the patient's trajectory after crisis through communication, validation, and clear safety-netting. By integrating physical assessment skills with trauma-informed communication, lawful decision-making, and practical safety planning, paramedics can respond to self-harm and suicidality in ways that protect life, preserve dignity, and support recovery while also protecting their own professional wellbeing and accountability.

Finally, these cases affect clinicians. Repeated exposure, perceived system gaps, and fear of adverse outcomes can contribute to moral distress and burnout. Safe care includes attending to the psychological safety of staff through supervision, peer support, and reflective learning.

Further learning materials

Multiple-choice questions

MCQ1: *Definitions*: Which statement best reflects current understanding of self-harm in pre-hospital care?

A. Self-harm always indicates suicidal intent

B. Self-harm is limited to cutting behaviours

C. Self-harm may occur with or without suicidal intent

D. Self-harm is primarily attention-seeking

Correct answer: C

Rationale: Self-harm is a heterogeneous behaviour that can function as emotion regulation, communication of distress, or suicide attempt, so intent must be assessed rather than assumed.

MCQ2: *Epidemiology*: Which group has the highest reported prevalence of self-harm in the UK?

A. Men aged over 60

B. Girls aged 11–16

C. Boys aged 11–16

D. Adults aged over 40

Correct answer: B

Rationale: UK epidemiology consistently reports the highest rates of self-harm in early adolescent girls, making this a key at-risk group for recognition and early intervention.

MCQ3: *Risk factors*: Which factor is most strongly associated with repetition of self-harm?

A. Female sex

B. Socioeconomic status alone

C. Previous history of self-harm

D. Physical fitness

Correct answer: C

Rationale: A prior episode of self-harm is the strongest predictor of repetition in the future and should heighten vigilance and safety planning.

MCQ4: *Pre-hospital priorities*: When attending a patient following self-harm, what is the paramedic's first priority?

A. Completing a suicide risk score

B. Establishing a psychiatric diagnosis

C. Ensuring scene safety and managing time-critical physiology

D. Developing a long-term care plan

Correct answer: C

Rationale: Pre-hospital care prioritises clinician/patient safety and time-critical physiological threats before psychosocial formulation or longer-term planning.

MCQ5: *Overdose management*: Which statement regarding paracetamol overdose is correct?

A. Symptoms always appear within the first hour

B. Normal observations exclude serious toxicity

C. Early treatment is critical to prevent liver failure

D. Capacity assessment is unnecessary if the patient is calm

Correct answer: C

Rationale: Paracetamol toxicity can be initially asymptomatic, and timely antidote treatment is essential to prevent hepatic injury and liver failure.

MCQ6: *Capacity and refusal*: Which principle is correct when a patient who has self-harmed refuses care?

A. Suicidal intent automatically removes capacity

B. Capacity is global and permanent

C. Capacity is decision-specific and time-specific

D. Refusal must always be respected regardless of risk

Correct answer: C

Rationale: Under the Mental Capacity Act, capacity must be assessed for the specific decision at the specific time, particularly where refusal carries serious risk.

MCQ7: *Risk assessment tools*: Current NICE guidance advises that suicide risk scales should:

A. Be used to predict future suicide

B. Determine discharge decisions

C. Replace clinical judgement

D. Not be used to stratify future suicide risk

Correct answer: D

Rationale: NICE advises against using risk scales to predict or stratify future suicide risk, emphasising holistic clinical assessment and formulation instead.

MCQ8: *Therapeutic approach*: Which communication strategy is most appropriate when managing self-harm?

A. Challenging the patient's beliefs

B. Neutral, validating, non-judgemental language

C. Avoiding discussion of intent

D. Focusing only on physical injury

Correct answer: B

Rationale: Calm, validating, non-judgemental communication reduces escalation, supports engagement, and enables safer assessment and decision-making.

Guided clinical reasoning questions

Immediate priorities: Safety and time-critical care:

Q1: *Scene safety*: Is the scene safe for clinicians, the patient, and others (e.g. sharps, ligatures, aggression, intoxication, unsafe environment)?

Q2: *Immediate risk of further harm*: Is the patient likely to self-harm again during your attendance (e.g. means available, escalating distress, intent expressed)?

Q3: *Physiological urgency*: What is the most time-critical physical risk right now (e.g. overdose, bleeding, head injury, airway compromise)?

Q4: *Key time points*: What is the timeline of events (e.g. time of self-harm/ingestion, discovery, help-seeking, current mental state trajectory)?
Rapid formulation: Understanding the 'why' and the 'why now':

Q5: *Precipitating factors*: What changed in the last hours/days that led to this episode?

Q6: *Function of self-harm*: What does the patient say the self-harm achieved (e.g. relief, numbness, punishment, communication, control)?

Q7: *Suicidal intent*: Was the act intended to end life, reduce distress, or both? How certain is the patient about wanting to die *right now*?

Q8: *Hopelessness and entrapment*: Does the patient describe feeling there is 'no way out' or that nothing will improve?
Suicide risk and protective factors (dynamic, not predictive):

Q9: *Current intent*: Does the patient still intend to die? If yes, is it active plans, means, time-frame, or passive 'wish I wouldn't wake up'?

Q10: *Plan and means*: Is there a specific plan, and access to lethal means at home or on scene?

Q11: *Lethality and medical severity*: How medically serious is the method used? What is the likely trajectory if untreated?

Q12: *Protective factors*: What is keeping the person alive today (e.g. relationships, values, responsibilities, future plans, faith, pets, treatment engagement)?

Q13: *Future orientation*: Can the patient identify any reason to accept help, even if small (e.g. 'not tonight', 'speak to GP', 'phone a friend')?

Capacity and consent in the context of self-harm:

Q14: *Decision to be assessed*: Is the patient consenting to assessment and observation? If not, what is the nature of the refusal?

Q15: *Capacity (MCA 2005)*: Can the patient (a) understand relevant information (e.g. what has happened and the likely consequences)?, (b) retain that information long enough to decide?, (c) use/weigh it as part of the decision-making process?, (d) communicate the decision?

Q16: *Influencing factors*: Could capacity be compromised or fluctuating due to intoxication, delirium, severe anxiety, psychosis, trauma response, severe depression, or cognitive impairment?

Q17: *Proportionality*: If considering restricting liberty, is the intervention necessary, proportionate, and the least restrictive option available?
Communication and de-escalation: What you do and say:

Q18: *Engagement*: What approach will most likely reduce shame and increase safety (e.g. privacy, tone, non-judgemental language, pacing)?

Q19: *Validation*: Have you acknowledged distress and meaning – 'It sounds unbearable' – without endorsing self-harm?

Q20: *Choice and collaboration*: What options can you offer that preserve autonomy (e.g. ED vs. crisis alternative, family contact, staying with patient while calling support)?

Q21: *If refusal persists*: Have you explored (a) what the patient fears about hospital?, (b) what would make help acceptable?, (c) whether they can agree to a 'short-term safety step' (e.g. assessment now and reconsider later)?

Disposition planning: Conveyance, referral, or safety plan:

Q22: *Clinical threshold*: What is the minimum safe next step given medical risk and expressed intent?

Q23: *Alternatives to ED*: Are any locally available crisis pathways viable now (e.g. mental health triage car, crisis team, crisis café/hub, urgent GP, community mental health)?

Q24: *Safety planning*: If not conveyed, what concrete safety actions can be agreed before leaving (e.g. remove/reduce means, supervision, crisis contact plan)?

Q25: *Safeguarding*: Are there children, vulnerable adults, domestic abuse, neglect, or coercive control concerns requiring escalation?

Q26: *Documentation*: What must be recorded to ensure continuity and legal defensibility (e.g. assessment, capacity rationale, options offered, patient's words, plan, and safety-netting)?

Teamwork and support:

Q27: *Clinical advice*: Who can you contact for senior support (e.g. clinical hub, mental health practitioner line, toxicology/poisons advice)?

Q28: *Handover*: What does the receiving team need to know to act safely (e.g. timeline, method, intent, capacity, risks/protective factors, safeguarding)?

Q29: *Aftercare for clinicians*: What support do you and your crewmate need after this call (e.g. debrief, reflection, follow-up)?

Reflective questions for learners

Q1: How might your own emotional reactions influence decision-making when a patient refuses care after self-harm?

Q2: What strategies help you balance respect for autonomy with your duty to preserve life in high-risk situations?

Q3: How can trauma-informed communication reduce escalation and improve patient safety during these encounters?

Q4: In Maria's case, what factors would most influence your assessment of capacity and proportionality of action?

Q5: How might your interaction as the first clinician affect the patient's willingness to engage with future mental health support?

Q6: What support do you need after managing a high-risk self-harm or suicidality call?

Teaching commentary

This chapter highlights the reality that self-harm and suicidality are among the most complex and emotionally demanding presentations encountered in pre-hospital care. Unlike many biomedical emergencies, these situations rarely offer clear thresholds or definitive answers. Instead, paramedics are required to integrate clinical assessment, communication skills, ethical reasoning, and legal frameworks within unpredictable and time-pressured environments.

A central teaching point is that risk cannot be predicted with certainty. The emphasis therefore shifts from attempting to categorise patients as 'low' or 'high' risk towards dynamic, person-centred clinical reasoning that focuses on immediate safety, current intent, protective factors, and proportionate decision-making. Learners should recognise that effective care often lies in *how* the assessment is conducted as much as *what* decisions are made. The chapter also reinforces the importance of understanding and applying the Mental Capacity Act in real-world contexts. Refusal of care following self-harm should prompt careful exploration rather than automatic acceptance or coercion. Capacity assessments must be specific, defensible, and revisited where distress, intoxication, or mental illness may impair decision-making.

Finally, learners should appreciate the significant impact of paramedic behaviour on patient experience and engagement with future care. Compassionate communication, collaborative safety planning, and clear handover practices can reduce stigma, promote trust, and potentially alter the patient's longer-term trajectory. Equally, recognising the emotional burden of this work and seeking appropriate support are an essential component of safe and sustainable paramedic practice.

References

Asurlekar, A. (2025). Handover practices for psychiatric admissions: A retrospective review of communication gaps. *BJPsych Open, 11*, S180. Available at: https://doi.org/10.1192/bjo.2025.10469

Beale, C., Lee-Davey, J., Lee, T., and Ruck Keene, A. (2024). Mental capacity in practice, part 2: Capacity and the suicidal patient. *BJPsych Advances, 30*(1), 11–20. https://doi.org/10.1192/bja.2022.82

Beckman, K. (2018). *Self-harm in youth – predicting mental illness, social marginalisation and suicide.* Thesis, Karolinska Institute. https://openarchive.ki.se/articles/thesis/Self-harm_in_youth_predicting_mental_illness_social_marginalisation_and_suicide/26907352?file=48950263 (accessed 9 October 2025).

Bettis, A., Liu, R., Walsh, B., and Klonsky, E. (2020). Treatments for self-injurious thoughts and behaviors in youth: Progress and challenges. *Evidence-Based Practice in Child and Adolescent Mental Health, 5*(3), 354–364. https://doi.org/10.1080/23794925.2020.1806759

Bjureberg, J., Dahlin, M., Carlborg, A., Edberg, H., Haglund, A., and Runeson, B. (2021). Columbia-Suicide Severity Rating Scale Screen Version: Initial screening for suicide risk in a psychiatric emergency department, *Psychological Medicine, 52*(16), 1–9. https://doi.org/10.1017/S0033291721000751

Bohman, B. (2023). Clinicians' perceptions and practices of diagnostic assessment in psychiatric services. *BMC Psychiatry, 23*, 191. https://doi.org/10.1186/s12888-023-04689-w

Cave, E. (2017). Protecting patients from their bad decisions: Rebalancing rights, relationships, and risk. *Medical Law Review, 25*(4), 527–553. https://doi.org/10.1093/medlaw/fww046

Chesin, M., Galfavy, H., Sonmez, C., Wong, A., Oquendo, M., Mann, J., et al. (2017). Non-suicidal self-injury is predictive of suicide attempts among individuals with mood disorders. *Suicide and Life-Threatening Behavior, 47*(5), 567–579. https://doi.org/10.1111/sltb.12331

Craigie, J., and Bortolotti, L. (2014). Rationality, diagnosis, and patient autonomy in psychiatry, in J. Sadler, K. Fulford, and C. van Staden (eds.) *The Oxford Handbook of Psychiatric Ethics*, vol. 1. Oxford: Oxford University Press. https://www.ncbi.nlm.nih.gov/books/NBK361400/

Cummins, T.M., English, O., Minnis, H., Stahl, D., O'Connor, R.C., Bannister, K., et al. (2021). Assessment of somatosensory function and self-harm in adolescents. *JAMA Network Open, 4*(7), e2116853. https://doi.org/10.1001/jamanetworkopen.2021.16853

Department for Constitutional Affairs (2007). *Mental Capacity Act 2005: Code of Practice.* https://www.gov.uk/government/publications/mental-capacity-act-code-of-practice (accessed 5 October 2025).

Department of Health (2015). *Mental Health Act 1983: Code of Practice.* https://www.gov.uk/government/publications/code-of-practice-mental-health-act-1983 (accessed 5 October 2025).

Department of Health and Social Care (DHSC) (2023). *Suicide prevention in England: 5-year cross-sector strategy.* https://www.gov.uk/government/publications/suicide-prevention-strategy-for-england-2023-to-2028/suicide-prevention-in-england-5-year-cross-sector-strategy#providing-effective-and-appropriate-crisis-support (accessed 9 October 2025).

Dúason, S., Gunnarsson, B., and Svavarsdóttir, M. (2021). Patient handover between ambulance crew and healthcare professionals in Icelandic emergency departments: A qualitative study. *Scandinavian Journal of Trauma, Resuscitation and Emergency Medicine, 29*, 21. https://doi.org/10.1186/s13049-021-00829-x

Duncan, E., Best, C., Dougall, N., Skar, S., Evans, J., Corfield, A., et al. (2019). Epidemiology of emergency ambulance service calls related to mental health problems and self harm: A national record linkage study. *Scandinavian Journal of Trauma, Resuscitation and Emergency Medicine, 27*, 34. https://doi.org/10.1186/s13049-019-0611-9

Ferguson, M., Rhodes, K., Loughhead, M., McIntyre, H., and Procter, N. (2022). The effectiveness of the safety planning intervention for adults experiencing suicide-related distress: A systematic review. *Archives of Suicide Research, 26*(3), 1022–1045. https://doi.org/10.1080/13811118.2021.1915217

Fernandes De Oliveira v. Portugal (2019). European Court of Human Rights (Application no. 78103/14). https://hudoc.echr.coe.int/eng/#{%22itemid%22:[%22001-189426%22]} (accessed 5 October 2025).

Fontalis, A., Prousali, E., and Kulkarni, K. (2018). Euthanasia and assisted dying: What is the current position and what are the key arguments informing the debate? *Journal of the Royal Society of Medicine, 111*(11), 407–413. https://doi.org/10.1177/0141076818803452

Ford, J., Thomas, F., Byng, R., and McCabe, R. (2020). Use of the Patient Health Questionnaire (PHQ-9) in practice: Interactions between patients and physicians. *Qualitative Health Research, 30*(13), 2146–2159. https://doi.org/10.1177/1049732320924625

Goreis, A., Prillinger, K., Bedus, C., Lipp, R., Mayer, A., Nater, U.M., et al. (2023). Physiological stress reactivity and self-harm: A meta-analysis. *Psychoneuroendocrinology, 158*, 106406. http://doi.org/10.1016/j.psyneuen.2023.106406

Hammarbäck, S., Holmberg, M., Wiklund Gustin, L., and Bremer, A. (2023). Ambulance clinicians' responsibility when encountering patients in a suicidal process. *Nursing Ethics, 30*(6), 857–870. https://doi.org/10.1177/09697330221149102

Harmer, B., Lee, S., Rizvi, A., et al. (2024). *Suicidal ideation.* https://www.ncbi.nlm.nih.gov/books/NBK565877/ (accessed 10 October 2025).

Howe, E. (2011). Should psychiatrists self disclose? *Innovations in Clinical Neuroscience, 8*(12), 14–17.

Human Rights Act 1998, c. 42. https://www.legislation.gov.uk/ukpga/1998/42/contents (accessed 5 October 2025).

Hunt, G., Marsden, R., and O'Connor, N. (2011). Clinical handover in acute psychiatric community mental health settings. *Journal of Psychiatric and Mental Health Nursing, 19*(4), 310–318. https://doi.org/10.1111/j.1365-2850.2011.01793.x

Iversen, H., Riley, H., Råbu, M., and Lorem, G.F. (2025). Building and sustaining therapeutic relationships across treatment settings: A qualitative study of how patients navigate the group dynamics of mental healthcare. *BMC Psychiatry, 25*, 424. https://doi.org/10.1186/s12888-025-06874-5

Joint Royal Colleges Ambulance Liaison Committee (JRCALC) (2022). *Joint Royal Colleges Ambulance Liaison Committee and Association of Ambulance Chief Executives Clinical Guidelines 2022*. Bridgwater: Class Professional Publishing.

Joint Royal Colleges Ambulance Liaison Committee (JRCALC) (2025). *JRCALC clinical guidelines update*, July. https://jrcalc.org.uk/publication-date-july-2025/ (accessed 11 December 2025).

King's College NHS Foundation Trust v. C and V [2015] EWCOP 59 (MacDonald J). https://www.39essex.com/our-thinking/cases/kings-college-nhs-foundation-trust-v-c-and-v/

Kool, N., van Meijel, B., Koekkoek, B., van der Bijl, J., and Kerkhof, A. (2014). Improving communication and practical skills in working with inpatients who self-harm: A pre-test/post-test study of the effects of a training programme. *BMC Psychiatry, 14*, 64. https://doi.org/10.1186/1471-244X-14-64

Leather, J., Keyworth, C., Kapur, N., Campbell, S., and Armitage, C. (2023). Implementation of national guidance for self-harm among general practice nurses: A qualitative exploration using the capabilities, opportunities, and motivations model of behaviour change (COM-B) and the theoretical domains framework. *BMC Nursing, 22*, 452. https://doi.org/10.1186/s12912-023-01360-3

Lever, G., Dowding, D., Jeyasingham, D., and Armitage, C. (2025). Health and social care professionals' awareness and implementation of NICE guidelines on self-harm: A rapid review of the literature. *BMJ Open, 15*, e093883. https://doi.org/10.1136/bmjopen-2024-093883

Mann, J., Michel, C., and Auerbach, R. (2021). Improving suicide revention through evidence-based strategies: A systematic review. *American Journal of Psychiatry, 178*(7), 611–624. https://doi.org/10.1176/appi.ajp.2020.20060864

Marchant, A., Turner, S., Balbuena, L., Peters, E., Williams, D., Lloyd, K., et al (2020). Self-harm presentation across healthcare settings by sex in young people: An e-cohort study using routinely collected linked healthcare data in Wales, UK. *Archives of Disease in Childhood, 105*(4), 347–354. https://doi.org/10.1136/archdischild-2019-317248

McCabe, A. (2023). Management of self-harm. *Emergency Medicine Journal, 40*(7), 472–473. https://doi.org/10.1136/emermed-2023-213283

McCann, T., Savic, M., Ferguson, N., Bosley, E., Smith, K., Roberts, L., et al. (2018). Paramedics' perceptions of their scope of practice in caring for patients with non-medical emergency-related mental health and/or alcohol and other drug problems: A qualitative study. *PLoS One, 13*(12): e0208391. https://doi.org/10.1371/journal.pone.0208391

Mental Capacity Act 2005, c. 9. https://www.legislation.gov.uk/ukpga/2005/9/contents (accessed 5 October 2025).

Mental Health Act 1983, c. 20. https://www.legislation.gov.uk/ukpga/1983/20/section/62 (accessed 5 October 2025).

Michail, M. (2021). How can we work together to keep you safe? A simple and effective intervention that can save lives. *British Journal of General Practice, 71*(710), 409. https://doi.org/10.3399/bjgp21X716909

Moldawsky, R. (2020). Is the psychiatric history losing its relevance? *Permanente Journal, 24*(4). https://doi.org/10.7812/TPP/19.186

Mughal, F., and Clarke, L. (2023). NICE self-harm 2022 guideline: Implications for ambulance staff. *British Paramedic Journal, 8*(2), 57–58. https://doi.org/10.29045/14784726.2023.9.8.2.57

Muzaffar, S. (2011). 'To treat or not to treat'. Kerrie Wooltorton, lessons to learn. *Emergency Medicine Journal, 28*, 741–744. https://doi.org/10.1136/emj.2010.100750

Najafi Kalyani, M., Fereidouni, Z., Sarvestani, R., Hadian Shirazi, Z., and Taghinezhad, A. (2017). Perspectives of patient handover among paramedics and emergency department members; A qualitative study. *Emergency (Tehran), 5*(1), e76. https://pubmed.ncbi.nlm.nih.gov/29201958/ (accessed 9 October 2025).

National Institute of Health and Clinical Excellence (NICE) (2022). *Self-harm: Assessment, management and preventing recurrence* (NG225). London: NICE. https://www.nice.org.uk/guidance/ng225 (accessed 10 October 2025).

National Institute of Health and Clinical Excellence (NICE) (2025). *Clinical knowledge summary: Self-harm.* https://cks.nice.org.uk/topics/self-harm/ (accessed 10 October 2025).

NHS England (2025). *Staying safe from suicide.* https://www.england.nhs.uk/long-read/staying-safe-from-suicide/ (accessed 9 October 2025).

Nowland, R., Steeg, S., Quinlivan, L., Cooper, J., Huxtable, R., Hawton, K., et al. (2019). Management of patients with an advance decision and suicidal behaviour: A systematic review. *BMJ Open, 9*, e023978. https://doi.org/10.1136/bmjopen-2018-023978

O'Keeffe, S., Suzuk,i M., Ryan, M., Hunter, J., and McCabe, R. (2021). Experiences of care for self-harm in the emergency department: Comparison of the perspectives of patients, carers and practitioners. *BJPsych Open, 7*(5), e175. https://doi.org/10.1192/bjo.2021.1006

Olié, E., Catanzaro, T., Malestroit, M., Guija, J., Giner. L., and Courtet, P. (2023). The capacity to consent to treatment is altered in suicidal patients. *Annals of General Psychiatry, 22*, 35. https://doi.org/10.1186/s12991-023-00459-w

Opland, C., and Torrico, T. (2024). *Psychotherapy and therapeutic relationship.* https://www.ncbi.nlm.nih.gov/books/NBK608012/ (accessed 5 October 2025).

Oquendo, M., and Bernanke, J. (2017). Suicide risk assessment: Tools and challenges. *World Psychiatry, 16*(1), 28–29. https://doi.org/10.1002/wps.20396

O'Rourke, M., Jamil, R., and Siddiqui, W. (2023). *Suicide screening and prevention.* https://www.ncbi.nlm.nih.gov/books/NBK531453/ (accessed 9 October 2025).

Owen, G., Gergel, T., Stephenson, L., Hussain, O., Rifkin, L., and Keene A. (2019). Advance decision-making in mental health: Suggestions for legal reform in England and Wales. *International Journal of Law and Psychiatry, 64*, 162–177. https://doi.org/10.1016/j.ijlp.2019.02.002

Park, L.J. (2020). Using the SBAR handover tool. *British Journal of Nursing, 29*(14). https://doi.org/10.12968/bjon.2020.29.14.812

Parker, L., Prior, S., Van Dam, P., and Edwards, D. (2022). Altruism in paramedicine: A scoping review. *Healthcare, 10*(9), 1731. https://doi.org/10.3390/healthcare10091731

Phillips, J. (2024). Paramedic role in emergency mental healthcare. *Journal of Paramedic Practice, 16*(5), 204–211. https://doi.org/10.12968/jpar.2024.16.5.204

Pretorius, T., and Padmanabhanunni, A. (2024). Examining the unidimensionality of the PHQ-9 with first responders: Evidence from different psychometric paradigms. *African Journal of Psychological Assessment, 6*, a165. https://doi.org/10.4102/ajopa.v6i0.165

Rahman, M., Dhira, T., Sarker, A., and Mehareen, J. (2022). Validity and reliability of the Patient Health Questionnaire scale (PHQ-9) among university students of Bangladesh. *PLoS One, 17*(6), e0269634. https://doi.org/10.1371/journal.pone.0269634

Rees, N., Porter, A., Rapport, F., Hughes, S., and John, A. (2018). Paramedics' perceptions of the care they provide to people who self-harm: A qualitative study using evolved grounded theory methodology. *PLoS One, 13*(10), e0205813. https://doi.org/10.1371/journal.pone.0205813

Reeves, K., Vasconez, G., and Weiss, S. (2022). Characteristics of suicidal ideation: A systematic review. *Archives of Suicide Research, 26*(4), 1736–1756. https://doi.org/10.1080/13811118.2021.2022551

Romeu, D., Guthrie, E., and Mason S. (2023). Understanding prehospital care for self-harm: Views and experiences of Yorkshire Ambulance Service clinicians. *Emergency Medicine Journal, 40*(7), 482–483. https://doi.org/10.1136/emermed-2022-212983

Royal College of Psychiatrists (2020) *Self-harm and suicide in adults*, CR229, July. https://www.rcpsych.ac.uk/improving-care/campaigning-for-better-mental-health-policy/college-reports/2020-college-reports/cr229 (accessed 9 October 2025).

Salvi, J. (2019). Calculated decisions: Columbia-Suicide Severity Rating Scale (C-SSRS). *Emergency Medical Practice, 21*(5), CD3–CD4. https://pmc.ncbi.nlm.nih.gov/articles/PMC7974826/ (accessed 9 October 2025).

Schaffer, D.H., Murray, B.P., and Khazaeni, B. (2026). *Acetaminophen toxicity.* Treasure Island, FL: StatPearls. https://www.ncbi.nlm.nih.gov/books/NBK441917/#article-17075.s19

Van de Velde, E., Vandewiele, H., Van Hecke, A., Eeckloo, K., and Malfait, S. (2024). Bedside handovers in mental health care: An explorative review. *Archives of Psychiatric Nursing, 51,* 10–16. https://www.psychiatricnursing.org/article/S0883-9417(24)00069-4/fulltext (accessed 15 October 2025).

Xiao, S., Ge, Q., Wang, T., Zhang, M., Hu, A., and Zhang, X. (2025). Psychometric characteristics of the Chinese version of the Columbia-Suicide Severity Rating Scale among people with mental health diagnosis. *BMC Psychiatry, 25,* 803. https://doi.org/10.1186/s12888-025-07187-3

Zamir, A., Tickle, A., and Sabin-Farrell, R. (2022). A systematic review of the evidence relating to disclosure of psychological distress by mental health professionals within the workplace. *Journal of Clinical Psychology, 78*(9), 1712–1738. https://doi.org/10.1002/jclp.23339

Zayed, M.G., Williams, V., Glendenning, A., Bulger, J., Hewes, T., Porter, A., et al. (2020). Care-pathways for patients presenting to emergency ambulance services with self-harm: National survey. *Emergency Medicine Journal, 37*(12), 752–755. https://doi.org/10.1136/emermed-2019-208967

9 Acute behavioural disturbance and substance-related presentations: Assessment, safety, and intervention

Ashley Stewart, Paula Gardner, and Jo Augustus

Introduction

Acute behavioural disturbance (ABD) and substance-related presentations represent some of the most complex, high-risk, and ethically challenging scenarios encountered in pre-hospital care. These presentations sit at the intersection of acute mental distress, physiological instability, substance intoxication or withdrawal, and heightened environmental risk, often requiring rapid clinical judgement under conditions of uncertainty. This chapter explores the historical and conceptual origins of ABD, examines its contested terminology, and situates current UK practice within evolving clinical, legal, and ethical frameworks. By integrating pathophysiology, assessment strategies, and multidisciplinary approaches, the chapter aims to support paramedics in delivering safe, proportionate, and evidence-informed care while prioritising patient dignity, staff safety, and least-restrictive intervention.

Historical context

To understand the concept of acute behavioural disturbance in its contemporary form, it is necessary to examine the historical origins and subsequent evolution of related terminology. The term 'excited delirium' was originally used in the late nineteenth and early twentieth centuries to describe febrile, agitated, and disoriented patients in medical settings. However, from the 1980s onwards, its use expanded within certain regions of the United States to describe deaths occurring during encounters between law enforcement and individuals exhibiting extreme agitation, often in the context of intoxication or mental illness (McGuinness and Lipsedge, 2022).

Over subsequent decades, 'excited delirium' became increasingly applied to cases involving sudden death following physical restraint in public or custodial settings. Importantly, multiple reviews have identified that the term was used inconsistently, lacked clear diagnostic criteria, and was frequently invoked retrospectively, often in the absence of definitive pathological evidence (McGuinness and Lipsedge, 2022; Physicians for Human Rights, 2022). This raised significant concerns regarding its scientific validity and clinical usefulness.

A further concern highlighted in the literature is the disproportionate application of the term to deaths involving racially minoritised individuals, particularly Black and Hispanic men, during encounters with law enforcement (Physicians for Human Rights, 2022). This pattern prompted widespread critique that the term functioned less as a medical explanation and more as a post-hoc label used to account for deaths occurring in the context of restraint, thereby obscuring the roles of environmental stressors, physiological compromise, and restraint-related harm.

As a result, 'excited delirium' came to be viewed by many professional bodies as a socially constructed concept lacking an adequate evidence base and carrying significant risk of reinforcing structural inequities. High-profile cases including those of George Floyd, Daniel Prude, Angelo Quinto, and Eric Parsa further intensified scrutiny of the term's use and contributed to calls for its abandonment (Physicians for Human Rights, 2022). It is important to note that neither excited delirium nor acute behavioural disturbance is recognised as a certifiable cause of death within the UK.

There is now broad consensus across healthcare and human rights organisations that 'excited delirium' should not be used in clinical or forensic practice. In response, UK services have increasingly adopted the term acute behavioural disturbance to describe presentations of severe agitation, delirium, and physiological instability requiring urgent medical intervention. While this terminology represents a move away from historically problematic language, it remains an umbrella descriptor rather than a diagnosis, and its use continues to attract debate regarding clarity, consistency, and potential unintended consequences.

Understanding this history matters for paramedics today because the language used to describe agitation shapes clinical judgement, inter-agency responses, and thresholds for intervention; awareness of the contested origins of these terms supports more accurate assessment, reduces the risk of bias, and reinforces the primacy of patient safety, proportionality, and ethical care.

Definitions

Currently, the term acute behavioural disturbance is used in the UK to describe severe presentations of agitation, delirium, and disordered behaviour, with associated physiological compromise (Humpries et al., 2025). Whilst ABD has become the preferred term within UK practice, it remains a highly contentious topic (Stark, 2024). Many argue that lack of clarity, understanding, and consensus has led to ABD becoming meaningless as a concept (Tracy, 2024). This is further supported by Humphries et al. (2024) and Tracy (2024), who highlight that there is no widely accepted definition of ABD and that terminology is used inconsistently, creating confusion in recognition, assessment, and management across multidisciplinary healthcare teams.

It is important for clinicians to understand that ABD is not a formal diagnosis, rather an umbrella term to describe clinical presentations of severe agitation (Stark, 2024). Acute behavioural disturbance includes a range of clinical conditions which result in altered psychological and physiological states of agitation. However, often these causes remain unknown or poorly understood (Humpries et al., 2025; Stark, 2024). Regardless, it is vital to understand that the clinical presentation of ABD is life-threatening and should be considered a time-critical emergency (Humphries et al., 2025; McGugan, 2001; Strömmer et al., 2020).

Despite ongoing debate around its usefulness as a concept, the term acute behavioural disturbance now features in both Royal College of Emergency Medicine (RCEM, 2024) and Maudsley Prescribing (Taylor et al., 2025) guidelines. Acute behavioural disturbance currently remains a recognised umbrella term (across ambulance and police services) and should still be used by frontline emergency providers to facilitate multi-agency communication and response to this medical emergency effectively (Gorton et al., 2022; Humphries et al., 2024). Due to its dangerous nature, a presentation of ABD will usually involve a coordinated response by the police and ambulance services.

At present, there is a lack of validated criteria available on which to base practice guidelines in the UK (Humphries et al., 2024; Stark, 2024). This has resulted in guidelines being created using dated research on 'excited delirium', a concept not recognised within UK practice (Humphries et al., 2025; Obasogie, 2021). Research priorities include further data collection and research, the need to review UK terminology surrounding ABD, and consider if a shift away from the term – and towards a new definition – is needed. National and international consensus on best practice (recognition criteria, assessment, treatment, and management) is also urgently needed to further guide UK practice and improve quality care provisions (Lindridge et al., 2025).

Current consensus in the UK

Recently in a UK first, a landmark multidisciplinary modified Delphi study was conducted to review ABD guidelines (Humpries et al., 2024). Key stakeholders came together across eight organisations, including the National Police Chiefs' Council, the Royal College of Emergency Medicine, Ambulance services, and the Faculty of Forensic and Legal Medicine to create new consensus guidelines on acute behavioural disturbance (Humpries et al., 2024).

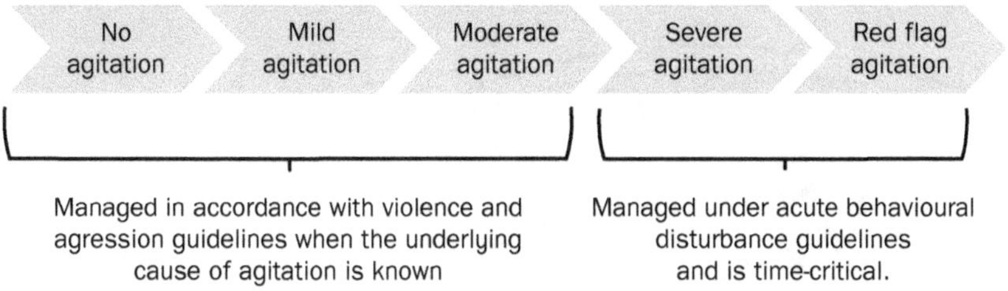

Figure 9.1: The agitation guidelines as a spectrum presentation of agitation (adapted from Humphries et al., 2024).

This consensus study provided a clear, unified, and evidence-based framework for the recognition and management of ABD. Key conclusions drawn from the study include:

- Clear consensus that ABD is not a separate entity to agitation.
- ABD should be incorporated within agitation guidelines and be considered a spectrum presentation of agitation (see Figure 9.1).
- There is no benefit to having separate guidelines for agitation and ABD.
- 'Agitation spectrum'-based guidelines would allow for improved recognition, assessment, and management of ABD.
- New terminology such as 'red flag agitation' to describe severely agitated patients at the greatest risk of deterioration and who may require specialist care should be considered.

Recognition of acute behavioural disturbance: 'Red flag agitation'

Recognition of ABD can be challenging, and currently no clear diagnostic criteria exist. Despite this, early recognition of ABD and having a clear understanding of its life-threatening, time-critical nature are key to effective care (RCEM, 2024). At present, RCEM best practice guidelines (2024) recommend identification of ABD through recognition of clinical features (Figure 9.1) and exclusion of other potential differential diagnoses (Figure 9.2).

Humpries et al. (2024) suggest that recognition should focus on a triad of consensus features that include tactile hyperthermia (being hot to touch), presenting with constant or near-constant activity, and extreme agitation or aggression. For ABD to be considered, the patient should present with at least two of these features (Faculty of Forensic and Legal Medicine, 2019). The presence of all three features is not needed.

Many additional signs and symptoms occur as a result of consensus feature pathophysiology. Without consensus features being present, these signs and symptoms are not sufficient in identifying ABD. Robust history-taking (understanding preceding events and identifying risk factors) and patient assessment remain key to building an accurate clinical picture of ABD. If

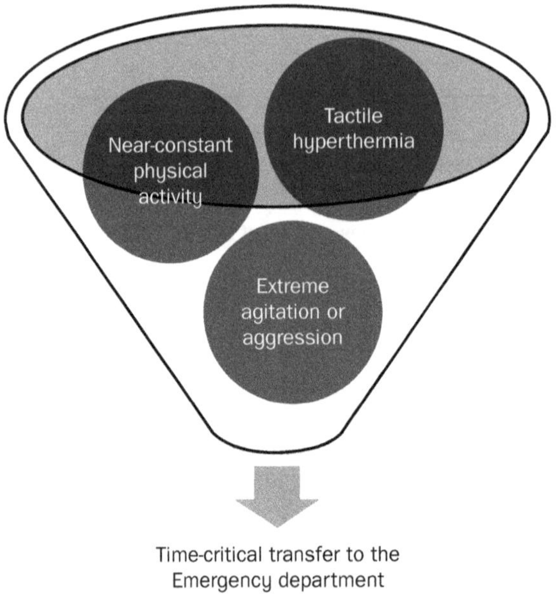

Figure 9.2: The triad of ABD (adapted from Gorton et al., 2022).

clinicians have identified ABD through a combination of consensus features, additional features, and clinical picture, then the situation should be treated as a life-threatening emergency with the focus on life-saving interventions and time-critical transfer to definitive care.

Additional clinical features of ABD include:

- does not fatigue
- naked/inappropriately clothed
- rapid breathing (tachypnoea)
- exhibiting exceptional strength
- sweating profusely
- increased pain threshold/tolerance
- not responsive to the presence of others (e.g. the police)
- violent behaviour
- tachycardia
- aggression with no identifiable cause
- exhibiting bizarre behaviour
- panic, paranoia, hypervigilance

Patients with ABD are at considerable risk of developing metabolic acidosis, hyperkalaemia, rhabdomyolysis, disseminated intravascular coagulation, and ultimately death. Furthermore, whilst paramedics should aim to identify, differentiate, and treat the underlaying cause, it is vital that delays to definitive treatment are avoided if ABD is declared. Clinicians must be aware that failure to recognise ABD can be fatal.

Case study: A call to police custody

Case study: Narrative

In the early hours of the morning, a paramedic crew is placed on standby when a Category 2 call is received:

> *'45-year-old male – intoxicated and severely agitated. Currently being detained in police custody'.*

On arrival at the custody suite, the crew is met by the custody sergeant, who appears visibly anxious and expresses appreciation for their attendance. While escorting the clinicians to the location where the individual is being detained, the sergeant provides an update on the situation.

Approximately one hour earlier, police officers had encountered the man wandering along the side of a motorway. He appeared confused, agitated, and paranoid. Officers were initially able to calm him and persuaded him to attend the police station for safety and further assessment. However, once in the police vehicle, his agitation escalated significantly. As the station was only a short distance away, officers were able to transport him there quickly. Since arrival, his behaviour has deteriorated further; he has become increasingly agitated and aggressive, reportedly striking his head against the walls, shouting, and removing his clothing. Officers had briefly restrained him in order to place him safely in a cell. At the time of the paramedics' arrival, custody staff were monitoring him via CCTV, with officers positioned outside the cell. The sergeant reiterates her relief at the clinicians' attendance.

As the crew walks down the corridor towards the cell, loud shouting and screaming can be heard. The CCTV feed shows the patient thrashing and pacing continuously around the confined space. Through the cell viewing hatch, the clinicians observe that he is diaphoretic, tachypnoeic, and displaying marked agitation. One of the paramedics attempts verbal engagement through the hatch in an effort to build rapport and initiate de-escalation; however, the patient does not respond coherently. Instead, he repeatedly shouts, *'You would like that, wouldn't you?'*

The custody officer reiterates that the team will provide whatever assistance is required to manage the situation safely. This scenario raises immediate clinical questions: does this presentation meet the criteria for red flag agitation/ABD, what time-critical physiology must be anticipated, and how should the paramedics work lawfully and safely alongside police custody staff? The sections below uses this case as a reference point for recognition, risk management, escalation, restraint/sedation planning, and documentation.

On-scene clinical reference

In this case, the patient's near-constant activity, diaphoresis, tachypnoea, and paranoid, agitated shouting should prompt early consideration of red flag agitation. These features indicate a potentially time-critical emergency requiring rapid escalation and structured management.

The following framework, aligned with the Joint Royal Colleges Ambulance Liaison Committee (JRCALC, 2025), outlines key priorities in the pre-hospital management of ABD.

1. **Immediate priorities:** Begin with a dynamic scene risk assessment. Request police and specialist clinical support early where required, and do not enter unsafe environments without adequate resources. Actively identify red flag agitation features.
2. **Recognise ABD as a time-critical emergency:** Near-constant activity, extreme agitation, tactile hyperthermia, rapid breathing, diaphoresis, paranoia, and delirium should be treated as life-threatening, even where the underlying cause is unclear.
3. **De-escalation (where safe):** Use calm, clear communication, minimise environmental stimulation, assign one lead communicator, and reassess continuously. De-escalation is an ongoing process rather than a single intervention.
4. **Containment and environment:** Remove hazards where possible. Use containment rather than restraint when safe to do so. Maintain continuous observation and avoid prone positioning.
5. **Restraint (if required):** Restraint should only be used for a clear clinical purpose, applying the minimum force for the shortest duration necessary. Coordinate with trained personnel and document justification carefully.
6. **Sedation/pre-rapid tranquilisation:** Escalate early to critical care or specialist teams where indicated. Intramuscular routes are often preferred for safety. The aim is to calm the patient, not induce unconsciousness, and to reduce time to effective sedation when clinically required.
7. **Post-sedation care:** Reassess using ABCDE: Airway, Breathing, Circulation, Disability, Exposure. Initiate active cooling, oxygen, intravenous fluids as appropriate, and continuous ECG and end-tidal carbon dioxide ($EtCO_2$) monitoring. Expedite transfer to definitive care.
8. **Legal and ethical principles:** Most patients with severe ABD will lack capacity due to delirium. Act in the patient's best interests, ensuring actions are necessary, proportionate, and the least restrictive option available. Maintain clear contemporaneous documentation.

Misidentification of ABD

It is vital that paramedics can accurately differentiate between aggressive/violent individuals, differential causes, and people who are experiencing ABD

(Peel, 2022). Acute behavioural disturbance cannot be diagnosed in patients who have agitation without delirium, or delirium without agitation (JRCALC, 2025). Misidentification can lead to inappropriate transfer of aggressive individuals to the emergency department and the 'medicalisation' of police matters. Likewise, misidentifying an individual experiencing ABD as a violent/aggressive offender can have severe consequences such as delaying definitive care or failure to initiate care at all. While all UK police custody staff should be trained in recognising ABD, some may need support and guidance from healthcare professionals to recognise and differentiate between presentations accurately. Applied to this case, the custody context increases the risk of mislabelling the presentation as 'violent non-compliance'; clinicians should actively test for delirium features and physiological red flags.

Substance misuse: The leading cause

Evidence suggests that substance misuse, including intoxication and withdrawal, is the most common cause of ABD (RCEM, 2023). Numerous post-mortem investigations have found drug use, particularly stimulants such as cocaine, to be most linked to death following an episode of ABD (Stevenson and Tracy, 2021). Additional drugs cited to cause ABD include cannabis, phencyclidine (PCP), methamphetamine, lysergic acid diethylamide (LSD), novel psychoactive substances, including synthetic cannabinoids (spice), together with abrupt cessation of antipsychotic medication. However, data also show that drug dose concentrations of these substances tend to be well below the toxic level required to cause poisoning and death (Tracy, 2024). By the time of death, drug concentrations in blood or tissue may not reflect levels during the behavioural disturbance. Urinary toxicology screening tests for novel psychoactive substances are unreliable and can result in false-negative results. Furthermore, it is important to acknowledge that ABD deaths are multifactorial (hyperthermia, acidosis, arrhythmia) and toxicology alone cannot determine causation, only support association. In custody settings, stimulant intoxication or withdrawal should be assumed possible until excluded; however, normal toxicology later does not rule out severe physiological collapse during the event.

Pathophysiology of ABD

The pathophysiology of ABD is complex and not yet fully understood (Stark, 2024; Tracy, 2024). Despite this, several hypotheses explaining ABD pathology have been considered in recent years (Stevenson and Tracy, 2021; Humphries et al., 2024). The most prominent hypothesis suggests that ABD is likely to be due to a combination of genetic susceptibility, dopamine-mediated pathways, catecholamine surge, hyperthermia, and metabolic acidosis (Stevenson and Tracy, 2021; Strömmer et al., 2020; McGugan, 2001). A notable occurrence in ABD is the impairment of normal homeostatic loops that should ordinarily

Table 9.1: The interplay between pathophysiological processes

Mechanism	Exacerbates	Results
Hyperthermia	Metabolic acidosis	Muscle breakdown, dehydration
Catecholamine surge	Hyperthermia and acidosis	Cardiac instability
Metabolic acidosis	Catecholamine sensitivity	Arrhythmia, cardiac arrest
Dopamine dysregulation	Catecholamine surge	Psychosis, agitation
Genetic susceptibility	All of the above	Increased risk of fatal outcome

limit these processes (Stevenson and Tracy, 2021; Strömmer et al., 2020). It is important to understand that these pathophysiological processes are often interconnected (Strömmer et al., 2020; Humphries et al., 2024) (see Table 9.1).

Genetic susceptibility

Research suggests that certain individuals may be more predisposed to developing ABD than others. Variants in genes (polymorphisms) such as catechol-*O*-methyl-transferase and monoamine oxidase A variation may affect how quickly catecholamines and dopamine are metabolised, prolonging sympathetic responses. Inherited differences in the dopamine D2 receptor (DRD2) genes can also affect the density and sensitivity of receptors. If receptors are too sensitive, this can lead to a person becoming more reactive to stress or stimulant drugs, which in turn would lead them to become more agitated during sympathetic (fight) responses.

Dopamine-mediated pathways

Dopamine is a key neurotransmitter (and hormone) made in the brain. Dopamine plays a role in several physiological functions, including regulating movement, thermoregulation, regulating mood/emotions, and regulating heart rate, kidney function, and blood vessel function. Excessive dopamine release (or hypersensitivity to dopamine receptors) can be caused by stimulant drugs, psychiatric disorders, novel psychoactive substances, and genetics, and result in unregulated/elevated levels of dopamine. This hyperdopaminergic state leads to paranoia, agitation, psychosis, and hyperthermia. Subsequently, this amplifies the body's sympathetic response and increases the production of catecholamines: adrenaline, noradrenaline, and dopamine. If the body cannot compensate for these increases through homeostasis, this process will continue, and the patient becomes at risk of hyperthermia and metabolic acidosis.

Catecholamine surge

Catecholamines are a group of hormones – adrenaline, noradrenaline, and dopamine – that are produced in the adrenal glands and play a key role in the body's sympathetic (fight or flight) and parasympathetic (rest and digest) responses. Stress, fear, agitation, and dopamine overactivity lead to the prolonged sympathetic response we see in ABD presentations. This in turn increases heart rate, vasoconstriction, and contractility of the heart. This results in reduced electrical stability of the heart with excess sympathetic outflow being linked to prolonged QT intervals, arrythmias (such as ventricular fibrillation), and increases in metabolic acidosis. This combination of processes is thought to result in a 'stunning' of the myocardium and cause stress-induced heart failure (takotsubo cardiomyopathy). This process is often compounded by restraint-induced exertion and metabolic acidosis. If catecholamine surge is not suppressed or reversed, the patient will become at risk of circulatory collapse and cardiac arrest.

Hyperthermia

Homeostasis of body temperature is the process known as thermoregulation. The hypothalamus acts as the body's thermostat and uses negative feedback mechanisms to regulate internal temperatures. In healthy individuals, normal internal body temperatures should remain stable between 36.7°C and 37.5°C. However, during states of severe agitation (and restraint), vast amounts of heat are produced due to significant increases in muscular activity. This relates to the consensus feature of near-constant activity resulting in prolonged and intense muscular activity and subsequent raising of body temperature aka tactile hyperthermia. However, clinicians should be aware that peripheral temperature measurements (ear) can be inaccurate, and assessment for tactile hyperthermia may be more valuable. Furthermore, it is important to note that muscles act as 'thermal reservoirs' and release stored heat long after physical exertion has increased. This can cause a state of 'sustained hyperthermia', which clinicians should be aware of. As previously mentioned, dopamine also causes thermo-dysregulation and increases hyperthermia. This prolonged hyperthermic state causes worsening agitation, metabolic acidosis, and rhabdomyolysis.

Metabolic acidosis

Metabolic acidosis can be defined as a clinical disturbance characterised by an increase in plasma acidity (McGugan, 2001; Strömmer et al., 2020). The numerous processes leading to metabolic acidosis in ABD include:

- Prolonged physical exertion, due to agitation and/or restraint leading to increased production of lactate acid.
- Dehydration and renal impairment, which impair the body's ability to metabolise and clear acid.
- Use of stimulant drugs also increases acid accumulation within the body.

These mechanisms, along with mechanisms previously mentioned, cause life-threatening metabolic acidosis. When patients become acidotic, hyperventilation occurs as a compensatory mechanism to reduce levels of CO_2 in the blood and return blood pH levels to normal. This mechanism is sometimes referred to as 'blowing off CO_2' in practice. However, if this compensatory response is inadequate or impaired due to exhaustion or restraint, then the uncompensated metabolic acidosis can lead to multi-organ failure and cardiac arrest (Strömmer et al., 2020; Stevenson and Tracy, 2021; Peel, 2022).

Summary

Understanding these interconnected pathophysiological mechanisms can lead us to the hypothesis that ABD could be conceptualised as a 'final common pathway' to death from many underlying causes and processes (Stevenson and Tracy, 2021). A key consideration for clinicians is that restraint significantly worsens physiological stress and accelerates all the pathways mentioned. This is thought to be why many individuals die suddenly during or shortly after periods of restraint. In practical terms, the patient described in the case study is at risk of rapid deterioration, particularly if prolonged restraint or delay to sedation is allowed to occur.

Guided clinical reasoning questions: Acute behavioural disturbance/red flag agitation

Address the questions below to structure thinking about custody in the case study and similar high-risk red flag agitation presentations. Use them to guide reflection rather than as a linear checklist.

Recognition and risk

Q1: What features suggest this presentation sits at the severe end of the agitation spectrum rather than simple aggression or intoxication?

Q2: Which consensus features of ABD/red flag agitation are present (e.g. near-constant activity, tactile hyperthermia, extreme agitation)?

Q3: What alternative diagnoses must be actively considered and excluded (e.g. hypoglycaemia, hypoxia, head injury, infection, psychosis)?

Safety and environment

Q4: Is the scene currently safe for the patient, clinicians, police, and bystanders?

Q5: Are there environmental hazards that increase risk: traffic, heights, sharps, confined spaces?

Q6: Should clinicians withdraw and wait for additional resources, and if so, why?

Pathophysiology and time-critical risk

Q7: What pathophysiological processes are most likely occurring in this patient (e.g. hyperthermia, catecholamine surge, metabolic acidosis)?

Q8: How might restraint, exertion, or delay worsen these processes?

Q9: What indicators suggest the patient is at imminent risk of collapse or cardiac arrest?

Decision-making and intervention

Q10: Have de-escalation strategies been attempted and documented where safe to do so?

Q11: Is restraint being used for a clear and defensible purpose?

Q12: Has early specialist support (e.g. police, critical care, senior clinician) been requested?

Q13: Does the patient have capacity to engage in decisions about care at this time?

Ethical, legal, and team considerations

Q14: Are interventions necessary, proportionate, and the least restrictive option?

Q15: Is the multidisciplinary team working collaboratively with shared situational awareness?

Q16: What documentation is essential to justify actions taken?

Reflection

Q17: How did team communication influence safety and outcomes?

Q18: What aspects of this incident were most ethically or emotionally challenging?

Q19: What learning can be transferred to future ABD/agitation cases?

Management: Scene safety and containment

Management of ABD within the pre-hospital environment can be challenging. Pre-hospital clinicians will often find themselves in chaotic and dangerous situations when managing ABD ('red flag agitation'). Following an ABCDE approach, it is vital that clinicians implement scene safety strategies to minimise risk to patients, bystanders, relatives, clinicians, and police officers. Key safety considerations should include:

- Carry out dynamic risk assessments and secure the scene as quickly as possible. Clinicians should wait for police support if there is any perceived threat to safety.
- The use of personal protective equipment and body armour should be considered by clinicians prior to attending the scene.
- Decisions should remain dynamic. If clinicians identify threats to safety after entering a scene, and police are not present, then it is acceptable to withdraw and move to a safe distance. Always consider entry and exit points and ensure safe exit points are available.
- Be aware that patients experiencing severe agitation will lose their ability to interact with their environment safely and will have no comprehension of risk.
- Rapid recognition of ABD/red flag agitation is key. Requesting specialist support early (police and critical care) will minimise time to sedation, thus reducing the window of risk.
- Be aware of physical and sharps-related injuries. The risk of injury increases significantly during restraint practices. Clear communication and a coordinated approach can minimise this risk. Intramuscular administration may be the preferred and safest route.
- Staff who have not undertaken approved restraint training should not be asked to restrain patients.
- Transfer of an ADB patient without sedation presents an extreme risk to both clinicians and the patient. Sedation is key to safe transfer. Transfer with restraint can be considered if sedation cannot be achieved. A dynamic risk assessment should always be undertaken prior to transporting an ABD patient.
- If resources allow, appoint a 'safety person' with the role to observe and clinically monitor the patient with a hands-off approach.

For the case study in this chapter, the confined cell environment supports containment, but it does not remove the need for rapid clinical escalation, observation, and a plan to minimise restraint time. Containing ABD patients within a safe environment is a key step in maintaining safety and minimising periods of physical restraint. Clinicians should be aware of hazards such as motorways, heights, broken glass/objects, and potential weapons. If possible, containing a patient in an area safe from these hazards may be beneficial. In police custody settings, empty cells can be a good location for containment. If this is undertaken, it is important that continual monitoring of the patient occurs. Restraining individuals to stop them being violent, when containment is available, should always be avoided.

Table 9.2: Key differences between containment and restraint (adapted from NICE, 2015)

	Containment (seclusion)	Restraint
Definition	Strategies used to **maintain safety and stability** through environmental, relational, or procedural means	The application of physical, mechanical, or chemical means to deliberately limit a person's movement or behaviour to prevent harm to themselves or others
Primary aim	To restore a sense of security and reduce escalation	To restore a sense of security and reduce escalation
Underlying principle	'Holding' the patient psychologically (offering safety and predictability)	'Holding' the patient physically (limiting their capacity for harm)
Ethical implications	Supports autonomy and dignity; uses the least restrictive means	Restricts autonomy; must be justified by imminent risk of harm
Legal governance	Governed by good practice guidelines, e.g. NICE (2015), MHA Code of Practice (Department of Health, 2015)	Legally regulated under Mental Health Act, Mental Capacity Act, and Human Rights legislation (especially Article 5 ECHR – deprivation of liberty)
Documentation	Record of interventions, rationale, and de-escalation attempts required	Must document justification, duration, staff involved, and post-event review

Seclusion is defined in accordance with the Mental Health Act 1983 Code of Practice: 'the supervised confinement of a patient in a room, which may be locked. Its sole aim is to contain severely disturbed behaviour that is likely to cause harm to others' (NICE, 2015: 63).

Temperature control

Acute behavioural disturbance causes uncontrolled hyperthermia leading to multi-organ failure and death. Numerous studies have reported a strong correlation between internal body temperatures over 42°C and very poor outcomes regarding morbidity and mortality (McGugan, 2001). Therefore, early cooling to regain normothermia is imperative. Patient temperatures should be assessed, and managed, as soon as it is practical and safe to do so. Pre-planning these interventions can be beneficial if resources are available. Clinicians should be mindful that active and passive cooling treatments should not result in delays to definitive care. Cooling methods are outlined below.

Passive cooling

- Removing clothing (maintaining dignity and respect).
- Reducing environmental temperatures: turning on the air conditioning in the ambulance, for example.
- Evaporative cooling via wet exposed skin in an air-conditioned ambulance: fans can also be used to increase evaporative cooling.

Active cooling

- Applying ice packs (when available) to vascular areas such as the neck, axilla, and groin.
- Applying wet sheets or blankets to a patient who has had clothing removed.
- Administration of cold intravenous fluids.

Antipyretics, such as paracetamol, lower the thermoregulatory set point within the hypothalamus during episodes of fever. However, this set point remains normal in the hyperthermia associated with ABD (McGugan, 2001). Therefore, antipyretics do not have a role in ABD temperature management.

De-escalation

De-escalation remains a first-line intervention within the pre-hospital management of ABD callouts. If there is no immediate risk to life, de-escalation strategies should be attempted before considering restraint and sedation (see Table 9.3). NICE guidelines recommend all health organisations provide staff with training on de-escalation.

It is important to understand that de-escalation should be a continuous process throughout the duration of treatment. Verbal de-escalation and effective teamwork with police have been found to be effective in most possible ABD cases (JRCALC, 2025). A two-year audit by the London Ambulance Service also found 62% of ABD callouts to be managed using de-escalation and standard care. However, it is important to consider that many of these calls would likely not have been ABD/red flag agitation presentations, rather conditions of varying agitation with known cause. These findings highlight the impracticality of aiming to define ABD in practice and support the case for agitation-based terminology and guidance. Whilst the effectiveness of de-escalation for 'true' ABD, or more appropriately 'red flag agitation' may be contested, it remains an important step in ensuring a stepwise approach and ensures that subsequent restraint and sedation are justified (Humphries et al., 2025). Accurate recording of de-escalation can also provide reassurance to relatives in cases where an adverse outcome leads to investigations.

Table 9.3: De-escalation strategies (adapted from JRCALC, 2025; NICE, 2015)

Category	Strategy
Scene safety and environment	Dynamic risk assessment
	Control environment
	Positioning for safety
Team coordination	Assign lead communicator
	Role briefing
	Police collaboration
	Leadership and followership
Verbal and non-verbal communication	Clear calm tone
	Empathy and reassurance
	Active listening
	Offer simple choices
Behavioural techniques	Avoid confrontation
	Respect personal space
	Set limits clearly
	Allow time and patience (if appropriate)
Medical considerations	Assess for medical cause
	Monitor from distance
	Sedation (if appropriate)
Post-incident actions	De-brief and documentation
	Handover
	Staff welfare

Restraint

Three forms of restraint exist in the context of acute behavioural disturbance: physical/manual restraint, mechanical restraint, and pharmacological restraint (sedation). These processes are discussed below. The three key purposes of restraint are: (1) to facilitate transportation, (2) to reduce the risk of harm to the individual and rescuers, and (3) to facilitate the administration of life-saving medication.

Restraint is often unavoidable within the context of pre-hospital ABD management and is usually required for safe sedation. If de-escalation attempts are ineffective, restraint may be needed to facilitate sedation. It must be clear that restraint should only be used to achieve a definitive purpose. Levels of applied force must be justifiable, appropriate, reasonable, and proportionate to the specific situation. Restraint must only be applied for the minimum amount of time possible (Faculty of Forensic and Legal Medicine, 2019; Gorton et al., 2022; Humphries et al., 2024). Clinicians must be aware of the associated risks of physical restraint. These include:

- Respiratory compromise due to positional asphyxia, particularly if restrained in a prone position or with pressure on the neck, chest, or back.
- Acceleration of pathophysiological pathways which hasten cardiovascular collapse and cardiac arrest.
- Physical injury to patient, police officers, and medical professionals.
- Legal implications and breach of human rights should unjustified or disproportionate levels of restraint be used.

Decision-making regarding the use of restraint, pre-rapid tranquilisation, and sedation is complex. Paramedics should share these decisions with specialist teams. Increasing consensus and implementation of 'agitation scale' guidelines within ambulance trusts are beneficial in supporting decision-making and providing proportionate and justified treatments.

Mechanical restraint

Mechanical restraint involves the use of authorised equipment, such as handcuffs or restraining belts, which can be applied effectively by appropriately trained staff such as police officers. The main purpose of mechanical restraint is to safely immobilise or restrict the movement of the service user (NICE, 2015). Correct application is vital, and inappropriate use results in unnecessary harm to the patient or can exacerbate the situation. For example, handcuffs restraining the arms to the rear of the body are more likely to cause respiratory compromise than arms placed in front of the body (JRCALC, 2025).

Chemical restraint

Chemical restraint can be defined as the use of prescribed medication that is administered for the purpose of controlling or subduing disturbed/violent behaviour, where it is not prescribed for the treatment of a formally identified physical or mental illness (NHS England, 2021; Zeller, 2017; NICE, 2015). Whilst this concept appears frequently in current guidelines, it does not accurately reflect the use of sedative medications in the context of ABD and agitation.

There is also debate around the use of the term 'chemical restraint'. Whilst this term has been – and remains to be – used within research and practice, many argue that the term has negative connotations and should be replaced. Zeller (2017) suggests that medicines are not commonly referred to as 'chemicals' and calling psychiatric medicines 'chemicals' differentiates them from other medicines and implies that agitation deserves punishment or subjugation as opposed to healing. Sedation is the most appropriate and preferred term.

Pre-rapid tranquilisation and sedation

Pre-rapid tranquilisation (PreRT) can play a key role in the treatment and management of severe agitation resolved by de-escalation techniques. It is defined as the use of parenteral (usually intramuscular or intravenous) medication, if oral medication is not appropriate, when urgent sedation with medication is required (NICE, 2015). It is important to note that PreRT and sedation are often used interchangeably in current practice to describe this process (Gorton et al., 2022; Humphries et al., 2024). The purpose of PreRT is threefold (adapted from Gorton et al., 2022):

1 To reduce further harm to the patient through prevention of further self-harm, accidental injury, hypoxia, metabolic acidosis, or catecholamine production.
2 To reduce the risk of harm to others.
3 To do no harm – by prescribing safe regimes and monitoring physical health.

The key aim of PreRT is to calm the patient – 'making them tranquil' – without significantly reducing their level of consciousness, although this is a risk of the procedure and may occur if the patient is already severely physiologically compromised (JRCALC, 2025). The use of PreRT for ABD and agitation on the severe scale of the spectrum has been associated with reduced mortality (Strömmer et al., 2020).

There are currently three types of medications used for PreRT: benzodiazepines, antipsychotics, and dissociative agents. At present there is a lack of high-quality evidence to clearly determine which is most suitable. However, there is a growing body of evidence to support the use of ketamine (dissociative anaesthetic) as a first-line agent in PreRT (RCEM, 2024). Once severe agitation has settled, the use of titrated intravenous bazinaprines can aid in maintaining the sedated state.

Ketamine used at appropriate doses can reliably terminate agitation in 3–5 minutes. Intramuscular ketamine has been recommended in the ED setting due to its predictable dose–response relationship and efficacy (Hopper et al., 2015; Riddell et al., 2017). The evidence base for the use of intramuscular ketamine in pre-hospital practice is also growing (Stevenson and Tracy, 2021). Calver (2010) found that standardised intramuscular protocols for ABD resulted in reduced time to ABD control, reduced numbers of adverse reactions, and reduced risk of injury to staff (Calver et al., 2010; Riddell et al., 2017).

Paramedics must be aware that PreRT procedures are reserved for specialists such as critical care paramedics and HEMS teams. Early recognition of ABD and early requests for attendance are key considerations for clinicians. Reducing 'time to sedation' may significantly improve outcomes and prevent rapid deterioration and death. Decision-making regarding PreRT is complex and more likely to be administered to patients who lack capacity, remain severely agitated, despite de-escalation measures, and who remain at risk to themselves and others. Specialist teams will likely have sedation assessment tools and frameworks.

Once a shared decision has been made to sedate, a pre-sedation plan should be clearly created by all members of the team. The plan should consider (adapted from Humphries et al., 2025):

1 Appoint roles (restraint team, clinical observer, sedation team, intravenous access, clinical assessment).
2 Communicate intended plan.
3 Anticipate problems.
4 Consider restraint options.
5 Plan intravenous access.
6 Plan for time-critical transport to appropriate care (resuscitation) and pre-alert: ATMIST (Age, Time, Mechanism, Injuries, Signs, Treatment) or SBAR (Situation, Background, Assessment, Recommendation).
7 Communicate the decision to relax restraint clearly.

Following sedation, initial management should include primary survey (ABCDE approach), oxygen therapy, intravenous fluids, cooling measures, pain relief, and continuous physiological monitoring. Physiological monitoring should include: basic observations (heart rate, respiratory rate, SpO_2, temperature, and blood pressure), end-tidal CO_2 monitoring, cardiac monitoring, and continuous clinical observation and reassessment.

Intravenous fluid resuscitation

The use of intravenous fluids to treat hypovolaemia (hyperthermia-induced), rhabdomyolysis, and acidosis should be considered if safe to do so (likely post-sedation). However, transport to definitive care should not be delayed for fluid therapy; instead, this can be considered and initiated en route.

Holistic considerations

Management of acute behavioural disturbance must extend beyond immediate containment and physiological stabilisation to include a holistic appreciation of the individual's wider context, vulnerabilities, and longer-term needs. Patients presenting with ABD are frequently experiencing a convergence of biological stress, psychological distress, substance use, trauma, and social adversity, which may include homelessness, marginalisation, previous adverse encounters with authorities, or unmet mental health needs. Paramedics should remain mindful that delirium, fear, and loss of control can profoundly affect behaviour and communication, and that apparent hostility may represent distress rather than intent. A holistic approach therefore requires trauma-informed communication, careful consideration of capacity, safeguarding awareness, and collaboration with police and mental health services to ensure continuity of care beyond the immediate crisis. Attention must also be given to the well-being of clinicians involved; exposure to violence, restraint, and high-stakes decision-making can contribute to moral distress, and structured debriefing and peer support should be considered an essential component of safe, sustainable practice.

Capacity

Delirium is a hallmark feature of ABD and therefore most patients within this cohort will lack mental capacity. However, it is important that clinicians are competent in mental capacity assessment and ensure capacity is assessed and documented accurately. This is particularly important when treating vulnerable patients. There has been growing concern amongst mental capacity specialists regarding the use of the Mental Capacity Act 2005 as an excuse not to provide care for vulnerable patients. It is important to understand that ABD patients are vulnerable and therefore at risk of stigmatisation, bias, judgement, and inappropriate use of the MCA by clinicians. This is fundamentally important when assessing capacity for patients presenting with varying levels of delirium/agitation.

Paramedic self-care and psychological safety

Managing acute behavioural disturbance places paramedics at heightened risk of psychological harm due to repeated exposure to violence, restraint, ethical uncertainty, and potential adverse outcomes. Trauma-informed practice must therefore be extended not only to patients but also to clinicians. Psychological safety is supported when paramedics are encouraged to recognise the emotional impact of these incidents, access timely debriefing, and discuss uncertainty or distress without fear of blame or judgement. Embedding reflective practice, peer support, and supportive leadership within ambulance services helps mitigate moral injury, compassion fatigue, and burnout. Recognising self-care as a professional responsibility rather than an individual weakness is essential to sustaining safe, ethical, and compassionate paramedic practice over time.

Lessons from the case: Police custody and red flag agitation

Recognise early: near-constant activity + diaphoresis + tachypnoea + paranoia = treat as time-critical.

Police custody: police custody does not mean the presentation is non-medical. Avoid defaulting to behavioural explanations; always consider delirium and medical drivers.

Escalate fast: reduce 'time to sedation' by early specialist/critical care request.

Minimise restraint harm: avoid prone positioning; shortest duration, clear purpose, coordinated team roles.

Prioritise physiology: cooling, oxygenation, monitoring (including $EtCO_2$ where available), rapid transport.

Document defensibly: red flags observed, de-escalation attempted, rationale for restraint/sedation, proportionality/legal basis.

Conclusion

Acute behavioural disturbance represents one of the most dangerous and ethically complex emergencies encountered in pre-hospital care. This chapter has demonstrated that ABD is not a discrete diagnosis, but a critical state of severe agitation, delirium, and physiological collapse, arising from diverse underlying causes including substance misuse, mental illness, and acute medical pathology.

Contemporary UK practice is rightly shifting away from the historically flawed concept of excited delirium towards agitation-spectrum models and the emerging recognition of red flag agitation. This reframing supports earlier recognition, clearer decision-making, and safer multidisciplinary responses. For paramedics, effective management depends on prioritising time-critical physiology, minimising restraint-related harm, and facilitating rapid access to sedation and definitive care when indicated. Equally important is the ability to work collaboratively with police and specialist teams, applying legal frameworks proportionately and transparently. Ultimately, safe ABD management is not defined by control, but by early recognition, decisive intervention, compassionate practice, and protection of life for patients, clinicians, and all those involved.

Further learning materials

Multiple-choice questions

MCQ1: *Terminology and diagnosis*: Which statement best reflects current UK understanding of acute behavioural disturbance (ABD)?

A. ABD is a formally recognised medical diagnosis

B. ABD is synonymous with excited delirium

C. ABD is an umbrella term describing life-threatening agitation with physiological compromise

D. ABD only applies to substance-related presentations

Correct answer: C

Rationale: In UK practice, ABD is not a formal diagnosis but a descriptive umbrella term for severe agitation with physiological compromise and risk of sudden collapse.

MCQ2: *Historical context*: Why has the term 'excited delirium' been widely rejected in UK clinical practice?

A. It refers only to psychiatric illness
B. It lacks a consistent evidence base and has been applied in racially biased ways
C. It is outdated but clinically accurate
D. It is recognised as a cause of death in the UK

Correct answer: B

Rationale: The term 'excited delirium' lacks consistent scientific validation and has been criticised for biased application, leading UK guidance to move towards agitation-spectrum terminology.

MCQ3: *Recognition of red flag agitation*: Which combination most strongly supports recognition of ABD/red flag agitation?

A. Verbal aggression and refusal of care
B. Delirium alone without agitation
C. Near-constant activity, extreme agitation, tactile hyperthermia
D. Intoxication with stable behaviour

Correct answer: C

Rationale: Near-constant activity, extreme agitation, and tactile hyperthermia are consensus red flag features associated with life-threatening ABD rather than simple aggression.

MCQ4: *Risk and urgency*: Why should ABD be treated as a time-critical medical emergency?

A. Patients are unpredictable and violent
B. It primarily requires police management
C. It is associated with rapid physiological collapse and sudden death
D. It always resolves with de-escalation

Correct answer: C

Rationale: ABD is linked to hyperthermia, catecholamine surge, metabolic acidosis, and arrhythmia, which can progress rapidly to cardiac arrest if untreated.

MCQ5: *Misidentification*: What is a key risk of misidentifying ABD as simple aggression?

A. Increased use of mental health services
B. Unnecessary sedation

C. Delay to life-saving medical intervention

D. Over-documentation

Correct answer: C

Rationale: Misidentifying ABD as behavioural aggression may delay recognition of physiological deterioration and postpone life-saving medical intervention.

MCQ6: *Pathophysiology*: Which pathophysiological process plays a central role in ABD?

A. Parasympathetic dominance

B. Dopamine-mediated catecholamine surge

C. Hypothermia and bradycardia

D. Reduced muscular activity

Correct answer: B

Rationale: Excess dopamine activity drives a catecholamine surge, amplifying sympathetic stress responses and contributing to hyperthermia, acidosis, and cardiac instability.

MCQ7: *Restraint*: Which statement best reflects best practice regarding restraint in ABD?

A. Restraint should be used early to control behaviour

B. Restraint worsens physiological stress and should be minimised

C. Prone restraint is safe if brief

D. Restraint removes the need for sedation

Correct answer: B

Rationale: Physical restraint increases exertion, acidosis, and cardiovascular stress, and therefore should be used only when necessary and for the shortest duration possible.

MCQ8: *Temperature management*: Why are antipyretics ineffective in ABD-related hyperthermia?

A. They act too slowly

B. They worsen agitation

C. The hypothalamic set point is not raised

D. They cause hypotension

Correct answer: C

Rationale: ABD-related hyperthermia results from excessive heat production and failed thermoregulation, not a raised hypothalamic set point, making antipyretics ineffective.

MCQ9: *Sedation*: What is the primary aim of pre-rapid tranquilisation (PreRT) in ABD?

A. To induce unconsciousness

B. To punish violent behaviour

C. To calm the patient and reduce physiological risk

D. To replace police restraint

Correct answer: C

Rationale: The aim of PreRT is to safely calm the patient, reduce physiological stress, and enable definitive care, rather than to induce unconsciousness.

MCQ10: *Capacity and ethics*: Which statement is most accurate regarding capacity in ABD?

A. All agitated patients lack capacity

B. Capacity is irrelevant in emergencies

C. Delirium often impairs capacity and best-interest decisions may be required

D. Capacity cannot be assessed in police custody

Correct answer: C

Rationale: Delirium commonly impairs decision-making capacity in ABD, requiring lawful best-interest decision-making where necessary and proportionate.

Reflective questions for learners

Q1: How can agitation-spectrum thinking help you avoid both over-medicalising aggression and missing life-threatening ABD?

Q2: What early signs would prompt you to escalate and request specialist support rather than persist with de-escalation alone?

Q3: How do restraint decisions interact with physiology, ethics, and human rights in ABD cases?

Q4: In multi-agency settings, how can paramedics advocate effectively for urgent medical care while maintaining collaborative working with police?

Q5: What aspects of ABD management do you find most ethically or emotionally challenging, and why?

Q6: How can post-incident debriefing and reflection support your psychological safety after managing high-risk agitation?

Teaching commentary

Acute behavioural disturbance represents a convergence of medical emergency, ethical complexity, and operational risk. This chapter has emphasised that ABD is not a diagnosis, but a time-critical physiological and behavioural emergency that requires early recognition, decisive action, and coordinated multi-agency working.

A key learning point is the shift away from rigid labels towards agitation-spectrum thinking. Students should understand that 'red flag agitation' signals a patient at high risk of rapid deterioration, where delays to sedation, prolonged restraint, or failure to manage hyperthermia and acidosis can be fatal. Clinical reasoning must therefore prioritise time, physiology, and safety over attempts at diagnostic certainty.

The chapter has also highlighted the risks of medicalising criminal behaviour or, more dangerously, failing to recognise a medical emergency. Paramedics play a pivotal role in bridging this gap, supporting police colleagues, and advocating for urgent medical intervention when required.

Finally, learners should recognise the moral and emotional burden of managing ABD. High-risk restraint decisions, exposure to violence, and fear of adverse outcomes can contribute to moral injury. Safe practice includes not only protecting patients, but also ensuring clinician safety, support, and reflective learning.

References

Calver, L.A., Downes, M.A., Page, C.B., Bryant, J.L., and Isbiter, G.K. (2010). The impact of a standardised intramuscular sedation protocol for acute behavioural disturbance in the emergency department. *BMC Emergency Medicine, 10*, 14. https://doi.org/10.1186/1471-227X-10-14

Department of Health (2015). *Mental Health Act 1983: Code of Practice.* https://assets.publishing.service.gov.uk/media/5a80a774e5274a2e87dbb0f0/MHA_Code_of_Practice.PDF

Faculty of Forensic and Legal Medicine (2019). *Acute behavioural disturbance: Guidance for clinicians.* London: Royal College of Emergency Medicine.

Gorton, A., Kalk, N., Payne-James, J., Rix, K., Shelley, S., Stark, M., et al. (2022). *Acute behavioural disturbance: Guidelines on management in police custody.* London: Faculty of Forensic and Legal Medicine, Royal College of Emergency Medicine. https://fflm.ac.uk/wp-content/uploads/2022/10/ABD-Guidelines-on-Management-in-Police-Custody-Oct-2022.pdf

Hopper, A.B., Vilke, G.M., Castillo, E.M., Campillo, A., Davie, T., and Wilson, M.P. (2015). Ketamine for acute agitation in the emergency department. *Journal of Emergency Medicine, 48*(6), 712–71. https://doi.org/10.1016/j.jemermed.2015.02.019

Humphries, C., Aw-Yong, M., Cowburn, P., Deakin, C., Grundlingh, J., Rix, K., et al. (2025). *Acute behavioural disturbance in emergency departments: Best practice guideline*, Version 3. London: Royal College of Emergency Medicine. https://rcem.ac.uk/wp-content/uploads/2025/05/Acute_Behavioural_Disturbance_in_Emergency_Departments_May2025_V3.pdf

Humphries, C., Kelly, A., Sadik, A., Walker, A., and Smith, J. (2024). Consensus on acute behavioural disturbance in the UK: A multidisciplinary modified Delphi study to determine what it is and how it should be managed. *Emergency Medicine Journal, 41*(1), 4–12. https://doi.org/10.1136/emermed-2023-213335

Joint Royal Colleges Ambulance Liaison Committee (JRCALC) (2025). *JRCALC clinical guidelines update,* July. https://jrcalc.org.uk/publication-date-july-2025/

Lindridge, J., Edwards, T., and Blackwood, L. (2025). Decision-making and acute behavioural disturbance (ABD): A qualitative thematic analysis of perspectives on decision-making by UK ambulance paramedics. *BMC Emergency Medicine, 25*(1), 135. https://doi.org/10.1186/s12873-025-01297-7

McGugan, E.A. (2001). Hyperpyrexia in the emergency department. *Emergency Medicine, 13*(1), 116–120. https://doi.org/10.1046/j.1442-2026.2001.00189.x

McGuinness, J., and Lipsedge, M. (2022). 'Excited delirium', acute behavioural disturbance, death and diagnosis. *Psychological Medicine, 52*(9), 1601–1611. https://doi.org/10.1017/S0033291722001076

National Institute for Health and Care Excellence (NICE) (2015). *Violence and aggression: Short-term management in mental health, health and community settings* (NG10). London: NICE. https://www.nice.org.uk/guidance/ng10/chapter/Recommendations (accessed 16 December 2025).

National Institute for Health and Care Excellence (NICE) (2024). *Delirium: Prevention, diagnosis and management in hospital and long-term care* (CG103). London: NICE. https://www.nice.org.uk/guidance/cg103

NHS England (2021). *Use of restrictive practices in health and care settings.* London: NHS England.

Obasogie, O.K. (2021). Excited delirium and police use of force. *Virginia Law Review, 107*(8), 1545–1620. https://virginialawreview.org/articles/excited-delirium-and-police-use-of-force/

Peel, M. (2022). Acute behavioural disturbance: Recognition, assessment and management. *Emergency Nurse.* https://doi.org/10.7748/en.2022.e2126

Physicians for Human Rights (2022). *'Excited delirium' and deaths in police custody.* New York: Physicians for Human Rights. https://phr.org/wp-content/uploads/2022/03/PHR-Excited-Delirium-Report-March-2022.pdf

Riddell, J., Tran, A., Bengiamin, R., Hendey, G.W., and Armenian, P. (2017). Ketamine as a first-line treatment for severely agitated emergency department patients. *American Journal of Emergency Medicine, 35*(7), 1000–1004. https://doi.org/10.1016/j.ajem.2017.02.026

Royal College of Emergency Medicine (RCEM) (2023). *Best practice guideline: Acute behavioural disturbance in emergency departments*, Version 2. London: RCEM. https://rcem.ac.uk/wp-content/uploads/2023/10/Acute_Behavioural_Disturbance_in_Emergency_Departments_Oct2023_V2.pdf (accessed 16 December 2025).

Royal College of Emergency Medicine (RCEM) (2024). *Red-flag agitation and acute behavioural disturbance: Best practice guidance.* London: RCEM.

Stark, M. (2024). Acute behavioural disturbance – what do we mean?' *Pathology, 56*(suppl. 1), S12. https://doi.org/10.1016/j.pathol.2023.12.049

Stevenson, R., and Tracy, D.K. (2021). Acute behavioural disturbance: A physical emergency psychiatrists need to understand. *BJPsych Advances, 27*(5), 333–342. https://doi.org/10.1192/bja.2020.67

Strömmer, E.M.F., Leith, W., Zeegers, M.P., and Freeman, M.D. (2020). The role of restraint in fatal excited delirium: A research synthesis and pooled analysis. *Forensic Science, Medicine and Pathology, 16,* 680–692. https://doi.org/10.1007/s12024-020-00291-8

Taylor, D., Barnes, T.R.E., and Young, A.H. (2025). *The Maudsley Prescribing Guidelines in Psychiatry* (15th edition). Hoboken, NJ: Wiley-Blackwell.

Tracy, D.K. (2024). Acute behavioural disturbance: What's in a name?' *BJPsych Open*, *10*(2), e38. https://doi.org/10.1192/bjo.2024.5

Zeller, S.L. (2017). *The end of chemical restraints: Expert opinion.* https://www.psychiatryadvisor.com/home/practice-management/the-end-of-chemical-restraints-expert-opinion/

10 Conclusion: Integrating evidence, compassion, and policy into paramedic mental health practice

Jo Augustus

The chapters in this book have demonstrated that mental health is not a peripheral component of paramedic practice, but a central and defining feature of contemporary emergency and urgent care. Across the life course, from childhood through older adulthood, people experiencing mental distress frequently find themselves in contact with ambulance services, often at moments of profound vulnerability. Paramedics therefore occupy a unique position at the intersection of health, social care, and public safety. As the Right Care, Right Person (RCRP) policy reshapes crisis response nationally, this role is strengthened further, placing paramedics at the forefront of health-led interventions and compassionate crisis resolution (NHS England, 2023).

This book has also shown that mental health presentations are deeply complex, shaped by the interaction of biological, psychological, social, and structural factors. A key theme throughout has been the importance of holistic assessment, drawing on frameworks such as the bio-psycho-social model and Bronfenbrenner's ecological systems theory. These approaches remind us that every person has a story behind their crisis: trauma histories, relationship patterns, cultural identities, financial pressures, discrimination, chronic illnesses, or experiences of exclusion. Understanding these broader contexts enables paramedics to interpret behaviour more accurately, respond more skilfully, and support people more humanely. Mental health care requires more than a checklist; it requires curiosity, compassion, and a willingness to see beyond the boundaries of a single moment.

A further recurring theme is the moral and professional imperative of equality, diversity, and inclusion (EDI). Social movements such as Black Lives Matter have exposed significant inequalities in mental health systems, including disproportionate rates of detention, reduced access to psychological support, and higher levels of coercive practice for racialised communities. Paramedics, as highly visible frontline responders, have a responsibility to challenge these inequities through culturally safe, anti-discriminatory, and trauma-informed practice. This includes examining personal biases, being attentive to cultural norms, and recognising that distress may be rooted in experiences of marginalisation rather than pathology alone. Inclusive practice is therefore not only ethical, it is also clinically essential.

Another major theme is the emotional labour of paramedic mental health work. Evidence from international studies demonstrates that pre-hospital clinicians frequently experience psychological distress, burnout, and symptoms of PTSD related to repeated exposure to trauma, suicide, violence and high-stakes, risk negotiation. The Health and Care Professions Council Standards of Proficiency (2023) rightly place wellbeing as a core professional responsibility, highlighting the need for reflective practice, supervision, and emotional support. Throughout the book, the case studies have illustrated how challenging and emotionally charged mental health cases can be, underscoring the need for organisational cultures that prioritise clinician wellbeing as a determinant of patient safety.

Looking to the future, the profession faces opportunities and challenges. The growing emphasis on community-based alternatives to hospital, digital triage tools, crisis response vehicles, and integrated care systems creates new spaces in which paramedics can lead and innovate. However, these developments must be accompanied by investment in education, workforce support, and evidence-driven practice. The following recommendations summarise the key priorities for advancing both practice and research.

Recommendations for clinical practice

Strengthening mental health care within paramedic practice requires a commitment to person-centredness, reflective decision-making, and interdisciplinary collaboration. Paramedics should embrace a trauma-informed ethos that places dignity, safety, and empowerment at the centre of every interaction. This approach helps to de-escalate crisis, build trust, and prevent re-traumatisation. Clinicians must also deepen their understanding of the bio-psycho-social influences on distress, recognising how physical health problems, trauma histories, cultural identity, and social disadvantage influence presentation and risk.

Legal literacy is another essential component of high-quality practice. The implementation of Right Care, Right Person (NHS England, 2023) requires paramedics to be more confident in assessing risk, evaluating capacity, and determining when police involvement truly meets the threshold of necessity. The Mental Health Act and Mental Capacity Act frameworks should be routinely applied in a manner that prioritises the least restrictive, most therapeutic option. Meaningful multidisciplinary working remains fundamental, as paramedics often form part of a wider system that includes crisis teams, liaison psychiatry, GPs, approved mental health professionals, and social care.

Key practice priorities include:

- Embedding trauma-informed, person-centred care into every mental health encounter.
- Enhancing holistic assessment skills using bio-psycho-social and ecological frameworks.
- Strengthening confidence in risk formulation, capacity assessment, and safety planning.
- Ensuring legal and ethical decision-making remains transparent, defensible, and compassionate.
- Improving interdisciplinary communication to support seamless handover and continuity of care.
- Cultivating reflective practice and prioritising clinician wellbeing as a safety issue.

Recommendations for future research

Future research must reflect the evolving reality of paramedic mental health practice. As ambulance services take on greater responsibility for crisis response, robust evidence is needed to evaluate the effectiveness, safety, and equity of emerging models of care. Research should explore not only clinical outcomes but also patient experience, cultural safety, workforce sustainability, and the impact of system design on vulnerable populations.

There is a particular need for research into the effectiveness of paramedic-led mental health interventions, especially in the context of non-conveyance decisions and community-based alternatives to hospital. As RCRP reconfigures pathways, it is essential to understand how paramedics can make nuanced, relationally informed decisions that balance autonomy, safety, and access to appropriate support. Research into health inequalities is also vital: the profession must better understand why certain communities experience poorer mental health outcomes and disproportionate crisis involvement, and how paramedics can play a role in addressing these disparities.

Priority areas for future research include:

- Evaluating outcomes of paramedic-led crisis response models, including mental health cars and joint response units.
- Exploring health inequalities in emergency mental health care and the impact of RCRP on different populations.
- Developing validated tools for mental health triage, risk formulation, and non-conveyance.
- Investigating the impact of mental health education, simulation, and reflective practice on clinical competence.

- Examining workforce wellbeing, burnout prevention, and organisational culture in mental health contexts.
- Assessing the role of digital decision-support tools and AI in enhancing crisis assessment and safety.

Closing reflection

This book has argued that the paramedic profession is at a pivotal moment. As mental health becomes an increasingly prominent aspect of urgent care, paramedics are uniquely placed to offer compassionate, evidence-based, and contextually aware support to individuals in crisis. The shift towards health-led crisis response, championed through NHS England policy, represents an opportunity to strengthen patient-centred practice and reduce unnecessary criminalisation. However, this opportunity brings responsibility: to understand the full complexity of human distress, to engage with patients as partners in care, and to cultivate the emotional resilience necessary for this challenging work.

The future of paramedic mental health practice will depend on the profession's ability to embrace reflective, ethically grounded, and research-informed approaches. By doing so, paramedics can help reshape emergency mental health care into a system defined by compassion, collaboration, and justice – one that not only responds to crisis but also affirms the dignity and humanity of every person who seeks help.

References

Health and Care Professions Council (HCPC) (2023). *Standards of Proficiency: Paramedics*. London: HCPC. https://www.hcpc-uk.org/globalassets/standards/standards-of-proficiency/paramedics.pdf (accessed 25 November 2025).

NHS England (2023). *National Partnership Agreement: Right Care, Right Person*, 26 July. https://www.gov.uk/government/publications/national-partnership-agreement-right-care-right-person (accessed 25 November 2025).

Index

Abbaspour, S. 2, 9
ABCDE model 141–2
ABD (*see* Acute behavioural disturbance)
Abd-Allah, F. 53
Abdoli, A. 53
Abdoli, N. 17, 20
Abner, S. 86
Abohashem, S. 88
Abu-Gharbieh, E. 53
Accardo, A.L. 21, 23, 24
Acosta, L. 117
ACS (*see* Acute coronary syndromes)
Activities of daily living (ADLs) 92
Acute behavioural disturbance (ABD)
  case study 217
  current consensus in 214–15
  definitions 213–14
  historical context 212–13
  management, scene safety and containment
    capacity of 231
    chemical restraint 228
    de- escalation 226–7
    holistic 230–1
    intravenous fluid resuscitation 230
    mechanical restraint 228
    pre- rapid tranquilisation and sedation 229–30
    restraint 227–8
    temperature control 225–6
  misidentification of 218–19
  on- scene clinical reference 218
  paramedic self- care and psychological safety 231–2
  pathophysiology of
    catecholamine surge 221
    dopamine- mediated pathways 220
    genetic susceptibility 220
    hyperthermia 221
    metabolic acidosis 221–2
  red flag agitation, recognition of 215–17
  substance misuse 219
Acute coronary syndromes (ACS) 138
Adams, F. 17, 22–4
ADHD (*see* Attention- deficit/hyperactivity disorder)
Adkins-Jackson, P.B. 53, 55
ADLs (*see* Activities of daily living)
Adroma, M. 117
Akbari, A. 85
Akello, J. 117
Aktas, G. 88, 93
Alabdali, A. 9
Alcazar-Gonzales, J. 21
Aldosoky, W. 88
Al-Dossary, S. 54
Al-Dwaikat, T. 54
Alexopoulos, G.S. 87
Alghamdi, A. 9
Alharbi, M. 9
Alhasan, D. 93
Ali, A.M. 54
Alisic, E. 18, 23
Aljerian, N. 9
Alkhamees, A.A. 54
Alladi, S. 53, 55, 57, 72, 74
Allard, S. 118
Allohidan, F. 9
Alshibani, A. 9
Altamura, M. 55, 56
Alzheimer's disease 55
AMHP (*see* Approved mental health professionals)
Amitay, E.L. 94
Amjad, H. 58
Anderson, D. 54, 58, 59, 60, 68, 69, 70, 71, 72, 74
Anderson, J.K. 113
Anderson, R.J. 86
Anderson, R.M. 55
Andrade, J. 113, 114
Angus, S.A. 141
Antepartum haemorrhage (APH) 117
Anxiety 23–4
APH (*see* Antepartum haemorrhage)
Approved mental health professionals (AMHPs) 167
Arean, P. 86

Armenian, P. 229
Armitage, C. 191, 193, 197, 198
Arnold, L. 125
Ashkenazy, E. 18, 19, 22
Ashworth, H. 91
Asthma 87
Asurlekar, A. 197
Atif, K. 2, 9
Attems, J. 56, 57
Attention- deficit/hyperactivity disorder (ADHD) 20, 34–7
Attrill, L. 59
Auerbach, R. 196
Augustus, J. 3, 4, 85, 113, 180, 212, 239
Autoimmune and inflammatory conditions 88–9
Aw-Yong, M. 219, 220, 226, 230
Ayubi, E. 95
Azcoaga-Lorenzo, A. 85
Azevedo, N.F. 121

Babu Sandilyan, M. 55
Bacaro, V. 21
Backes, C.H. 120
Bacon, A.M. 113, 114
Badr, J. 105
Baggs, A.E. 18, 19, 22
Bains, G.S. 93
Balbuena, L. 181
Banerjee, S. 59
Bannister, K. 183
Baptie, G. 113, 114
Barati, M. 95
Barbato, E. 141
Barnea, E.R. 118
Barnes, P.J. 135, 147, 149, 150
Baron, S.L. 136
Baron-Cohen, S. 17
Barratt, A. 21
Barrere, C. 69
Bashirian, S. 95
Bass, M. 91
Bateman, B.T. 118
Baud, J. 23, 24, 26
Beach, E. 120, 121
Beale, C. 199, 200
Beason-Held, L.L. 56
Beckman, K. 195
Bedekar, K. 137
Bedford, J. 118
Bedson, A. 120, 121
Bedus, C. 183
Beeson, L.E. 115
Begum, F. 118
Behavioural and psychological symptoms of dementia (BPSD) 59–60, 69
Bell, K. 21
Beller, E. 17
Bellgrove, M.A. 20, 24, 26
Benarroch, E.E. 56, 57
Bengiamin, R. 229
Benton, M. 114, 119
Berardino, G. 55, 56
Berendsen, A.J. 139
Bernanke, J. 195
Berring, L.L. 91
Berry, C. 141
Berry, S.N. 123, 124, 125
Bervoets, J. 22, 23
Besser, L.M. 53, 55
Best, C. 194
Bettis, A. 192
Betts, D.E. 23
Beyer, F. 95
Beyeza-Kashesya, J. 118
Bhattacharyya, T. 139
bio- psycho- social (BPS) model
  adapting for paramedic practice 12–14
  holistic assessment, importance of 12
  reflection tool 15
Bipolar disorder 161–2
Bish, M. 2
Bitsika, V. 21, 23
Bjureberg, J. 196
Black, M.H. 22, 23
Black, S. 60, 67, 70, 120, 121
Blackwood, L. 214
Blaskowitz, M.G. 20
Bliekendaal, W. 20, 23, 25, 26
Bloch, C. 24
Bloomer, M.J. 142, 148
Blutinger, E. 54, 58, 72, 74
Boerman, L.M. 139
Boeve, B.F. 55, 56
Bohman, B. 193
Bond, L. 25
Booth, L. 54, 61, 69
Bortolotti, L. 199
Bosley, E. 192, 198
Botha, M. 22
Boulton, E. 95

Bounds, C.G. 93
Bowden, S.L.J. 19, 24, 25, 26, 61, 69
Bower, J. 56, 57
Boyle, M. 117
BPSD (*see* Behavioural and psychological symptoms of dementia)
Bradley, S. 26
Brandão, T. 54, 60, 69
Brandling, J. 60, 67, 70
Brauckmann, V. 88, 93
Breast cancer 139
Bremer, A. 192, 193, 194, 197, 199
Brice, S. 20, 24, 25
Bridgman, H. 89, 94, 102
Briggs, H. 93, 104
Brikell, I. 20, 24, 26
Brimdyr, K. 120, 121
Brinton, R.D. 135, 147, 149, 150
Brites, R. 54, 60, 69
Bronfenbrenner, U. 4, 5, 239
Bronfenbrenner's ecological systems model 5–7
Brooks, L.A. 142, 148
Brown, J. 20, 21, 23
Brown, P.C.M. 20, 24
Brown, S. 180
Brown, T. 91
Bryant, A. 118
Bryant, J.L. 229
Buckman, J.E.J. 20, 21, 23
Bulger, J. 197, 198
Bunting, D. 93
Burgess, W. 137
Burghof, L. 24
Burrow, E. 121
Buswell, M. 60, 67, 70
Butson, C.R. 21
Byng, R. 196
Bynum, J.P.W. 58
Byrne, R.A. 141
Bystrova, K. 121

C- SSRS (*see* Columbia- suicide severity rating scale)
Cadwell, K. 120, 121
Calver, L.A. 229
Camerucci, E. 56, 57
Campbell, B. 54, 58, 59, 60, 67, 68, 69
Campbell, S. 193, 198
Campillo, A. 229
Campos, A. 93
Cancer 89, 138–9
Capstick, A. 54, 67, 69, 70, 71, 72
Carcausto-Zea, M. 21
Carcel, C. 135, 148
Cardiovascular disease (CVD) 87–8, 138
Cardona, F. 21
Carfoot, S. 121
Carias, K.V. 21
Carlborg, A. 196
Carlin, J.B. 121
Carrero, J-J. 135, 147, 149, 150
Caruso, R. 89
Carvalho, A.F. 114
Cascio, C.J. 25
Castillo, E.M. 229
Catanzaro, T. 200
Catts, H.W. 20
Cave, E. 200
Cerri, S. 117
Chaganti, S. 56
Chainarong, N. 118
Chakkarapani, A.A. 120
Chan, B.S. 56
Chandraharan, E. 118
Chapin, L.A. 58
Chapman, R. 17, 22
Charlton, R. 20, 21, 23
Chen, C. 56
Chen, M. 56
Chen, Q. 87, 117
Cheng, G. 56
Chesin, M. 194, 195
Chester-Jones, M. 118
Cheston, R. 60, 67, 70
Chieffo, A. 141
Children and young people (CYP)
  case study 29–31
  clinical presentations in 23–9
  legal, ethical, and professional issues 38
  neurodevelopmental disorders 19–23
  pre- hospital environment 18
  self- care and emotional labour 37–8
  systems pressures 39
  trauma- informed practice 19
Chirico, A. 25
Choonara, E. 54, 58, 60, 67, 69, 70
Christopher, L. 54, 71, 72, 73
Chronic kidney disease (CKD) 89
Chronic obstructive pulmonary disease (COPD) 87

Chronic respiratory diseases 87
Chung, P.J. 20
Civieri, G. 88
CKD (*see* Chronic kidney disease)
Claar, V. 54
Clarke, L. 191, 197
Clarke, S. 93, 104
Claßen, P.C. 89
Clegg, L.M. 113
Clouse, R.E. 86
Cohn, E.G. 25, 26
Colebatch, J.G. 56
Collier, L. 59
Collins, P. 118
Collis, R. 120
Columbia- suicide severity rating scale (C- SSRS) 195
Compton, D.L. 20
Conley, A.C. 25
Cooper, C. 20, 21, 23, 54
Cooper, J. 199
COPD (*see* Chronic obstructive pulmonary disease)
Corfield, A. 194
Cortese, S. 20, 24, 26
Costafreda, S.G. 53, 55, 57, 72, 74
Costanzo, F. 25
Coughlan, J.J. 141
Coughlin, S.S. 87
Courtet, P. 200
Courtney-Pratt, H. 54, 58, 59, 60, 67, 68, 69
Cowburn, P. 219, 220, 226, 230
Cowling, T. 94
Craigie, J. 199
Crane, L. 17, 22, 23, 24
Criado Perez, C. 135, 147, 149, 150
Crimmins, G. 113, 124
Crocq, M. 19
Cullen, A. 72
Cummins, T.M. 183
CVD (*see* Cardiovascular disease; Cardiovascular diseases)
CYP (*see* Children and young people)

Dagnan, D. 19, 20, 22, 25, 26
Dahhou, M. 118
Dahlen, H.G. 120
Dahlin, M. 196
Dasgupta, A. 139
Dastgir, S. 120
Davie, T. 229
Davies, J. 85
Davis, P.G. 121
D'Cruz, D. 89, 91, 102
de Bock, G.H. 139
De Deyn, P.P. 55, 56
de Puget, V.G. 22, 23
De Silva, M. 54, 71, 72, 73
De Waal, B. 54, 71, 72, 73
Deakin, C. 219, 220, 226, 230
Debby, V.D. 55, 56
Deborah, M.R. 23, 25
Deevongkij, K. 118
Delcomyn, C.L. 91
Dementia
  advancements in pre- hospital 71–2
  assessing mental capacity 61
  assessment and non- pharmacological de- escalation strategies 60
  behavioural and psychological symptoms of 59–60
  case study 62–8
  characterised by 53
  communication techniques for individuals 68–9
  de- escalation and behavioural management strategies 69
  environmental cues and routine observations 59
  epidemiology and impact 53–4
  ethical considerations 69–70
  evolving role of 71
  implications for paramedic practice 74–5
  interdisciplinary collaboration 70
  legal and professional responsibilities 70
  pathophysiology and types of 55–7
  policy and healthcare system changes 72–3
  pre- hospital care for 75
  red flags prompting conveyance 60–1
  safety and risk considerations 58–9
  training and education needs 72
DeMeo, D.L. 135, 147, 149, 150
den Ruijter, H.M. 135, 136, 138, 143, 148, 149
Dening, T. 55, 61
Denis, J-L. 105
Dennick, K. 86

Department of health and social Care (DHSC) 198
Derejczyk, J. 61
Dern, S. 18, 19, 22
Devall, A.J. 115
Dewison, N. 19, 22, 25, 26
Dhira, T. 196
DHSC (*see* Department of health and social Care)
Di Martino, D.D. 117
Diabetes mellitus 86
Dialysis 89
Dibb, B. 22
Dicker, B. 135
Dickson, D.W. 55, 56
Dickson, R. 121
Do, V. 115
Doherty, C.J. 141
Doherty, M. 26
Dominelli, P.B. 141
Donnellan, D. 121
Dougall, N. 194
Doust, J. 17
Dowding, D. 191, 197, 198
Downer, T. 67, 70
Downes, M.A. 229
Downey, C. 139
Downing, C. 180
Draper, J. 143, 147, 148
Du, J. 139
Dúason, S. 197
Duinmeijer, I. 20, 23, 25, 26
Dumas, L. 121
Duncan, E. 194
Dunne, C.P. 59, 61
Dunne, S.S. 59, 61
Dysmenorrhoea 137
Dyspnoea 87
Dyspraxia 21

Eating disorders 164–5
Eccleston, C. 54, 58, 59, 60, 67, 68, 69
Eclampsia 117
Ectopic pregnancy 115–16
Edberg, H. 196
Edge, D. 114, 119
EDI (*see* Equality, diversity, and inclusion)
Edison, P. 55
Edwards, D. 191
Edwards, T. 214
Eecklooe, K. 198
Ekström, A. 20, 25
El Baou, C. 20, 21, 23
Elser, H. 118
Elsherif, M.M. 21
Emond, K. 2
Endometriosis 137
Engel, G.L. 4, 12, 90
Engelborghs, S. 55, 56
England, E. 70
English, O. 183
Epilepsy 88
Equality, diversity, and inclusion (EDI) 2, 7–8, 239
Ergan, S.N. 20, 21
Ertle, E.M. 59, 60
Escobar, C. 54, 58, 72, 74
Escobar, M.F. 118
Eshghi, H. 2, 9
Espinoza, L.E. 87
Ethical decision- making 38
Evans, J. 194
Evans, N. 59
Evans, S. 55

Faedda, N. 21
Faisal, M. 54, 67, 69, 70, 71, 72
Fallot, R.D. 91
Falter-Wagner, C. 24
Farooqi, A. 86
Fazio, S. 54, 68, 69
Feakes, R. 61
Feldstein Ewing, S.W. 20, 24
Felker, A. 114, 116
Fereidouni, Z. 197
Ferguson, D.W. 89
Ferguson, E. 89, 94
Ferguson, M. 196
Ferguson, N. 192, 198
Fernandez Villalba, E. 121
Fernández-Fernández, F.A. 21
Ferrucci, L. 56
Fielding, C. 23, 25
Fields, L. 139, 140, 147
Findlay, H.J. 113
Firth, J. 85, 88, 114
Fisher, L. 86
Flanagan, B. 67, 70, 113, 116, 124
Fonseca, L.M.M. 121
Fontalis, A. 200
Foote, K.D. 21

Ford, E. 89
Ford, J. 120, 196
Fortin, M. 135, 147, 149
Fossey, M. 85
Francis, K.L. 113
Franke, B. 20, 24, 26
Frankland, J. 54, 67, 69, 70, 71, 72
Frawley, T. 25
Freedland, K.E. 86
Freeman, M.D. 214, 219, 220, 221, 222, 229
Freeston, M. 20, 24, 25
Frontotemporal dementia 56–7
Frost, D.M. 22
Fullana, J. 20
Furukawa, T.A. 114
Fuschi, D. 94

Galea, A. 85
Galfavy, H. 194, 195
Galiana, A. 18, 24
Gallagher, T. 26
Galletly, C. 85, 88
Gardner, A. 143
Gardner, P. 3, 4, 180, 212
Garratt, M. 23
Gavin, B. 25
Ge, Q. 196
George, K.M. 53, 55
Gergel, T. 199
Gerry, S. 118
Ghasemi, H. 17, 20
Ghodrati-Torbati, A. 2, 9
Ghosh, J. 115
Gill, C.E. 21, 24
Gill, J. 89
Gillespie-Lynch, K. 17, 22
Gillies, C. 86
Gilroy, S.P. 21, 24
Gilsanz, P. 87
Giner, L. 200
Giummarra, M.J. 18, 23
Glasgow, R.E. 86
Glass, D. 89
Glasziou, P. 17
Glendenning, A. 197, 198
Gliatto, P. 54, 58, 72, 74
Goadsby, G. 85
Goffman, E. 26
Goldstein, L.S.B. 55
Goldstein, R.D. 115
Goldstein, S. 93
Gonzalez-Calderon, G. 57
Goodarzi, F. 95
Goode, D. 91
Goodman, D.W. 20, 24, 26
Goodwin, L. 120, 121, 124
Goreis, A. 183
Gorton, A. 214, 216, 228, 229
Gosling, C. 54, 58, 59, 60, 68, 69, 70, 71, 72, 74
Gou, W.L. 117
Gouweloos, J. 18, 23
Gräff, P. 88, 93
Grantz, K.L. 118
Grassi, L. 89
Graves, B.W. 120, 121
Graviotto, H.G. 57
Green, L. 118
Green, S. 115
Greer, C. 18, 22, 23, 25
Greiner de Magalhães, C. 21
Gremesty, G. 89
Grewal, S.S. 88
Gri, N. 94
Grigsby, A.B. 86
Grimsrud, E. 113–15, 125
Grimwood, T. 25
Groenewald, C. 115
Grossman, M. 57
Grossman, S. 91
Grundlingh, J. 219, 220, 226, 230
Gryglewska, B. 61
Guija, J. 200
Gullon-Scott, F. 21
Gundavarpu, S. 58
Gunduz, A. 21
Gunnarsson, B. 197
Guo, P.L. 117
Gupta, S. 120
Guribye, F. 22
Gurol-Urganci, I. 113
Guthrie, B. 135, 147, 149
Guthrie, E. 192, 197, 199

Hackett, R.A. 86, 93
Hadian Shirazi, Z. 197
Hadjichrysanthou, C. 55
Haft, S.L. 21
Haglund, A. 196
Halek, M. 59, 60
Haley, M.M. 120, 121
Hall, A. 95

Halliday, G. 55, 56
Hallit, S. 54
Hallyburton, A. 90
Hammarbäck, S. 192, 193, 194, 197, 199
Han, M.X. 54, 58, 59, 60, 68, 69, 70, 71, 72, 74
Hanley, M. 23, 25
Hanlon, E. 88
Hansen, J.P. 91
Hansen, S. 113, 116
Hardy, B.W. 21
Harmer, B. 194
Harper, G. 17, 22, 23, 24
Harris, M. 91
Harris, W. 54, 58, 59, 60, 67, 68, 69
Harrison, M.J. 25, 26
Hartman, C.A. 20, 24, 26
Harwood, R. 89, 91, 102
Hashemian, A.H. 17, 20
Hatch, B. 21
Havard, A. 135, 148
Hawdon, J. 113
Hawton, K. 199
Hazell, W. 93
Health and Care Professions Council (HCPC) Standards of Proficiency 9, 11, 12, 27–9, 38, 44, 45, 70, 171
Heath, M. 123
Helander, J. 22, 23
Hemingway, L. 54, 58, 59, 60, 68, 69, 70, 71, 72, 74
Henchie, A. 22, 26
Henderson, E.J. 72
Hendey, G.W. 229
Hendricks, E. 115
Hendriks, E. 115
Hennah, M. 54
Henriksen, L. 113, 114, 115, 125
Hessler, D. 86
Hewes, T. 197, 198
Heylen, A. 55, 56
Heyne, D.A. 21, 23
Hill, K.D. 120
Hill, M. 113, 116
Hill, R. 96
Hill-Jarrett, T.G. 53, 55
Hilton, S. 113
Hinsliff-Smith, K. 61
Hinson-Enslin, A.M. 87
Hipólito, J. 54, 60, 69
History- taking, in women's emergencies 142–3
Ho, I.S.S. 85
Hoban, R.A. 118
Hodgins, P. 85
Hoeft, F. 21
Hoffmann, S.H. 86
Hǒgh, P. 56
Holland, E. 85
Holm, T. 91
Holmberg, M. 192, 193, 194, 197, 199
Hooper, S.B. 120
Hopper, A.B. 229
Hopper, L. 113, 116
Horsbǒl, T.A. 86
Howard, L. 88, 90
Howe, E. 193
HPA (*see* Hypothalamic-pituitary-adrenal axis)
Hsu, B. 135, 148
Hu, A. 196
Hua, Y. 56
Huang, J. 58
Huang, W. 56
Hudasch, D. 88, 93
Huene, L. 123
Hughes, S. 182, 191, 192, 194, 195
Human, M. 115
Humphries, C. 214, 215, 219, 220, 226, 228, 229, 230
Hunt, B.J. 118
Hunt, G. 197
Hunter, B. 124
Hunter, J. 182, 192, 193, 197
Huntley, J. 53, 55, 57, 72, 74
Hussain, O. 199
Hutman, T. 17, 22
Huxtable, R. 199
Hvass, A.M.F. 123
Hvidhjelm, J. 91
Hypothalamic-pituitary- adrenal (HPA) axis 183
Hyun, J. 53, 55

IADLs (*see* Instrumental activities of daily living)
Ikhile, D. 89
Ingard, C. 22, 23
Ingham, B. 19, 22, 23, 24, 25, 26
Instrumental activities of daily living (IADLs) 92

Intellectual disability 20
Intent, plans, actions, protection (IPAP) 191
IPAP (*see* Intent, plans, actions, protection)
Isaacs, D. 25
Isail, O-M. 89
Isbister, G.K. 229
Iversen, H. 192, 193
Ivzori, Y. 17, 23

Jadzinski, P. 70
James, R.J.E. 89, 94
Jamil, R. 195
Janssen, L. 20, 23, 25, 26
Jardine, J. 113
Jasani, A. 54, 58, 72, 74
Jasper, B.A. 117
Jeffery, H.C. 115
Jeffrey, G. 135, 147, 150
Jelic, V. 56
Jeyasingham, D. 191, 197, 198
John, A. 182, 191, 192, 194, 195
Johnson, K.A. 21
Johnson, K.R. 20
Joint royal colleges ambulance liaison committee (JRCALC) 191
Jones, A. 124
Jones, D. 54, 67, 69, 70, 71, 72
Jones, S. 88, 90
Joseph, K.S. 118
JRCALC (*see* Joint royal colleges ambulance liaison committee)

Kadlaskar, G. 21
Kalisch, L.A. 23, 24, 26
Kalk, N. 214, 216, 228, 229
Kalokyri, A. 20
Kamlin, C.O. 121
Kanyon, S. 114, 116
Kapadia, V. 121
Kapp, S.K. 17, 22
Kapur, N. 193, 198
Kassam-Adams, R. 18, 23
Kazda, L. 21
Keene, A. 199
Kelly, A. 214, 228, 229
Kelly, M. 139
Kerkhof, A. 192
Kerley, C.I. 56
Key, A.P. 25
Keyworth, C. 193, 198
Khatatbeh, H. 54
Khazaeni, B. 184
Khoshravesh, S. 95
Khunti, K. 85
Kiely, P.D.W. 89, 94
King, P. 70
King, R. 67, 70
Kinghorn, G. 139, 140, 147
Kinnaird, E. 19, 24, 25
Kinney, H.C. 115
Kirkpatrick, B. 21, 24
Kissane, D. 89
Kiyak, S. 114
Kline, C. 54, 68, 69
Kloer, P. 22, 26
Klonsky, E. 192
Knapp, M. 85
Knight, M. 114, 116, 118
Koekkoek, B. 192
Koenen, K.C. 87
Kofoed-Enevoldsen, A. 86
Kolanowski, A. 59, 60
Kommer, A. 89
Kompoliti, K. 21, 24
Kool, N. 192
Kostev, K. 89
Kotnis, R. 114, 116
Koyanagi, A. 85, 88
Kramer, M.S. 118
Kulkarni, K. 200
Kunadian, V. 135, 136, 138, 143, 148, 149
Kunonga, T.P. 95
Kurtz, S. 143, 147, 148

Labenz, C. 89
Lamar, M. 53, 55
Lamaro, V. 137
Landolt, M.A. 18, 23
Lau, D.C.W. 94
Lawrence, K.A. 23, 24, 26
Lazzaro, G. 21
LBD (*see* Lewy body dementia)
Leader, G. 21, 24
Leather, J. 193, 198
Leccisotti, I. 55, 56
Lee, S. 194
Lee, T. 199, 200
Lee-Davey, J. 199, 200
Leffert, L.R. 118
Lehn, S.F. 86
Lehnhardt, F. 24

Leith, W. 214, 219, 220, 221, 222, 229
Leng, F. 55
Lepage, M. 121
Lepore, F. 18, 22, 23, 25
Lepping, P. 61
Leurent, B. 59, 60
Lever, G. 191, 197, 198
Levy-Carrick, N. 91
Lewis, T.R. 120
Lewy body dementia (LBD) 56
Li, C. 56
Li, H. 103
Li, X.L. 117
Li, Y. 56
Lim, W.H. 137
Lindridge, J. 214
Linton, S. 113, 116
Lipp, R. 183
Lipsedge, M. 213
Liston, R. 118
Lithander, F.E. 72
Liu, K.Y. 53, 55, 57, 72, 74
Liu, L. 56
Liu, R. 192
Livingston, G.H. 53, 55, 57, 72, 74
Llana Martin, I. 121
Lloyd, K. 181
Lloyd-Williams, M. 89
Locatelli, I. 20
Lofthouse-Jones, C. 70
Lombardi, E. 18, 22, 23, 25
Long- term conditions
  case study 97–101
  clinical presentation and pre- hospital assessment 90–101
  effective communication with patients and caregivers 101–2
  effective signposting and community integration 105
  emergency care to prevention 104
  ethical considerations 103–4
  multi- agency collaboration 103
  patient education and self- management support 102–3
  in pre- hospital care 86–9
  recognising and managing acute exacerbations of chronic illnesses 102
  remote monitoring and telemedicine 105
  specific markers of 93–4
  training and education needs 105–6
Longhitano, Y. 94
Lonigan, C.J. 20
Lopez Escobar, A. 121
Lord, B. 67, 70, 113, 124
Lord, K. 59, 60
Lorem, G.F. 192, 193
Loughhead, M. 196
Loughney, A. 120
Lozupone, M. 55, 56
Lucas, P. 54, 58, 59, 60, 67, 68, 69
Lukasse, M. 113, 114, 115, 125
Lundervold, A.J. 22
Lustman, P.J. 86

Maass, S.W.M.C. 139
Maden, M. 96
Maessen, S.E. 135
Mahoney, W.J. 20
Mahtani, K. 96
Mair, F.S. 135, 147, 149
Make every contact count (MECC) 104
Malel, Z.J. 118
Malestroit, M. 200
Malfait, S. 198
Malli, M. 21
Manias, E. 142, 148
Mann, J. 194, 195, 196
Mann, L.M. 141
Mao-Draayer, Y. 88, 93
MAPPA (*see* Multi- agency public protection arrangements)
MARAC (*see* Multi- agency risk assessment conferences)
Marchant, A. 181
Maria, S.J. 113
Marin Gabriel, M.A. 121
Marsden, R. 197
Marshall, J.E. 116
Marx, W. 114
Masellis, M. 57
Masharani, U. 86
Mason, S. 192, 197, 199
Massimo, L. 57
Massoni, L. 21
Mast, B.T. 59, 60
Maternity care
  case study 121–5
  clinical assessment 118–21
  continuous assessment 121
  newborn transition and initial assessment 120

pre- hospital setting, presentations relevant to 115–18
thermoregulation and skin- to- skin contact 120–1
Mathai, J. 136
Matthiesen, A-S. 121
Mauvais-Jarvis, F. 135, 147, 149, 150
Mavrides, E. 118
Mayer, A. 183
Mayor, J. 88, 93
Mazhar, M.K.A. 72
McAdam, H. 121
McAtee, R. 54
McCabe, A. 191
McCabe, R. 182, 192, 193, 196, 197
McCann, L. 72
McCann, T. 192, 198
McClelland, G. 120, 121
McCowan, S. 26
McDaid, D. 85
McDonald, K.E. 18, 19, 22
McGeechan, K. 21
McGugan, E.A. 214, 219, 221, 226
McGuinness, J. 213
McInnes, A. 137
McIntyre, H. 196
McKeith, I.G. 55, 56
McKenna, L. 120, 135
McKenna, L.G. 120
McLelland, G.E. 120, 135
McMillan, C.T. 57
McMullen, S. 94
McNally, S. 53, 59, 60, 69, 70
McNicholas, F. 25
McVilly, K.R. 26
McWilliams, D.F. 89, 94
MDT (*see* multidisciplinary team)
MECC (*see* Make every contact count)
Medical emergencies in eating disorders (MEED) 164
Medina-Rioja, R. 57
MEED (*see* Medical emergencies in eating disorders)
Mehareen, J. 196
Melby, V. 91
Mendola, P. 118
Menghini, D. 21, 25
Menopause and perimenopause 138
Mental health
bio- psycho- social model 4, 12–15
children and young people (CYP) 17–39
crisis assessment, skills required for 11–12
ecological systems theory 4–7
equality, diversity, and inclusion 7–8
key conceptual models 11
long- term conditions 85–106
in neurodivergent CYP 23–4
person- centred care 3–4
symptoms 3
women's health and wellbeing,gendered care 138–9
women's mental health 113–26
Merz, N.B. 135, 147, 149, 150
Metacognition 92
Mhyre, J.M. 118
Michael, T. 58
Michail, M. 196
Michel, C. 196
Miles, A. 113, 116
Miller, M. 21
Miller, P.K. 19, 22, 23, 24, 25, 26, 54, 61, 69
Mills, B. 113, 116
Mills, J.L. 118
Mink, J.W. 21
Minnis, H. 183
Miranada, J.J. 135, 147, 149
Miscarriage 115
Mitchell, A.J. 89
Moghaddam, N. 61
Moghekar, A. 56
Moldawsky, R. 193
Molina-Rodríguez, F.N. 21
Mollica, A. 55, 56
Molloy, L. 139, 140, 147
Molony, S. 54, 69
Moniz-Cook, E. 59, 60
Monticone, V. 94
Montminy, J. 69
Moore, H.L. 20, 24, 25
Moore, K. 25
Moore, Z. 121
Moretti, M.C. 55, 56
Morgans, A. 120, 135
Morgans, A.E. 120
Morley, C.J. 121
Moroianu, L-A. 89
Morris-Rosendahl, D. 19
Morriss, R. 86
Motulsky, A. 105
Mountain, G. 59, 60
Mughal, F. 191, 197

Mukadam, N. 54
Mullan, A.F. 56, 57
Mullan, J.T. 86
Muller, P. 113
Multi- agency public protection arrangements (MAPPA) 143
Multi- agency risk assessment conferences (MARAC) 143
multidisciplinary team (MDT) 167
Multiple sclerosis 88
Mumford, S.L. 118
Murray, B.P. 184
Musculoskeletal and bone health 139
Muslim, Z. 118
Muzaffar, S. 199

Naidoo, N. 54, 71–3
Najafi Kalyani, M. 197
Nakimuli, A. 117
Nakubulwa, S. 117
Namagembe, I. 117
Nassar, A.H. 118
Nater, U.M. 183
National Early Warning Score 2 (NEWS2) 118–19
National institute for health and care excellence (NICE) 18
National institute of health and clinical excellence (NICE) 190
Naylor, C. 85
NCDs (*see* Neurocognitive disorders)
Neely, L.C. 21, 23, 24
Neurocognitive disorders (NCDs)
  best practices for paramedics 68–71
  clinical presentation and pre- hospital assessment 58–61
  dementia (*see* Dementia)
  epidemiology and impact 53–4
  role of paramedics 54
Neurodevelopmental disorders
  attention- deficit/hyperactivity disorder (ADHD) 20, 34–7
  autism spectrum condition (ASC) 19–20
  child and adolescent developmental consideration 23
  co- occurrence and intersection 21
  dyspraxia 21
  intellectual disability 20
  neurodiversity paradigm 22–3
  specific learning disabilities (SLDs) 20–21
NEWS2 (*see* National Early Warning Score 2)
NICE (*see* National institute for health and care excellence; National institute of health and clinical excellence)
Nicholas, J. 57
Nichols, E. 53
Nicholson, W. 118
Nicolaidis, C. 18, 19, 22
Nissen, E. 120, 121
Nizami, I. 20
Nordby, E.S. 22
Nordgreen, T. 22
Norman, A. 113, 114
Nowland, R. 199
Nugent, L. 121
Nunes, B.P. 135, 147, 149
Nunes, O. 54, 60, 69

Ó Breasail, M. 72
Obasogie, O.K. 214
O'Connor, N. 197
O'Connor, R.C. 183
O'Connor, T. 121
Odendaal, H.J. 115
O'Donnell, C.P.F. 121
Oduola, S. 143
Oei, J.L. 121
Oeksengaard, A. 56
O'Keeffe, S. 182, 192, 193, 197
Okun, M.S. 21
Olié, E. 200
O'Meara, P. 2
O'Nions, E. 20, 21, 23
Opland, C. 192, 193
Oprescu, F. 67, 70
Oquendo, M. 194, 195
Orellana, C. 56
O'Rourke, M. 195
Ortega, M. 120
Ossenkoppele, R. 55
Out- of- hospital birth 116
Ovarian torsion 136–7
Owen, G. 199

Page, C.B. 229
Paggetti, A. 21
Pallisera, M. 20
Papadopoulou, A. 115
Paramedic management, self- harm

assessment tools 195–6
handover strategies 197–8
managing patients manifesting self-harm behaviours 192–4
onward psychiatric care 196
paramedic interventions, review of 197
pre- hospital assessment techniques and risk evaluation tools 190–2
predictive aspects of 194–5
referral pathways and interprofessional collaboration 198–9
risk assessment 195
suicidal ideation 194
suicide and self- harm 194
Paramedic practice
autistic adults in 33
case- based learning 10–11
clinical practice, recommendations for 240–1
evolution of 2–3
future research, recommendations for 241–2
mental health (*see* Mental health)
neuroaffirming approaches 31–2
paramedic wellbeing 9–10
professional considerations for 37–9
psychological assessment considerations 119–20
Parasiliti, M. 117
Paredes-Velazco, R. 21
Park, L.J. 197
Parker, L. 191
Parker, S. 95
Parkinson's disease 88
Parkinson's disease dementia 57
Parr, J.R. 20, 24, 25
Parsonage, M. 85
Parsons, C. 54, 58, 72, 74
Paslaru, A.M. 89
Passarello, N. 25
Patel, D.R. 20
Patel, R. 114, 116
Patient autonomy 103–4
Patient health questionnaire (PHQ) 196
Patrick, N.J. 23
Patrick, Y.W. 3, 4, 85, 113
Patton, D. 121
Paul, J. 89
Pavel, L.L. 89
Payne-James, J. 214, 216, 228, 229
Peel, M. 222
Peet, S. 20, 23, 25, 26
Pellicano, E. 17, 22, 23, 24
Pelvic inflammatory disease (PID) 137
Penner, M. 24
Penninx, B.W.J.H. 114
Person- centred care 3–4
Personality disorders 162–3
Peters, A. 54, 71, 72, 73
Peters, E. 181
Peters, S. 135, 148
Petpichetchian, C. 118
Petrova, T. 56
Pett, G. 120
Pezzuti, L. 21
Phillips, J. 192, 197, 198
PHQ (*see* Patient health questionnaire)
Phung, J. 24
Piccioni, A. 94
PID (*see* Pelvic inflammatory disease)
Piotrowicz, K. 61
Pires, C.T. 54, 60, 69
Pirlot, C. 24
Plesea-Condratovici, A. 89
PMDT (*see* Prehospital maternity decision tool)
Pocock, H. 70
Pollack, A.Z. 118
Pompei, G. 135, 136, 138, 143, 148, 149
Pontes, M.C.F. 21, 23, 24
Pontes, N.M.H. 21, 23, 24
Poole, L. 86, 93
Popit, S. 20
Porter, A. 182, 191, 192, 194, 195, 198, 199
Postpartum haemorrhage 118
Powell, L. 20, 24, 25, 26
Pre- eclampsia 117
Pre- hospital setting
appropriate communication strategies 191
appropriate referral 191
assessment of women's health 139–43
bias in 91
chronic care model 90
collaborative working 28
communication differences 25–6
decision- making in 27–8
diagnostic overshadowing 90–1
dysmenorrhoea 137
endometriosis 137

exacerbation, vital signs, and monitoring 91–2
functional independence 92, 95–6
gynaecological emergencies 136
medication review and compliance issues 96–7
menopause and perimenopause 138
mental health presentations 23–4
multidisciplinary team (MDT) 27
NICE guidelines relevant to CYP neurodevelopmental conditions 27
out- of- hospital birth and imminent birth 116
ovarian torsion 136–7
pelvic inflammatory disease 137
range of risk assessment strategies 191–2
safeguarding and risk assessment 26–7
sensory and environmental factors 24–5

Pre- rapid tranquilisation (PreRT) 229
Prehospital maternity decision tool (PMDT) 118
PreRT (*see* Pre- rapid tranquilisation)
Presentation of self 26
Prillinger, K. 183
Prine, L. 115
Pring, K. 21
Prior, S. 191
Procter, N. 196
Prousali, E. 200

Qamar, I. 88
Quigley, E. 26
Quigley, T. 114, 119
Quinlan, J.F. 139
Quinlivan, L. 199
Quitoriano, C.D. 58

Råbu, M. 192, 193
Rahman, M. 196
Rahman, R. 22, 26
Rahman, S. 89, 94
Rahmani, A. 17, 20
Ramachandran, S. 121
Ramasauskaite, D. 118
Ramsay, M. 70
Randall, D. 135, 148
Raponi, M.B.G. 121
Rapp, S.R. 21
Rapport, F. 182, 191, 192, 194, 195
Raymaker, D.M. 18, 19, 22
Raynor, M.D. 116
RCRP (*see* Right care, right person; Right Care, Right Person)
Rebegea, L.F. 89
Record- keeping 38
Redfern, O.C. 118
Reed, R. 113, 124
Rees, N. 93, 104, 182, 191, 192, 194, 195, 198, 199
Reeve, J. 96
Reeves, G.E.M. 89, 94, 102
Reeves, K. 194
Reid, C. 22, 26
Reid, H.E. 114, 119
Rhind, S. 113
Rhodes, K. 196
Riba, M.B. 89
Riddell, J. 229
Riecke, T. 88, 93
Rifkin, L. 199
Right Care, Right Person (RCRP) 2, 8–9, 160
Riley, H. 192, 193
Risk stratification tools 28
Rittenberg, E. 91
Rix, K. 214, 216, 228, 229, 230
Rizvi, A. 194
Roberts, A.L. 87
Roberts, L. 192, 198
Rockwood, K. 95
Rodin, G. 89
Rodriguez, C.M.T. 57
Rodríguez-Armendariz, E. 18, 24
Roehr, C.C. 120
Romani, M. 21
Romanik, W. 61
Romero Blanco, I. 121
Romeu, D. 192, 197, 199
Rosenbaum, S. 85, 88
Rosenberg, R. 115
Rosendahl, J. 125
Rosenkilde, S. 86
Ross, L. 54, 58, 59, 60, 68, 69, 70, 71, 72, 74
Rossello, X. 141
Rossetti, S. 21
Rost, M. 125
Round, J. 59, 60
Ruck Keene, A. 199, 200
Ruiz, A. 88, 93
Ruiz, M.T. 121

Runeson, B. 196
Rutter, H. 118
Ryan, A. 91
Ryan, M. 182, 192, 193, 197

Sabattini, E. 117
Sabin-Farrell, R. 193
Sadik, A. 214, 228, 229
Sahlén, B. 20, 25
Salari, N. 17, 20
Salvi, J. 196
Sampson, E.L. 59, 60
Samuelsson, C. 20, 25
Samus, Q.M. 58
Sanchez, R. 69
Sanders, S. 17
Sandgren, O. 20, 25
Sarker, A. 196
Sarvestani, R. 197
Savic, M. 192, 198
Schaffer, D.H. 184
Schei, B. 113, 114, 115, 125
Scheper, A. 20, 23, 25, 26
Schizophrenia and psychotic disorders
  assessment and risk formulation 160
  clinical presentation 159–60
  pre- hospital management 160–1
Schleicher, E.M. 89
Schlembach, D. 118
Schneider, M. 23
Schofield, P. 59
Scott, S. 59, 60
Scott, T. 4
Seebaluck, J. 56
Segers, J. 22, 23
Seidu, S. 86
Selbæk, G. 53, 55, 57, 72, 74
Self- harma and suicidality
  case study 183–90
  ethical, legal considerations 199–200
  impact on patients, families, healthcare 181–2
  paramedic management and treatment approaches 190–9
  pathophysiological and psychological 182–3, 182–90
  reasons for 180–1
  risk factors 181
Serod, K. 20
Serrano, C. 57
Severe and enduring mental illness (SMI) 87, 157
  associated risks and medical complications in SMI 165–70
  best practice for paramedics 167–8
  bipolar disorder 161–2
  case study 168–70
  complex health inequalities 158
  eating disorders 164–5
  future of mental health, paramedic practice 171
  impact of 159
  personality disorders 162–3
  schizophrenia and psychotic disorders 159–61
  treatments, interventions, and the role of 166–7
  understanding 158–61
Seymour, J. 61
Shared decision- making 38
Sharpley, C.F. 21, 23
Shaw, E. 94
Shaw, S.C.K. 26
Sheikh, Z. 114, 119
Shelley, S. 214, 216, 228, 229
Shelton, E.L. 120
Sherman, L.E. 17, 22
Shi, Y. 103
Shiga, A. 56
Shimizu, H. 56
Shiri, M.H. 17, 20
Siddiqi, N. 85, 88
Siddiqui, W. 195
Silva, M.P.C. 121
Silverman, J. 143, 147, 148
Silvers, J.A. 23
Singer, J. 17
Siskind, D. 85, 88
Skalska, A. 61
Skar, S. 194
Skou, S.T. 135, 147, 149
Slater, P. 91
Slaughter, J.L. 120
SLDs (*see* Specific learning disabilities)
Sloan, M. 89, 91, 102
SMI (*see* Severe and enduring mental illness)
Smith, J. 214, 228, 229
Smith, K. 120, 135, 192, 198
Smith, L. 120

Smith, M.D. 72
Snaedal, J. 56
Sneath, E. 93
Solmi, M. 114
Somatisation 24
Sondergaard, R. 91
Sonmez, C. 194, 195
Sorbara, M.G. 57
Sorrentino, P. 25
Sotiropoulos, J. 121
Spacey, A. 54, 61, 69
Specific learning disabilities (SLDs) 20–21
Speight, J. 86
Spencer-Smith, M. 23, 24, 26
Spiers, G.F. 95
Spradley, L. 54
Squance, M.L. 89, 94, 102
Stahl, D. 183
Stang, C.D. 56, 57
Stark, M. 214, 219, 228, 229
Steacy, L.M. 20
Steeg, S. 199
Stefanis, L. 56, 57
Steinmetz, J.D. 53
Stephenson, L. 199
Stevenson, R. 219, 220, 222, 229
Stewart, A. 212
Stewart, C. 19, 24, 25
Still births 115
Storch, E.A. 21
Stratton, L. 54, 68, 69
Streeter, A. 23, 25
Strömmer, E.M.F. 214, 219, 220, 221, 222, 229
Structured debriefing 37–8
Stuhec, M. 20
Sturt, J. 86
Suicidal ideation 24, 194
Sumner, J.A. 87
Suzuki, M. 182, 192, 193, 197
Svavarsdóttir, M. 197
Svensson, K. 120, 121
Swayambunathan, J. 139
Symonds, P. 89
Szczerbi?ska, K. 61

Tada, M. 56
Taghinezhad, A. 197
Tajik, R. 2, 9
Takeuchi, R. 56
Talleff, J.L. 87
Tal-Saban, M. 17, 23
Tanaka, H. 56
Tarantino, V. 25
Taylor, H. 60, 67, 70
Taylor, J. 55, 56
Tchanturia, K. 19, 24, 25
te Pas, A.B. 120
Teague, B. 143
Teimori, G. 2, 9
Telemedicine 105
Terry, N.P. 20
Thambisetty, M. 56
Theron, G. 118
Thomas, A. 22, 26
Thomas, F. 196
Thomas, R. 17
Thomasson, W. 54
Thornicroft, G. 88, 90
Thornton, C.E. 120
Thorsted, A.B. 86
Thwaites, R. 19, 22, 25, 26
Tickle, A. 193
Tierney, L. 54, 58, 59, 60, 67, 68, 69
Tippett, V. 93
Todd, V. 135
Tong, M. 117
Torrico, T. 192, 193
Touza Pol, P. 121
Toyoshima, Y. 56
Tracy, D.K. 214, 219, 229
Tran, A. 229
Trauma- informed assessment 139–40
Trauma- informed practice 19
Trostian, B. 139, 140, 147
Turcano, P. 56, 57
Turk, A. 96
Turner, S. 181
Tyler, M.P. 18, 23

Ubom, A.E. 118
Ure, A. 23, 24, 26
Uygur, H. 21, 24

Vallerand, D. 118
Valls, M. 20
Van Acker, F. 55, 56
Van Dam, P. 191
van de Hoef, T.P. 135, 136, 138, 143, 148, 149

Van de Velde, E. 198
Van Deerlin, V.M. 57
van der Bijl, J. 192
van der Kant, R. 55
Van Hecke, A. 198
van Marwijk, H. 89
van Meijel, B. 192
Vanacore, N. 21
Vandewiele, H. 198
VanOrmer, J. 23
Vargas-Salas, O. 21
Vasconez, G. 194
Vascular dementia 56
VAWG (*see* Violence against women and girls)
Vela-Romero, M. 18, 24
Venous thromboembolism (VTE) 116–17
Verhaak, P.F.M. 139
Vermeiren, Y. 55, 56
Vicari, S. 21
Vigliante, M. 21
Vilà, M. 20
Vilke, G.M. 229
Violence against women and girls (VAWG) 143
Viscioni, L. 117
Vogeley, K. 24
Völkel, M. 125
Vollset, S.E. 53
Voss, S. 60, 67, 70, 120, 121
VTE (*see* Venous thromboembolism)

Wagner, E.H. 90, 91
Wagner, R.K. 20
Walker, A. 214, 228, 229
Walker, H.C. 25
Walker, K. 113
Walker, L. 56, 57
Wallace, M.T. 25
Walsh, B. 192
Wang, A. 56
Wang, C. 88, 93
Wang, T. 196
Wang, X. 103, 135, 148
Warren, J.D. 57
Webster, K. 113
Weinmann-Menke, J. 89
Weintraub, D. 55, 56
Weiss, S. 194
Weisz, D.E. 120
Wejse, C.M. 123
Welch, C. 24
Welch, J. 17, 22, 23, 24
Welles-Nyström, B. 121
Wernet, M. 121
Wevrick, R. 21
White, N. 59, 60
Whitley, A.G. 120
Whitworth, G. 61
Widström, A. 120, 121
Widström, A-M. 121
Wiklund Gustin, L. 192, 193, 194, 197, 199
Williams, D. 181
Williams, J. 54, 58, 60, 67, 69, 70
Williams, V. 197, 198
Williamson, P. 121
Wilson, A.C. 20, 21, 24
Wilson, M.P. 229
Wincup, C. 89, 91, 102
Winning, A. 87
Winsor, T. 123
Witges, K. 94
Withanarachchie, V. 135
Wittkowski, A. 114, 119
Wolff, J.L. 58
Women's health and wellbeing
  adapted ABCDE framework for 141–2
  addressing research gaps 149
  advancing paramedic education 148–9
  assessment principles 143–8
  case study 144–8
  conditions encountered in pre-hospital care 136–8
  evolving role of paramedics 149–50
  focused history- taking in 142–3
  future directions and challenges 148–150
  integrating UK guidelines 143
  key signs,symptoms in women's emergency presentations 140–1
  mental health, psychosocial crises 138–9
  system- level integration and policy development 149
  workforce development 148–9
Wong, A. 194, 195
Wong, G. 96
Wong, M.M. 55
Woods, N. 137
Worbe, Y. 21

Xiao, S. 196
Xue, Y. 117

Yakoob, M.Y. 118
Yang, I.A. 93
Yang, X. 56
Yaseen, A. 93
Yohannes, A.M. 87
Young, A. 89, 94
Yuan, B. 103

Zaccone, E. 117
Zaguri-Vittenberg, S. 17, 23
Zamir, A. 193
Zanza, C. 94
Zayed, M.G. 197, 198
Zeegers, M.P. 214, 219, 220, 221, 222, 229
Zeller, S.L. 228
Zeng, R. 56
Zhang, M. 196
Zhang, X. 196
Zhao, D. 54, 58, 72, 74
Zimmerman, S. 69
Zlomke, K. 23
Zwiggelaar, R. 22, 26
Zwitserlood-Nijenhuis, M. 20, 23, 25, 26

www.ingramcontent.com/pod-product-compliance
Lightning Source LLC
La Vergne TN
LVHW010714061126
851857LV00014B/1178